# TESTIMONIALS

RE:  Dr. Rao Konduru's Publications
1. Permanent Diabetes Control
2. The Secret to Controlling Type 2 Diabetes
3. Reversing Obesity
4. Reversing Sleep Apnea
5. Reversing Insomnia
6. Drinking Water Guide                        www.drinkingwaterguide.com

TO WHOM IT MAY CONCERN
      Dr. Rao Konduru, PhD is a patient of mine who has suffered from chronic diabetes for most of his life; He also suffered from uncontrollable obesity, sleep apnea and chronic insomnia for the past 3 to 4 years. He has managed to reverse all of these conditions by taking non-pharmacological and science-based natural measures with great success. He has created 6 how-to user guides/books with regard to how he achieved this, and I recommend these books for anyone suffering from these conditions.

Sincerely,
Dr. Ali Ghahary, MD
Brentwood Medical Clinic
4567 Lougheed Hwy
Burnaby, British Columbia, Canada

---

RE: Permanent Diabetes Control (book)        www.mydiabetescontrol.com
Dr. Konduru is an intelligent and committed scientist who has learned to manage his diabetes and cardiovascular risk factors. This book represents a comprehensive and readable review that could help many people with diabetes.

Dr. Marshall Dahl
BSc, MD, PhD, FRCPC, Certified Endocrinologist
Faculty of Medicine
University of British Columbia
Vancouver, British Columbia, Canada

---

RE: Reversing Sleep Apnea (book)        www.reversingsleepapnea.com
Dear Rao,
I read your book this weekend and It Is an impressively comprehensive and extremely well-documented review of the broad spectrum of therapies available to treat and help relieve sleep apnea. You are to be heartily congratulated on a finely-researched and very practical work that will be accessible and useful to a wide audience of readers. I wish you every success.

Best regards,
 Mr. Martin R. Hoke
 President (Creator and Owner of Navage.com)
 RhinoSystems, Inc.
 Brooklyn Heights, OH-44131
 USA

---

# DRINKING WATER GUIDE

## The Quick-Reference Manual to Choosing Clean & Healthy Water

### DRINKING WATER GUIDE'S MESSAGE:

- Please do not drink tap water, well water, or bottled water. Please always drink distilled water as is the purest water.

- But distilled water quickly absorbs $CO_2$ from air and forms carbonic acid, making it acidic. So learn how to neutralize it or slightly alkalize it before drinking.

- World Health Organization cautioned that drinking distilled water without minerals in it is harmful to our health (minerals & electrolytes could leach out from body's reservres) so learn how to remineralize it.

- Distilled water that is either neutralized (pH=7) or slightly alkalized (pH=7 to 7.25), and remineralized up to a TDS level of 200 ppm is the healthy drinking water.

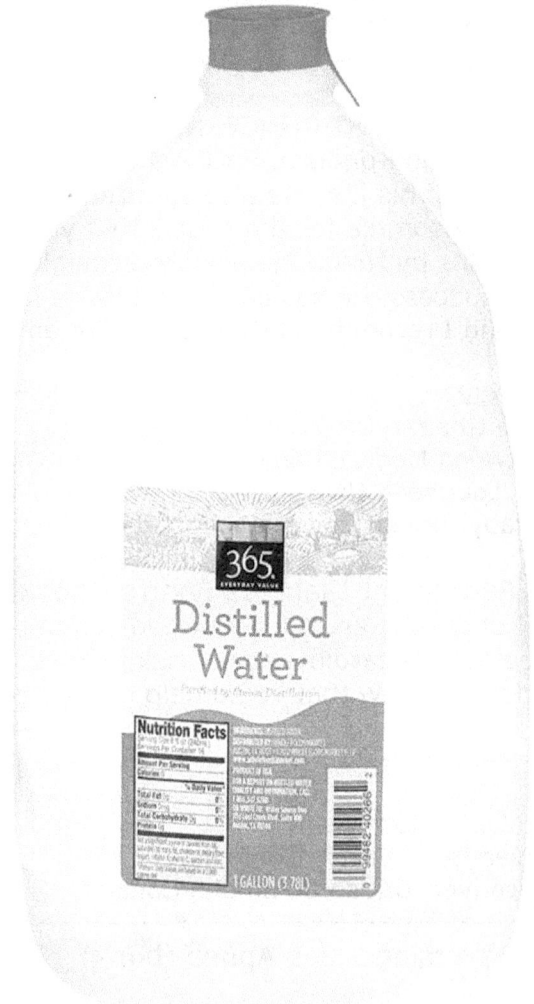

## www.DrinkingWaterGuide.com

Please refer to Chapter 14, Chapter 17, Chapter 18 & Chapter 19 to learn "How to remineralize and alkalize the purified water at home." There are many experiments conducted at home.

# DRINKING WATER GUIDE-II
## How to Remineralize and Alkalize the Purified Water at Home!

Drinking Water Guide-II was created with 8 important chapters "Chapter 1, Chapter 2, Chapter 3, Chapter 4, Chapter 14, Chapter 17, Chapter 18 & Chapter 19" of the complete book "Drinking Water Guide," which has 20 chapters and 540 pages.

## CHAPTER 1 & CHAPTER 20
🌐 If you want to learn about "The Big Bang Theory and The Origin of The Earth's Water," please read Chapter 1. Drinking Water Guide unveiled the origin of the Earth's water. The water we drink today is at least 4.54 billion years old, older than our palnet Earth.

## QUICK READ: PLEASE READ PAGES 76, 87 & 88
🌐 To learn quickly "How to Remineralize and Alkalize the Purified Water at Home," please read pages 76, 87 & 88 where you will find step-by-step instructions. By reading these 3 pages, you will be able to remineralize and alkalize the purified water at home like a layperson.

🌐 If you have basic scientific background, please read and practice all scientific experiments presented in Chapter 17 and Chapter 18. Make your own purified water using a ZeroWater Pitcher. And learn how to alkalize and remineralize the zero water at home as explained in Chapter 14.

| | | DRINKING WATER GUIDE |
|---|---|---|
| | | The Quick-Reference Manual to Choosing Clean & Healthy Water [The Original Book With 20 Chapters & 540 Pages] |
| ✓ | CHAPTER 1 | THE ORIGIN OF THE EARTH'S WATER |
| ✓ | CHAPTER 2 | DRINKING WATER FACTS & STATISTICS |
| ✓ | CHAPTER 3 | IMPORTANCE OF DRINKING WATER |
| ✓ | CHAPTER 4 | TYPES OF DRINKING WATER |
| | CHAPTER 5 | TAP WATER |
| | CHAPTER 6 | BOILED WATER |
| | CHAPTER 7 | BOTTLED WATER |
| | CHAPTER 8 | SPRING WATER |
| | CHAPTER 9 | WELL WATER |
| | CHAPTER 10 | DEMINERALIZED WATER OR DEIONIZED WATER |
| | CHAPTER 11 | REVERSE OSMOSIS WATER |
| | CHAPTER 12 | DESALINATED WATER |
| | CHAPTER 13 | DISTILLED WATER |
| ✓ | CHAPTER 14 | ZERO WATER, BRITA AND PUR FILTRATION SYSTEMS |
| | CHAPTER 15 | ATMOSPHERIC WATER GENERATORS |
| | CHAPTER 16 | HOW TO SANITIZE REUSABLE WATER BOTTLES |
| ✓ | CHAPTER 17 | REMINERALIZATION OF THE PURIFIED WATER |
| ✓ | CHAPTER 18 | ALKALINE WATER |
| ✓ | CHAPTER 19 | DRINKING WATER GUIDE IN A NUTSHELL |
| | CHAPTER 20 | THE ORIGIN OF THE EARTH'S WATER (Continued) |

# ATTENTION READERS: There Are 3 Books

**1. Drinking Water Guide** is the 540-page thick book loaded with all 20 chapters. This book describes about all kinds of drinking water available for human consumption (Tap Water, Boiled Water, Bottled Water, Spring Water, Well Water, Demineralized Water, Reverse Osmosis Water, Desalinated Water, Distilled Water, Water from ZeroWater, Brita or PUR pitchers & Water from Atmospheric Water Generators), their defects, and appropriate "RECOMMENDATIONS" on how to rectify those defects, and how to drink clean and healthy water in order to protect your health. In the 2nd part of the book, in Chapter 17, Chapter 18 & Chapter 19, this book teaches "How to Remineralize and Alkalize the Purified Water at Home Correctly and Precisely." There are more than 10 Scientific Experiments Conducted at Home. If you know how to use the TDS meter, digital kitchen scale & digital pH meter, you can easily remineralize and alkalize the purified water at home.

**2. Drinking Water Guide-II** is the 256-page compacted version, compiled with 8 important chapters (Chapter 1, Chapter 2, Chapter 3, Chapter 4, Chapter 14, Chapter 17, Chapter 18 & Chapter 19). This book is created for those people who cannot afford to purchase the complete book Drinking Water Guide (Paperback). In Chapter 1, this book teaches "The Formation of Our Universe, Stars, Our Milky Way Galaxy, Our Solar System, Our Sun, Our Earth & Our Moon!" based on scientific research findings. In Chapter 2, Chapter 3, Chapter 4, Chapter 14, you will learn about the importance of drinking water, types of drinking water, and how to drink purified water that is properly remineralized and slightly alkalized. If genuine RO water and distilled water are not available in the market, this book suggests that a consumer must switch to zero water. Make your own purified water using a ZeroWater pitcher. And learn how to alkalize and remineralize the zero water at home. Everything is explained clearly in Chapter 14. Just by reading the instructions provided in 2 pages only, you will be able to remineralize and alkalize the purified water (RO water, distilled water, or zero water) like a layperson. In Chapter 17 & Chapter 18, there are more than 10 Scientific Experiments Conducted at Home. Any reasonable person with minimal scientific background will be able to read and understand these experiments.

**3. The Origin of the Earth's Water** is the 166-page compacted version, compiled with 6 important chapters (Chapter 1, Chapter 2, Chapter 3, Chapter 4, Chapter 14 & Chapter 20). This book is created for those people who are interested on reading the scientific findings about how the planet Earth possessed that much liquid water. In Chapter 1 and Chapter 20, this book teaches "The Formation of Our Universe, Stars, Our Milky Way Galaxy, Our Solar System, Our Sun, Our Earth & Our Moon!" based on scientific research findings. In Chapter 2, Chapter 3, Chapter 4, Chapter 14, you will learn about the importance of drinking water, types of drinking water, and how to drink purified water that is properly remineralized and slightly alkalized. If genuine RO water and distilled water are not available in the market, this book suggests that a consumer must switch to zero water, and must learn how to alkalize and remineralize the zero water at home. Everything is explained clearly in Chapter 14. Just by reading the instructions provided in 2 pages only, you will be able to remineralize and alkalize the purified water (RO water, distilled water, or zero water) like a layperson.

**The Big Bang Theory** explained in Chapter 1 of the above-mentioned 3 books is the most relevant, most essential, and most important part. In order to understand "The Origin of the Earth's Water," a reader must understand the formation of our Universe, the formation of Stars and the formation of our Solar System, as explained in Chapter 1. This book also teaches in Chapter 1 that all those heavier elements of our periodic table, including all those minerals that we use today to remineralize and alkalize the purified water, were originally manufactured in the burning cores of collapsing stars by a process known as "stellar nucleosynthesis," even before our Solar System and our planet Earth were created. It is therefore of utmost importance to understand, as explained in Chapter 1, the formation of our Universe, the formation of Stars, and the formation our Solar System. All 3 books unveiled, based on scientific findings, the origin of our Earth's water, the age of our Earth's water, the age of our planet Earth, the age of our Sun, the age of our Solar System, and the age of our Milky Way, and the age of our Universe.

# DRINKING WATER GUIDE

## The Quick-Reference Manual to Choosing Clean & Healthy Water

DRINKING WATER GUIDE'S MESSAGE:

- Please do not drink tap water, well water, or bottled water of any kind directly without knowing how pure it is.

- Please always drink purified water (RO water, distilled water, or zero water), and learn how to remineralize and alkalize the purified water at home.

- Purified water that is either neutralized (pH=7) or slightly alkalized (pH=7 to 7.25), and remineralized up to a TDS (Total Dissolved Solids) level of 200 ppm is the healthy drinking water.

- MAKE YOUR OWN MINERAL WATER: This book teaches everything you need on "how to drink purified water that is remineralized up to 88 trace minerals in it, and slightly alkalized."

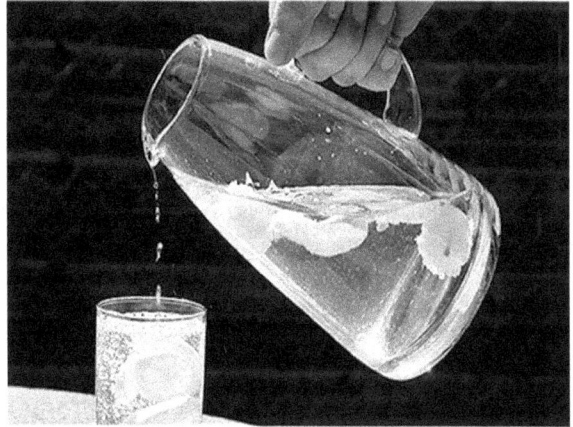

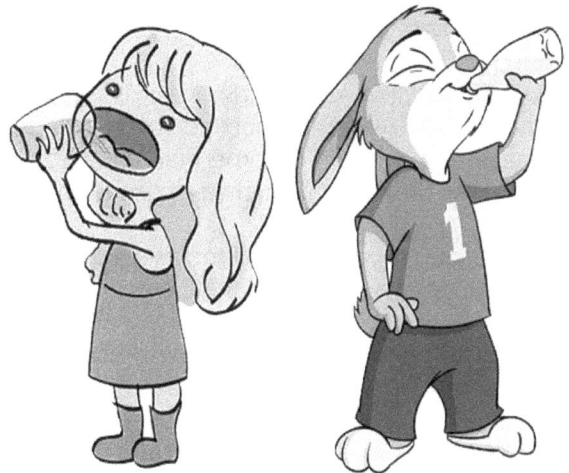

## www.DrinkingWaterGuide.com

◎ Please refer to Chapter 14, Chapter 17, Chapter 18 & Chapter 19 to learn "How to remineralize and alkalize the purified water at home." There are many experiments conducted at home.

# AMAZON REVIEWS: Drinking Water Guide
## The Quick-Reference Manual to Choosing Clean & Healthy Water

-------------------------------------------------------------------------------

Please do not ignore reviews. Please read all reviews thoroughly.
You can learn a lot by reading through the reviews below:

-------------------------------------------------------------------------------

Deanna Maio
*5.0 out of 5 stars*   Comprehensive Drinking Water Guide
Reviewed in the United States on February 17, 2020
Verified Purchase

NIKOLA TESLA said it all: "only a lunatic will drink unsterilized water". Very many people are still drinking unsterilized tap water and contaminated bottled water, jeopardizing their health, and developing strange diseases, and making many trips to hospitals and board-certified doctors. The tap water disaster incident that occurred in Flint, Michigan, USA in 2014 is a typical example of lead contamination that affected more than 100,000 residents.

This book describes about all kinds of drinking water available for human consumption, their defects, and appropriate "recommendations" in order to rectify those defects, and how to drink clean and healthy water in order to protect your health in the current day circumstances. This book Drinking Water Guide teaches many drinking water strategies:

(i) I must be wise and cautious all the time and should not take chances. I must not drink tap water, well water or bottled water of any kind, and make my own distilled water by purchasing and using a home distiller. Or, I must purchase RO water from a nearby supermarket, and I must always drink only purified water.

(ii) I would add very little Himalayan pink salt, Celtic sea salt or a few drops of ConcenTrace mineral drops to remineralize the purified water before drinking.

(iii) I would add a tiny bit of baking soda or a few drops of ConcenTrace mineral drops in order to improve the alkalinity and the presence of minerals in the purified water.

(iv) I would use pH strips or digital pH meter, monitor my drinking water pH, every now and then, and make sure that the purified water I drink is either neutralized (pH=7) or slightly alkalized (pH=7 to 7.5).

(v) I would use a TSD meter, and monitor the TDS level of my drinking water, and make sure that TDS level is always below 200 ppm. I will also research and find out the ideal TDS level that suits my body. I can do that by adjusting the tiny amount of Himalayan pink salt.

I am very grateful that I learned all the above-mentioned valuable information from this book "Drinking Water Guide". What an impressive book! I urge you to get this book without any hesitation.

-------------------------------------------------------------------------------

# AMAZON REVIEWS: Drinking Water Guide-II
## How To Remineralize and Alkalize The Purified Water At Home!

-------------------------------------------------------------------------

Peggie Tyson
*5.0 out of 5 stars*  Why remineralize and alkalize the purified water at home?
Reviewed in the United States on June 29, 2022
Verified Purchase

## Why remineralize and alkalize the purified water at home?

This book answered that question very clearly. World Health Organization (WHO) cautioned repeatedly long ago that drinking demineralized water (RO water, distilled water, zero water, or any other purified water) is harmful to our health because certain scientific investigations revealed the fact that minerals and electrolytes could leach out from body's reserves and cause strange diseases and many abnormalities if there are not enough minerals and electrolytes present in the drinking water. We therefore must learn how to precisely remineralize the purified water before drinking.

Also purified water quickly absorbs carbon dioxide ($CO_2$) from the surrounding air and forms carbonic acid, making it acidic. The pH of purified water may drop to as low as 5.6, making it dangerously acidic. We therefore must also learn how to neutralize (pH=7) or slightly alkalize (pH=7 to 7.25) the purified water before drinking.

HIMALAYAN PINK SALT, CELTIC SEA SALT, CONCENTRACE MINERAL DROPS & BAKING SODA: Himalayan pink salt contains 88 trace minerals in it, and attributes to many health benefits. Himalayan pink salt also contains six electrolytes "sodium, potassium, chloride, magnesium, phosphorus and calcium" in it. Our bodies desperately need all these 6 electrolytes. Celtic sea salt contains 72 trace mineral in it, and ConcenTrace mineral drops contains 73 trace minerals in it. All these products are claimed to have the essential electrolytes in them. Baking soda is the best alkalizing agent.

We can very easily remineralize the purified water to any desired TDS level by adding the precisely measured tiny amount of Himalayan pink salt, Celtic sea salt, ConcenTrace mineral drops. ConcenTrace mineral drops can be used to simultaneously remineralize and alkalize the purified water (RO water, Distilled Water, or Zero Water) at home. We can very easily alkalize the purified water by adding a trace amount (only a few kernels) of baking soda.

This awesome book presented many experiments conducted at home on how to remineralize and alkalize the purified water at home using TDS meter, digital kitchen scale and digital pH meter. And I am using those experiments.

-------------------------------------------------------------------------

----------------------------------------------------------------------------------

Anamaría Aguirre Chourio
*5.0 out of 5 stars* Best Drinking Water Guide to Live Healthy!
Reviewed in the United States on March 18, 2020
Verified Purchase

Drinking Water Guide-II would certainly benefit many people in the way we never have imagined. Everyone should listen to the most important message of this book "Please do not drink tap water, well water & bottled water. Please always drink purified water, and learn how to remineralize and alkalize the purified water at home." This book has guided me and taught me many healthy water-drinking habits, and I list some of them below:

(i) I purchased a Countertop Water Distiller (the same distiller recommended in this book), and I now make my own distilled water every day. No more tap water.

(ii) I also purchased ConcenTrace mineral drops from a health food store near me.

(iii) I also purchased a TDS meter (the same meter recommended in this book) from Amazon. I learned how to use it from this book.

(iv) ) I also purchased a Digital pH Meter (the same meter recommended in this book) from Amazon. I learned how to use it from this book.

(v) I have read Chapter 17, Chapter 18 & Chapter 19 several times. It was very easy to read and understand procedures. In Chapter 17, I read that: An adult must drink at least 8 cups or 2 liters of purified water, and so 16 drops of ConcenTrace mineral drops are required per day to remineralize the purified water to keep the TDS level under 200 ppm, and to keep the drinking water slightly alkalized.

(vi) Every day, when I wake up in the morning, I mix 16 drops of ConcenTrace mineral drops with 2 liters (8 cups) of distilled water, and I drink all 8 cups throughout the day. The water I drink thus is purified, remineralized up to 200 ppm, and slightly alkalized as well (this is perfectly healthy water).

The manufacturer of ConcenTrace mineral drops recommends 40 drops per day without specifying the total number of cups of water to be mixed with per day. But this book recommends that more than 16 drops per 2 liters of purified water would be unnecessary, and may develop life-threatening long-term side effects because of high sodium consumption (I fully agree!).

I am sure that these water-drinking habits would keep me in good health. I now know that I would not become a victim of contaminated drinking water (mostly tap water), and will not develop any strange diseases due to mineral deficiency, and my body's cells would not leach minerals like some scientists claim.

----------------------------------------------------------------------------------

--------------------------------------------------------------------------------

Amazon Customer
*5.0 out of 5 stars*  How to Remineralize Purified Water Like a Layperson?
Reviewed in India on October 2, 2022
Verified Purchase

I have read just 2-page instructions titled "How to Alkalize and Remineralize Like a Layperson?" very kindly provided in the beginning of Chapter 17. That information is enough for me to remineralize and alkalize the purified water.

## TRIAL AND ERROR PROCEDURE
(i) Every day I make "4 liters (16 cups)" of purified water using a zero water pitcher, and store it in a glass bottle. I add only a few kernels of Himalayan pink salt to this zero water, shake the glass bottle vigorously and monitor the TDS level using the TDS meter that comes "attached" with the zero water pitcher. The TDS level is usually close to 10 ppm.
(ii) I add a few more kernels of Himalayan pink salt, shake the glass bottle vigorously and monitor TDS level again. The TDS level is usually close to 20 ppm.
(iii) I add a few more kernels of Himalayan pink salt, shake the glass bottle vigorously and monitor TDS level again. The TDS level is usually close to 30 ppm. This is my desired TDS level.
(iv) I boil this remineralized zero water using a glass kettle, and refrigerate it before drinking.
(v) Every day I drink 10 to 16 cups of purified water (zero water) remineralized to a TDS level of approximately 30 ppm. Drinking lots of pure water helps me lose weight, and keeps my weight normal.
(vi) I do not try to alkalize the purified water (zero water), but I eat 1 lemon a day. That keeps my body at neutralized state (my urine pH close to 7). I will continue drinking this kind of purified and remineralized water for the rest of my life. I am sure this habit will keep my body healthy.

I am greatly indebted to this extremely important book "Drinking Water Guide-II: How to Remineralize and Alkalize the Purified Water At Home."

--------------------------------------------------------------------------------

Harish Garg
*5.0 out of 5 stars*  Extremely Important Guide to Remineralize and Alkalize the Purified Water!
Reviewed in India on July 27, 2022
Verified Purchase

Drinking Water Guide-II contains extremely important and beneficial information to remineralize and alkalize the purified water at home. I found it extremely useful and helpful.

(i) With the help of this book, I purchased a ZeroWater pitcher and started making my own zero water from tap water. Zero water is better than distilled water because the distilled water being sold in supermarkets is untrustworthy (as it could have scum in it). Zero water has a TDS level of zero so we must remineralize it before drinking according to World Health Organization (WHO).

(ii) With the help of this book, after reading the experiments conducted at home, I added a tiny pinch (only a few kernels) of Himalayan pink salt to zero water so that TDS level is approximately 20 ppm. I monitored TDS level of zero water using the TDS meter that comes with the ZeroWater pitcher.

(iii) With the help of this book, after reading the experiments conducted at home, I added a tiny pinch (only a few kernels) of baking soda so that the pH of the zero water would be approximately 7. I measured the pH level of zero water using a digital pH meter as explained in this book. I also learned how to use "pH drops" to measure zero water pH.

(iv) With the help of this book, after reading the experiments conducted at home, I often measure my urine pH using "pH paper for urine," and make sure that it is close to 7. That means my urine is neither acidic nor alkaline, but it is neutralized. Whenever my urine pH is more than 8, I discontinue adding baking soda to the zero water until my urine pH comes down close to 7.

I drink every day at least 8 cups of zero water that is remineralized and either neutralized or slightly alkalized. I learned all the aforementioned drinking water strategies from this great guidebook "Drinking Water Guide-II."

-----------------------------------------------------------------------------------------------

Anoop J.
*5.0 out of 5 stars*   Remineralization of the Purified Water is Simplified!
Reviewed in India on October 6, 2022
Verified Purchase

## REMINERALIZATION OF THE PURIFIED WATER IS SIMPLIFIED:
After I read this book's experiments conducted at home in Chapter 14 & Chapter 17,
I developed my own simplified method to remineralize the purified water as explained below.

I purchased a countertop water distiller, and I make my own distilled water enough for a week, every week, and I store it in glass bottles. Did you know the distilled water must be stored in glass bottles with lid?

Every day I pour about 4 liters of distilled water in a glass container with lid, and start adding Himalayan pink salt. I add only a few kernels of Himalayan pink salt, mix and shake the water bottle thoroughly, and monitor the TDS level using the TDS meter. If the TDS level is less than 50 ppm, I add a few more kernels of Himalayan pink salt, mix and shake the water bottle thoroughly, and monitor the TDS level again using the TDS meter. I repeat this procedure until the TDS level of distilled water reaches approximately 50 ppm. I drink at least 8 cups of this remineralized distilled water at 50 ppm.

The most fascinating fact is that I spend less than 2 minutes to remineralize the purified water at my home. Many people think that remineralization is a complex process, and don't even try to do it. The same procedure can be used to remineralize any kind of purified water (RO water, distilled water, or zero water) to any desired TDS level. Everybody in my family circle and many of friends adopted this procedure, and every day, they all make and drink the remineralized distilled water at 50 ppm.

--------------------------------------------------------------------------

kaitlyn Jeffries
*5.0 out of 5 stars* This Book Is Primer!
Reviewed in the United Kingdom on December 21, 2020
Verified Purchase

World Health Organization (WHO) reported and cautioned long ago that drinking demineralized water (which is the processed and purified water) is harmful to our health because the minerals could leach out from body's cells. Scientists suggested that this leaching effect can be diminished or minimized by remineralizing the purified water.

Many people don't know how to add the right amount of Himalayan pink salt, Celtic sea salt or ConcenTrace mineral drops in order to remineralize the purified water at home, but just use fingers, teaspoons, or even tablespoons without weighing precisely, and without knowing the exact quantity of the salt being consumed daily. Himalayan pink salt, Celtic sea salt or ConcenTrace mineral drops contain extremely high quantity of sodium. We must beware of that important information regarding the high sodium content.

Drinking Water Guide-II quotes that: The RDA (Recommended Daily Allowance) of sodium is 2,300 milligrams for healthy adults, and 1,500 milligrams for adults with a history of heart disease, who are over 51 years old or are African-American. We should never exceed this upper limit considering all foods and drinks being consumed daily.

Research showed that many people who overconsumed sodium chloride (NaCl) beyond the RDA developed and suffered from hypertension, osteoporosis, kidney stones, Menierre's Syndrome (ear ringing), insomnia, motion sickness, asthma, and a variety of cancers.

Both books Drinking Water Guide and Drinking Water Guide-II teach, with experiments conducted at home, how to remineralize the purified water (either RO water or distilled water) precisely and correctly without exceeding the upper limit of 200 ppm for the TDS (Total Dissolved Solids) level, which could save your life from serious health consequences. This book is primer on this particular topic!

--------------------------------------------------------------------------

KON
*5.0 out of 5 stars* I enjoyed this book very much!
Reviewed in the United States on December 13, 2019
Format: Kindle Edition

This book is extremely extraordinary, in the wake of perusing this book I am so intrigued. On account of the writer, I would prescribe this book to anybody. Many thanks to the author for giving us such a beautiful book.

--------------------------------------------------------------------------

-------------------------------------------------------------------------------

**stacy anderson**
*5.0 out of 5 stars* Learn How to Remineralize & Alkalize the Purified Water at Home!
Reviewed in the United Kingdom on June 8, 2021
Verified Purchase

At first I have read Chapter 17 and Chapter 18 thoroughly, and understood the contents. Then I practiced on "how to use TDS meter, digital kitchen scale and digital pH meter". It is very important to be proficient in using these items in order to remineralize and alkalize the purified water (RO water or distilled water) at home.

In Chapter 17, Table 17.14 gives the short-cut information on how much Himalayan pink salt or Celtic sea salt is to be added to remineralize 1 liter or 2 liters of the purified water. I just follow this table. My preferred TDS level in my drinking water is 50 ppm. So every day I add 100 mg of Himalayan pink salt to 2 liters of the purified water (RO water) as I drink 8 cups a day, and monitor the TDS level using TDS meter. That would keep the TDS level at 50 ppm.

If I eat one lemon a day, it would help keep my body at nearly neutralized state. If I want to slightly alkalize the purified water, I would add a tiny bit of baking soda to the purified water, and monitor the pH of my drinking water using a digital pH meter. I should make sure that pH is under 7.25. I must be cautious that drinking highly alkalized water every day is dangerous.

Alternatively, I would add ConcenTrace mineral drops to purified water (16 drops per 2 liters of purified water) which would both remineralize and alkalize the purified water at the same time without exceeding the upper limit. However, I must make sure that the TDS level is under 200 ppm, and pH level is between 7 and 7.25 (slightly alkalized) by adjusting the number of drops. I can drink this kind of healthy and nutritious purified water every day.

This book Drinking Water Guide-II has taught me "How to Remineralize and Alkalize the Purified Water at Home" very nicely and so I am greatly indebted to it.

-------------------------------------------------------------------------------

**radpaikr**
*5.0 out of 5 stars* Always Drink Purified Water That Is Remineralized & Slightly Alkalized!
Reviewed in India on June 7, 2021
Verified Purchase

I have read both books Drinking Water Guide & Drinking Water Guide-II, and learned many interesting drinking water strategies. Drinking Water Guide-II (which is the second part of the complete book Drinking Water Guide) is created for those people who cannot afford to purchase the complete book. After reading these 2 books, I made up my mind. I will never drink tap water anymore.

I can purchase purified water (RO water or distilled water) at the nearby supermarket, but drinking such water directly could make my immune system weak and could cause strange diseases as is cautioned by the World Health Organization long ago. So I decided to remineralize and slightly alkalize the purified water so that I would be completely safe.

I have adopted the following RULE, very nicely described, illustrated, and exemplified in the book:

The purified water that is either neutralized (pH=7) or slightly alkalized (pH=7 to 7.25), and remineralized up to a TDS (Total Dissolved Solids) level of 200 ppm is the healthy drinking water.

Every day, I make this kind of drinking water at home by adding Himalayan pink salt, Celtic sea salt, or ConcenTrace mineral drops to the purified water (RO water or distilled water). I add a tiny amount of baking soda or ConcenTrace mineral drops (a few drops) to adjust the drinking water pH. If you know how to do it, it takes only a few minutes a day to make the purified water that is remineralized and alkalized.

I recommend these two extremely useful books "Drinking Water Guide and Drinking Water Guide-II" to every household. Please do not drink tap water. Read these books.

-------------------------------------------------------------------------------------------------

Anurag Sharma
*5.0 out of 5 stars* Drink Distilled Water That is Slightly Alkalized & Remineralized!
Reviewed in India on October 7, 2021
Verified Purchase

By reading this book (Chapter 18), I have purchased an "Alkaline Water Pitcher" online from Amazon. Alkaline water pitcher does two jobs at a time: (i) it filters and removes all contaminants, toxins from tap water, and (ii) it adds minerals to the filtered water improving both pH level and TDS level. The final product from the pitcher is the alkalized mineral-rich water. This book taught me how to carefully select an "Alkaline Water Pitcher" to meet my specific needs and interests.

I have also purchased a TDS meter and Digital pH meter. I monitor the TDS level and pH level of my drinking water every now and then, and make sure that the water I drink is slightly alkalized and remineralized up to a TDS level of 200 ppm. I learned everything from this wonderful book. Do not hesitate to have this book at your home.

-------------------------------------------------------------------------------------------------

Travis Neff
5.0 out of 5 stars   Strongly recommenced
Reviewed in the United States on August 25, 2019
Format: Kindle Edition Verified Purchase

Explained very clearly and the way author explained. I really like this text book. They're also full of good information.

-------------------------------------------------------------------------------------------------

------------------------------------------------------------------------

**Rahul gupta**
*5.0 out of 5 stars* Always Drink Purified Water at Balanced pH Level!
Reviewed in India on October 7, 2021
Verified Purchase

This book "Drinking Water Guide-II" has taught me how to drink water at balanced pH level. I have heard that many people nowadays are drinking alkaline water every day, which is not a healthy drinking habit.

**THIS BOOK REMINDS US:** The pH of your stomach is always acidic and varies from 1.5 to 3.5, and sometimes your stomach pH reaches 4 or 5. The acids present in stomach are very important and essential for digestion, and to kill bacteria and viruses. Drinking alkaline water continuously makes it difficult to maintain the stomach pH in the acidic range.
**THIS BOOK CAUTIONS US:** Though the human body has an amazing ability to maintain a normal steady pH in the blood between 7.35 and 7.45, if you drink alkaline water at high pH of 9 or 10 all the time, it becomes very difficult for the body to maintain normal blood pH between 7.35 and 7.45.
You may develop alkalosis (a condition developed due to the presence of excess base), and this condition could affect the proper functioning of lungs, kidneys & liver. Read this book and learn your lesson!

------------------------------------------------------------------------

**Sunil Chandel**
*5.0 out of 5 stars* Drink Distilled Water That is Slightly Alkalized & Remineralized!
Reviewed in India on October 8, 2021
Verified Purchase
After I read this book "Drinking Water Guide-II," I learned how to purchase and use the TDS meter, Digital Kitchen Scale, and Digital pH meter. If I know how to use these instruments, everything becomes easy to remineralize and how to alkalize the purified water (RO water or distilled water) at home.

I now drink only distilled water purchased at the local pharmacy. I have implemented the following principle and make my own mineral water every day. Distilled water that is either neutralized or slightly alkalized, and remineralized up to a TDS level of 200 ppm is the healthy drinking water. I am deeply indebted to Drinking Water Guide-II.

------------------------------------------------------------------------

**kazoua vang**
5.0 out of 5 stars    Excellent book
Reviewed in the United States on December 15, 2019
Format: Kindle Edition
I absolutely would need to prescribe this to anybody intending to improve any bit of their life. Many thanks to the author for giving us such a beautiful book.

# DRINKING WATER GUIDE-II
## How to Remineralize and Alkalize the Purified Water at Home!
### Authored by Rao Konduru, PhD

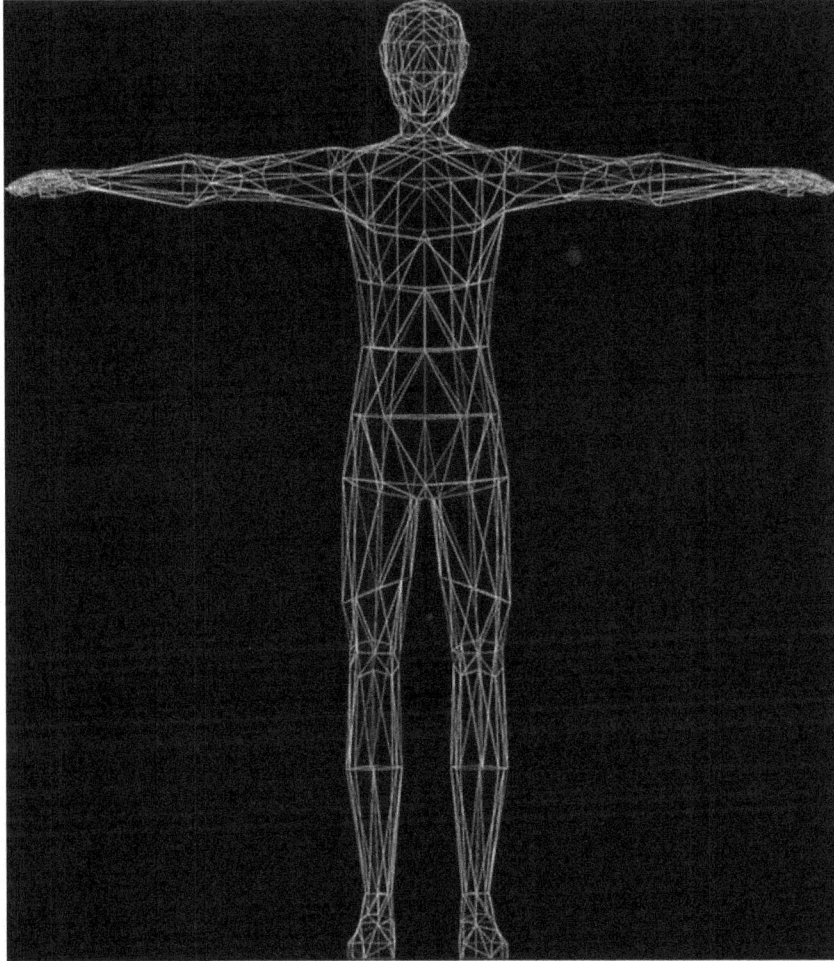

## THE AMAZING HUMAN BODY

● Did you know more than 99% of your amazing body's molecules are water molecules, and 55% to 60% of your body weight is water? You therefore should make sure that the water in your body is clean, healthy and nutritious, and more importantly one 100% free of contaminants. This book is designed to help you achieve that goal!

# DRINKING WATER GUIDE-II
## How to Remineralize and Alkalize the Purified Water at Home!

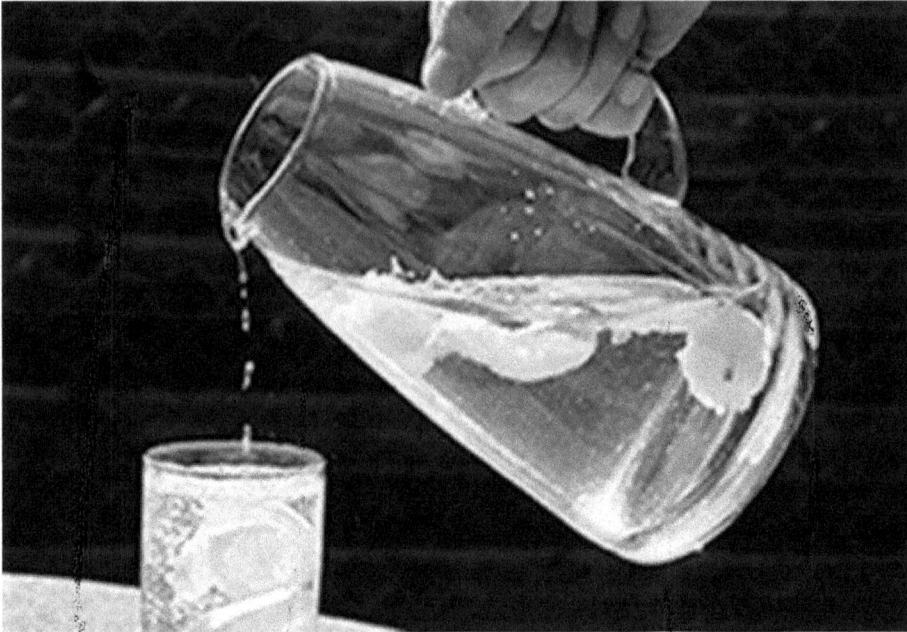

## DRINKING WATER GUIDE REMINDS YOU

- Please Do Not Drink Tap Water, Well Water, Or Bottled Water!
- Please Always Drink Purified Water: RO Water, Or Distilled Water!
- Expensive Water Purification Systems For Home Use Are Unnecessary!
- Purchase Purified Water from Local Vendors, Or Make Your Own!
- Learn How to Remineralize and Alkalize the Purified Water At Home!

## DRINKING WATER GUIDE TEACHES YOU

- Formation Of Our Universe, Our Milky Way Galaxy, Our Sun, Our Earth & Our Moon!
- How In Our Universe Our Earth Possessed That Much Liquid Water?
- How to Remineralize & Alkalize? Experiments Conducted At Home!
- How to Use Himalayan Pink Salt, Celtic Sea Salt & ConcenTrace Drops!
- How To Obtain Alkaline Water: There Are 10 Methods Discussed!
- Water Ionizers | Kangen Water | Hydrogen Water | Atmospheric Water
- How To Make Your Own Nutritious Alkaline & Mineral Water At Home!
- How To Adjust the Drinking Water pH and TDS to Any Desired Level!

**This Guide Will Help You Become A Drinking Water Expert!**
**Author: Rao Konduru, PhD**

# PREFACE: DRINKING WATER GUIDE-II

▶ **The Big Bang Theory** explained in Chapter 1 of this book "Drinking Water Guide-II" is the most relevant, most essential, and most important part. This book teaches that all those heavier elements of our periodic table, including all those minerals that we use today to remineralize and alkalize the purified water, were originally manufactured in the burning cores of collapsing stars by a process known as "stellar nucleosynthesis," even before our Solar System and our planet Earth were created. Stars are responsible for all the constituents of our planet Earth. It is therefore of utmost importance to understand, as explained in Chapter 1, the formation of our Universe, the formation of Stars, and the formation our Solar System.

## Drinking Water Guide-II is a 254-Page Book, and Teaches:

❧ All kinds of drinking water available for human consumption, their defects, and appropriate "RECOMMENDATIONS" on how to rectify those defects, and how to drink clean and healthy water in order to protect your health in the current day circumstances.

❧ How to purchase purified water in supermarkets at Refill Yourself Stations, or from local vendors, or how to make your own purified water by purchasing the appropriate units.

❧ How to remineralize and alkalize the purified water at home. In Chapter 14, Chapter 17 & Chapter 18, there are many **Experiments Conducted at Home** with easy-to-follow instructions on how to correctly and precisely remineralize the purified water by adding Himalayan pink salt, Celtic sea salt, or ConcenTrace mineral drops.
All you need are: TDS meter, digital kitchen scale, digital pH meter, and measuring spoons.

❧ Any reasonable person with minimal scientific background would be able to read and understand these experiments, and would be able to remineralize and alkalize the purified water.

❧ In Chapter 18, the book details how to make your own alkaline water at home using baking soda or ConcenTrace mineral drops, and how to purchase appropriate machines that make alkaline water.

❧ How to purchase and use Water Ionizers, Kangen water machines, Hydrogen water machines and RO water machines that produce alkalized and remineralized water at home. The topic about Atmospheric Water Generators is another highlight.

**Akaline Water:** Many people, mostly Kangen water fans, drink alkaline water every day which is not a healthy habit. Drinking Water Guide cautions that drinking too much alkaline water on a daily basis could shift the normal blood pH (between 7.35 and 7.45), and could develop alkalosis (presence of excess base), and this condition could affect the proper functioning of lungs, kidneys & liver. At the same time, this book recommends that drinking limited alkaline water periodically every now and then is healthy.

**Ionized Water, Kangen Water & Hydrogen Water:** This book teaches the basic principle behind the water ionizers, Kangen water machines and hydrogen water machines, and describes how these machines function.

**Hydrogen Water:** Hydrogen water is the latest wellness trend to hit the US, UK and Asian markets with benefits such as reducing inflammation, wrinkles, and bone loss, and some people believe that hydrogen water also helps metabolise fat and glucose faster than the regular water.

**Zero Water:** A consumer must be extremely careful in the current day market when purchasing and drinking purified water (RO water and distilled water), and must make sure that it is genuinely purified water. Distilled water being sold in supermarkets and by local vendors is untrustworthy. If genuine RO water and distilled water are unavailable, this book suggests that a consumer must switch to zero water. Make your own purified water using a ZeroWater pitcher. And learn how to remineralize and slightly alkalize the zero water at home. Please refer to Chapter 14 for complete details.

Drinking Water Guide-II is a must-have book by every household and every library of any community, school, college or university of every village, town or city around the world.
-- The Author

# COPYRIGHT

Book Title:     Drinking Water Guide-II
Sub-Title:      How to Remineralize and Alkalize the Purified Water at Home!
Author:         Rao Konduru, PhD (Also Called Dr. RK)
Publisher:      Prime Publishing Co.
Address:        720 – Sixth Street, Unit: 161
                New Westminster, BC, Canada, V3L 3C5
Website:        www.drinkingwaterguide.com
ISBN #          ISBN 9780973112078

This book "Drinking Water Guide-II" has been registered under ISBN Number "ISBN 9780973112078" with the National Library of Canada Cataloguing in Publication, Ottawa, Ontario, Canada. The original manuscript has been submitted to the Legal Deposits, Library and Archives Canada, Ottawa, Ontario, Canada. All rights reserved!

## WARNING

## DISCLAIMER

The author of this book titled "Drinking Water Guide-II" assumes no liability or responsibility including, without limitation, incidental and consequential damages, personal injury or wrongful death resulting from the use of any treatment method presented in this book. A person should have a thorough understanding on the potential risks of choosing and drinking purified water, alkaline water, hydrogen water, atmospheric water, or use of any filtration unit or water pitcher. Misusing the drinking water strategies without a clear concept on how to control pH and TDS (Total Dissolved Solids) could lead to adverse and serious side effects. More specifically, adding baking soda, pH booster drops, ConcenTrace drops, and/or any other mineral drops to purified water for remineralization in an attempt to prepare alkaline water requires experience and a thorough understanding on how to do it correctly. A reader should seek appropriate medical advice from a healthcare professional when using the methods illustrated in this book. All contents in this book are for educational purpose only, and do not in any way represent the professional medical advice.

## REGARDING THE REFERENCES

Please note that the hypelinks of the references provided in all chapters are not guaranteed to work. The owners of those websites might have changed the contents, and some of those websites might have even disappeared from the Internet. However the information collected from all the scientific articles and journal papers was found to be true and reliable at the time the literature search was performed.

# TABLE OF CONTENTS

# CHAPTER 1  THE ORIGIN OF THE EARTH'S WATER
### EARTH GOT ITS WATER EVEN BEFORE IT WAS BORN

# TABLE OF CONTENTS

## Did you know?
The oxygen we breathe today was originally created in the Stars
even before our Solar System was created!
The water we drink today was originally created in the stars-forming clouds
even before our Solar System was created!
When you look up at night, you are seeing factories called Stars!

# ATTENTION READERS!

## CHAPTER 1 CONTAINS THE PRECIOUS INFORMATION
### Drinking Water Guide Unveiled "The Origin of the Earth's Water" In Chapter 1 & Chapter 20.

☻ The primary element "hydrogen" was first created 380,000 years after the Big Bang, and thereafter it was abundantly available throughout our Universe. Stars formation commenced 400 million years after the Big Bang, and since then stars have been manufacturing heavier elements, including the very important oxygen, like factories in their burning cores, and have been dumping them in the interstellar medium via supernova explosions. More than 6 billion years ago, even before our Solar System and our Earth were created, the heavier element "oxygen" was created in the burning cores of collapsing stars in the interstellar medium.

☻ The abundantly available hydrogen and oxygen then commingled together under the appropriate climate conditions and formed ice-cold water molecules by the chemical reaction: $2 H_2 + O_2 = 2 H_2O$. Those ice-cold water molecules then entered into the space dust (also known as stardust) and interstellar gas in the interstellar medium, from a gigantic cloud of which our Solar System was created 6 billion years ago. The formation of our Solar System completed 4.54 billion years ago. And that is how our Earth inherited liquid water even before it was born. Our Earth was thus born with water, and the water we drink today is at least 4.54 billion years old, older than our Solar System.

☻ In order to understand "The Origin of the Earth's Water," a reader must understand, as explained in Chapter 1, the formation of our Universe, the formation of Stars, and the formation of our Solar System with a clear concept.

☻ This book also revealed, based on brilliant scientific findings, the age of our Earth's water, the age of our planet Earth, the age of our Sun, the age of our Solar System, the age of our Milky Way Galaxy, and the age of our Universe.

☻ **The Big Bang Theory Explained in Chapter 1** is the most relevant, the most essential, and the most intriguing part of this book. Stars are responsible for all the constituents of our planet Earth that are needed for the formation and survival of every human being, animal and plant. Did you know "the oxygen we breathe today was originally created in the Stars even before our Solar System was created, and the water we drink today was originally created in the stars-forming clouds even before our Solar System was created?" This book teaches that all those heavier elements of our periodic table, including the most important carbon, nitrogen, oxygen, phosphorus, sulfur, and other elements, and including all those minerals that we use today to remineralize and alkalize the purified water, were originally manufactured in the burning cores of collapsing stars by a process known as "stellar nucleosynthesis," even before our Solar System and our Earth were created. When you look up at night, you are seeing factories called stars.

☻ It is therefore of utmost importance to understand, as explained in Chapter 1, the formation of our Universe, the formation of Stars, and the formation our Solar System.

Please read and understand CHAPTER 1 with keen observation. You will enjoy it!

# AMAZING FACTS ABOUT OUR UNIVERSE, OUR STARS, OUR MILKY WAY GALAXY, OUR SOLAR SYSTEM, OUR SUN, OUR EARTH & OUR WATER!

The following scientific facts were endorsed by NASA (National Aeronautics and Space Administration) and many other space agencies around the world:

- **Our Universe is approximately 13.8 billion years old.** [1, 2, 3, 4, 5]
  The NASA's spacecraft known as Wilkinson Microwave Anisotropy Probe (WMAP) mission has precisely determined the age of our Universe.

- **Our Universe has trillion trillion stars.** [6, 7]
  There are 1,000,000,000,000,000,000,000,000 stars. There are $10^{24}$ stars. [6, 7]
  That's is a 1 followed by twenty-four zeros.
  This is a grossly rough estimate. The exact number of stars is unknown.

- **Our Universe is embedded with at least 2 trillion Galaxies.** There are $2 \times 10^{12}$ Galaxies. [8, 9, 10]
  **The Spiral-Shaped Milky Way Galaxy is one of them upon which we all live.**

- Our Milky Way Galaxy was born about 13.6 billion years ago. [11, 12, 13]

- Our Milky Way Galaxy has 100 billion stars on the lower end, and 400 billion stars on the upper end, totaling at least 500 billion stars. [14]

- Did you know every star represents a Solar System with planets orbiting around it?

- That means our Milky Way Galaxy so far has at least 500 billion Solar Systems. [14, 15, 16] Our Solar System is one of them.

- **Our Solar System (our Sun, our Earth & 7 other planets)** began its formation on our Milky Way Galaxy 6 billion years ago, and completed its formation 4.54 billion years ago. [55-60]

- **Did you know stars manufacture planets?** Our Sun (which is a star) manufactured 8 orbiting planets "Mercury, Venus, our Earth, Mars, Jupiter, Saturn, Uranus and Neptune" while in a spinning and swirling motion under gravity for one and half billion years. [55-60]

- The age of our planet Earth, our Sun & our Solar System was determined by radiometric dating, which is the most accurate and reliable technique to date older rocks. [65-71]

- **Did you know stars manufacture heavier elements like factories do?** When you look up at night, you are seeing factories called stars equipped with nuclear-fusion reactors! [39, 40, 41]

- Early stars were massive, short-lived and exploded into supernovae while manufacturing and dumping all those 117 heavier elements of our periodic table into the interstellar space from a gigantic cloud of which our Solar System was created! The SIX essential elements "Carbon, Hydrogen, Nitrogen, Oxygen, Phosphorus and Sulfur (CHNOPS)" are absolutely needed for the formation and survival of every human being, animal & plant. [40-45]

- **The size of our Sun is enormous:** Our Sun is 864,400 miles (1,391,000 km) across, 109 times our Earth's diameter, weighs about 333,000 times more than our Earth, 93 million miles (149.5 million km) away from our Earth, and our Sun is so humongous that even 1,300,000 Earths could fit inside of it. [61]

- **Our Sun has a lifespan of 9 to 10 billion years.** Which means our Sun will run out of nuclear fuel, extinguish or die after 4 to 5 billion years. When our Sun dies, our planet Earth, our Moon & 7 other planets will be engulfed with it and possibly vaporized. Afterwards our Sun will either become a white dwarf or explode into a supernova in which case a new star will born out of the debris. [62]

- **The water we drink today is at least 4.54 billion years old, older than our planet Earth, older than our Sun, and older than our Solar System.** Our planet Earth inherited up to 50% of its water (primordial water) from the interstellar medium even before it was born, and the remaining water came to our planet Earth by the bombardment of Asteroid (not Comets) during and after the early stages of our Solar System formation. Our ancestors' belief that Comets brought water to our planet Earth was later proved by our recent scientists to be a myth! [80-166]

**OUR UNIVERSE, OUR STARS, OUR MILKY WAY GALAXY, OUR SOLAR SYSTEM, OUR SUN, OUR PLANET EARTH & OUR MOON: How Were They Created?**

# FORMATION OF OUR UNIVERSE
**BIG-BANG THEORY: A THEORY BASED ON THE SCIENTIFIC FACTS**

## 1. Big Bang Theory: Can We Trust It?

No one knows for sure what triggered the Big Bang. But the discovery of Cosmic Microwave Background radiation in 1965 made the Big Bang theory the best theory of describing the origin and evolution of our Universe. With the aid of the NASA's highly sophisticated spacecraft known as the Wilkinson Microwave Anisotropy Probe (WMAP), ground-based telescopes, and brilliant scientific calculations, our astronomers, cosmologists, space researchers and scientists understood what exactly happened in the beginning stages of our Universe. [22]

● The most important finding was the afterglow of creation, light and radiation leftover from the Big Bang. This relic of the Big Bang pervades our Universe and is visible to microwave detectors as a birthmark, which allowed our scientists to piece together clues of our early Universe. [23, 24, 25]
● This "afterglow of creation" commonly known as the Cosmic Microwave Background radiation is the leftover heat from the fireball of the Big Bang in which our Universe was born 13.8 billion years ago. It provides a unique insight into our Universe's infancy as the world-renowned theoretical physicist and cosmologist late Dr. Stephen Hawking described it as our Universe's "baby photo," and said that it is the discovery of the century if not of all time. And another cosmologist, astrophysicist and Nobel Prize winner Dr. George Smoot said that "it is like seeing the face of the God—the Creator." [26]

After this discovery of the afterglow of creation of our Universe, surrounding light and radiation leftover from the Big Bang, more and more scientists and very many common people around the world started accepting and entrusting the Big Bang theory.

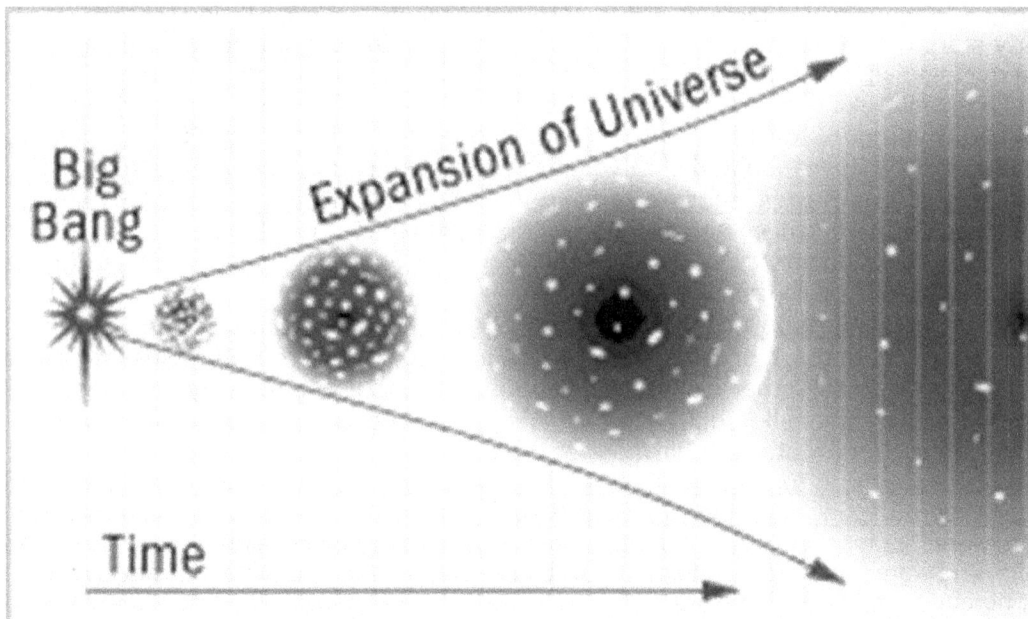

Figure 1.3  Our Universe has begun expanding like a magical balloon immediately after its birth.

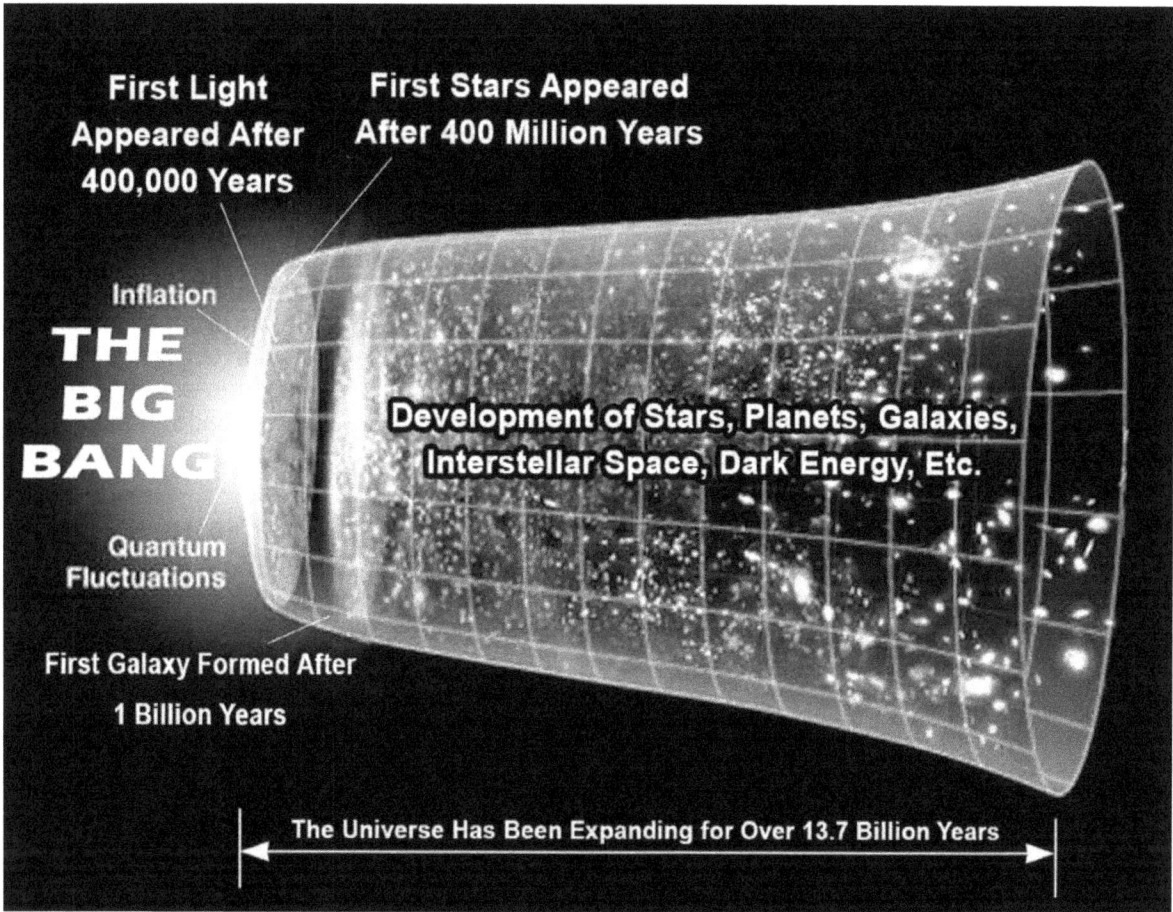
Figure 1.1 The formation of our Universe after the Big Bang.

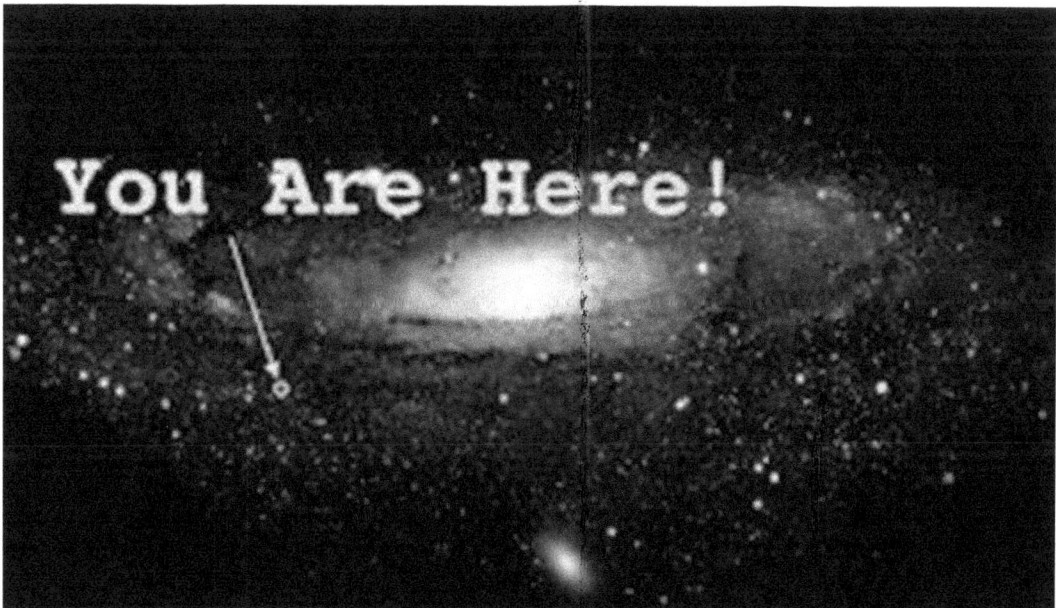
Figure 1.2 Location of our planet Earth on the spiral-shaped Milky Way Galaxy.

## 2. Big Bang Theory: What Does It Say?

Big Bang theory states that our Universe has begun its formation from an unimaginably hot and dense point of Singularity some13.8 billion years ago, and has started expanding unstoppably since then. The original temperature at the time of birth was infinite or at least 100 Nonillion degrees or $10^{32}$ degrees Kelvin. [27] When our just-born Universe was unimaginably so young, that is to say when it was only $10^{-34}$ second young — that is to say, when it was only a hundredth of a billionth of a trillionth of a trillionth of a second in age — Whew!— it underwent an incredible growth spurt or burst of expansion known as inflation in which period the space itself expanded exponentially faster than the speed of light, breaking the laws of physics. *The Big Bang was not a violent explosion, but it was a rapid and peaceful expansion*. During that period of a tiniest fraction of a second, our Universe doubled in size at least 90 or 100 consecutive times, going from a subatomic-sized to the golf-ball-sized instantaneously, and blew up the space like a giant magical balloon into several kilometers, and never stopped expanding thereafter. [23, 27]

## 3. Big Bang Theory: Singularity, Inflation & Primordial Soup

**a. Singularity:** A singularity means a point where some property is infinite. If you extrapolate the properties of our Universe to the very instant of the Big Bang, you will find that both the density and the temperature go to infinity. That compacted tiny point with infinite density from which our Universe expanded might have contained all the clues (all the mass, space and time that ever needed), from which the whole Universe emerged. This decision came from the observations of the NASA's WMAP's cosmic microwave background, which contained the afterglow of light and radiation leftover from the Big Bang. [23, 25]

**b. Inflation:** The initial stage of the Big Bang called "Cosmic Inflation" was so quick, as it lasted only $10^{-34}$ second. All the energy and heat from that explosion was shot out. And wherever that expansion of that peaceful explosion travelled with time, it automatically created space upon which our Universe lies. [25]

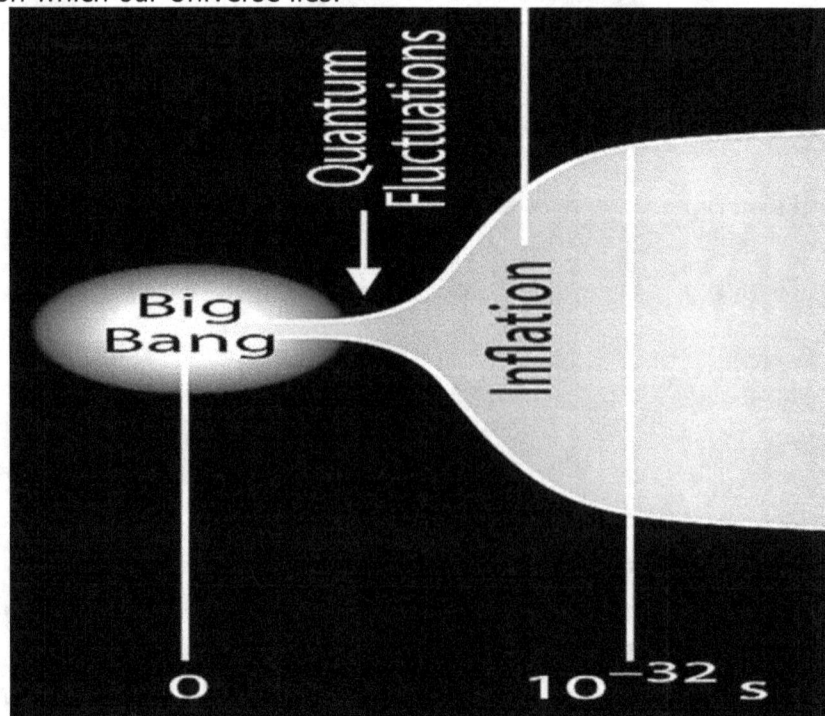

Courtesy of Steemit
Figure 1.4  The inflation ends when time = $10^{-32}$ second [25]

The temperature of our Universe at that instant was unimaginably 100 Nonillion degrees or $10^{32}$ degrees Kelvin. [27,28] During that time of Cosmic Inflation, matter and anti-matter annihilated each other, and as a result no matter existed. No atoms were generated yet, even though there was some surplus of quarks left behind. [29]

### c. Primordial Soup

Cosmologists believe that our newborn Universe existed as a hot and dense primordial soup, broth or plasma of highly energized matter, went through a burst of expansion like a giant magical balloon faster than the speed of light. At that incredibly high temperature and high pressure, matter was crushed into a soup of its constituent quarks, electrons and gluons (no atoms were formed yet). Our just-born Universe was found to be doubled its size at least 90 consecutive times in a span of $10^{-32}$ second. This phase of primordial soup, also known as **Cosmic Inflation**, ended when our Universe was only $10^{-32}$ second old. [25]

⦿ Everything in our Universe, including every person in this world, is made up of atoms. Science tells us that those atoms consist of nuclear particles called protons and neutrons in their hearts. These subatomic particles, in turn, are made up of building blocks known as quarks, which are glued together by particles aptly named gluons. [18] However, during the time of Inflation, our Universe was so hot that quarks were kept apart from gluons. The result would have been a hot dense mixture of quarks and gluons known as a quark-gluon plasma. During that state of primordial soup, atoms were not yet created, but all the matter existed in a special state of baryons (protons and neutrons), and at that instant our Universe was extended into only a few kilometers across. [30]

### d. Our Scientists Have Recreated the Big Bang's Primordial Soup Conditions, and Achieved a Temperature of 5.5 Trillion °K in A Giant Atom Smasher at CERN'S Large Hardon Collider!

CERN (Conseil Européen pour la Recherche Nucléaire), Geneva, Switzerland:[30, 31, 32, 33]

It is the European Organization for Nuclear Research, also called CERN in French language, that operates the largest particle physics laboratory in the world. On August 13, 2012, the scientists at CERN's Large Hadron Collider (LHC), Geneva, Switzerland, announced that they had achieved temperatures of over 5 trillion °K and perhaps as high as 5.5 trillion °K when they attempted to recreate the conditions of the Big Bang's "Primordial Soup" that represented the earliest moments following the Big Bang.
The giant 27 kilometer (16.7 mile) long particle accelerator is the most powerful in the world, and only it can generate the appalling energies needed to probe these earliest conditions of our Universe. The research team had been using the ALICE (A Large Ion Collider Experiment) experiment to smash together "lead ions" at 99% of the speed of light (Speed of light is 186,000 miles per second or about 300,000 Kilometers per second) to recreate a quark-gluon plasma – an exotic state of matter (Primordial Soup) believed to have filled our Universe just after the Big Bang during the time of inflation. The accelerator slammed the lead nuclei together at a record energy level of 5.02 tera electron Volts (TeV), or about 5 trillion electron Volts. When the nuclei collided at a slightly off center angle, they formed a football-shaped "droplet" of quark-gluon plasma as shown in the figure below. The whole scientific community marvelled by this groundbreaking achievement.

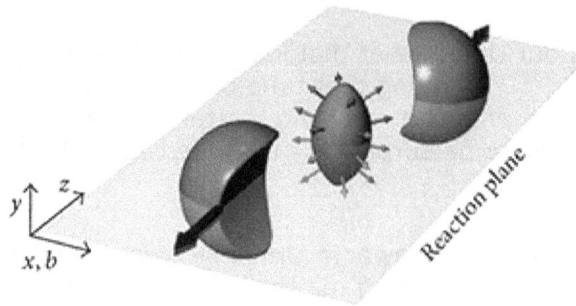

Courtesy of the University of Copenhagen, Denmark.
Figure 1.5  The formation of football-shaped quark-gluon plasma was recorded.
A temperature from 5 trillion °K to 5.5 trillion °K was also recorded.

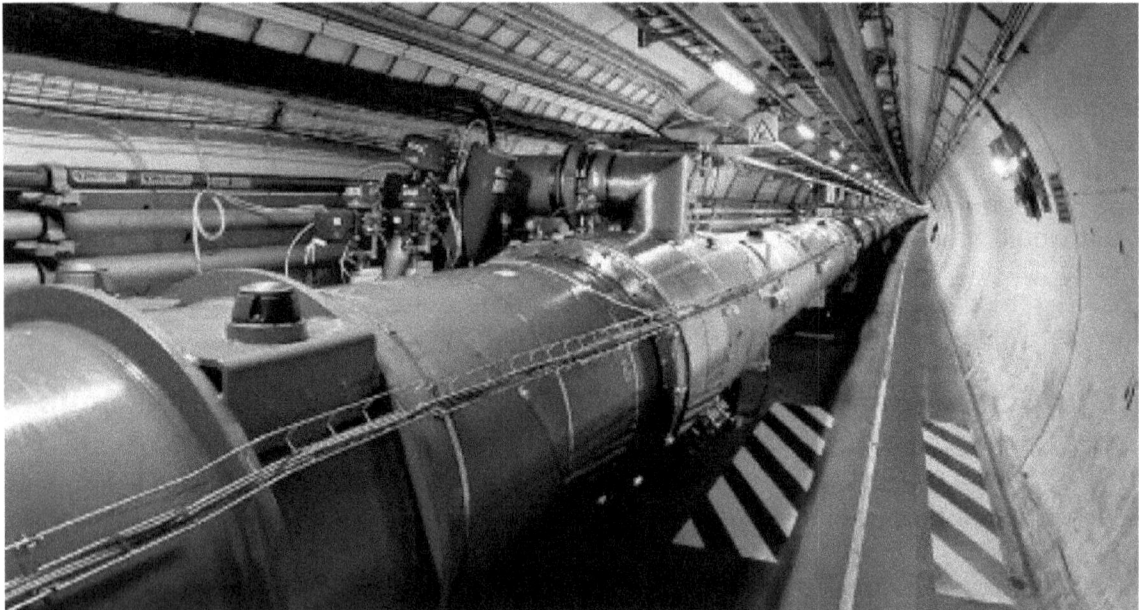

Courtesy of CERN, Geneva, Switzerland
Figure 1.6  Large Hardon Collider (LHC), Recreation of Early Universe, CERN, Geneva, Switzerland.
The giant 27 kilometer (16.7 mile) long particle accelerator.

## 4. Nearly One Second After the Big Bang, Our Universe Has Cooled Down, Temperature Dropped to 1 Billion Degrees Kelvin,

and the most fundamental particles such as quarks, electrons, photons and neutrinos just formed, but not yet bound together. [27, 28, 33]

⊕ Our Universe continued to expand not as quickly as during inflation, but at a much slower rate. As our Universe was further being cooled down and expanded, it was being governed by the four fundamental forces such as:
(i) the gravity,
(ii) the strong force,
(iii) the weak force, and
(iv) the electromagnetic force.

## 5. Nearly 3 Minutes After the Big Bang,
## The First Most Important Event Took Place:
## Hydrogen & Helium Nuclei Were Created!

⚬ Our Universe was still unimaginably hot, but there was an exponential drop in temperature. The temperature of our Universe dropped from 100 Nonillion degrees or $10^{32}$ degrees Kelvin to 1 billion degrees Kelvin or $10^9$ degrees Kelvin. That sudden drop in temperature caused a kind of cooling effect as the energy solidified into matter. That cooling process is analogous to the way how steam condenses to liquid droplets as water vapor cools in steam distillation, or how the water is being frozen into ice in the freezer [34, 35]. Those cooling conditions (both temperature and pressure) of our newborn Universe 3 minutes after the Big Bang perfectly suited for the quarks to coalesce and bound into hadrons such as protons and neutrons. It was called hadrons era. The protons and neutrons in turn combined to form nuclei of light elements such as hydrogen and helium. No neutral atoms were created yet. That was the first most important event that took place in the history of the Big Bang because:

Our visible Universe today is approximately composed of: [35]
  ▹ 90% Hydrogen (by mole fraction),
  ▹ 8% Helium (by mole fraction), and
  ▹ 2% Everything Else (by mole fraction).

## 6. Nearly 380,000 Years After the Big Bang,
## The Second Most Important Event Took Place:

The primary element "Hydrogen" was created, and thereafter hydrogen was abundantly available throughout our Universe. The nuclei of the light elements such as hydrogen, helium, lithium and beryllium attracted electrons, and formed neutral or stable atoms in a process known as "stellar nucleosynthesis."    The First Light Appeared!  { **LET THERE BE LIGHT!** }

⚬ During 300,000 to 380,000 years after the Big Bang, our Universe was still unbearably too hot for light to shine. Nearly 380,000 years after the Big Bang, the temperature of our Universe dropped to about 4000 degrees Kelvin, and then to 3000 degrees Kelvin. [36]

### ◌ RECOMBINATION PERIOD: [29, 37]

**REMEMBER!** About 3 minutes after the Big Bang, the quarks coalesced and bound into hadrons such as protons and neutrons. The protons and neutrons in turn combined to form nuclei of light elements such as hydrogen and helium. About 380,000 years after the Big Bang, our Universe was filled with a hot and dense fog of ionized gas. The nuclei of the light elements **hydrogen, helium, lithium and beryllium** attracted electrons, and formed neutral and stable atoms in a process called "**nucleosynthesis**". Hydrogen is the dominant primordial element created 380,000 years after the Big Bang, as our scientists now know that 90% of the Universe today is made made up of hydrogen. This process of particles pairing up in order to form stable atoms was called "Recombination", and that process actually started occurring approximately 240,000 to 300,000 years after the Big Bang, and intensified after 380,000 years. Our Universe went from being opaque to transparent at this point. Up to 300,000 years after the Big Bang, light had formerly been stopped from traveling freely because it would frequently scatter off the free electrons. About 380,000 years after the Big Bang, the free electrons were bound to protons in an attempt to form neutral atoms, and therefore the light was no longer being impeded. Even though our Universe became transparent relatively, our Universe at that point of time was not fully visible because THERE WERE NO STARS.

# FORMATION OF STARS

## 7. Nearly 400 Million Years After the Big Bang,
## The Third Most Important Event Took Place:

**The First Stars Appeared, and the Formation of Stars and Planets Continued Until Today!**

Nearly 400 Million Years After the Big Bang, our Universe already switched to cold weather, below freezing temperatures. The temperature dropped to and varied between − 213 °C and -254 °C (between 60 °K and 19 °K). [29]

### ◐ REIONIZATION PERIOD [27, 29, 37]

◉ Some Big Bang theorists believe that the first stars began their formation 200 million years after the Big Bang, but some other scientists believe that the first stars were clearly visible after 400 million years. However, NASA posted that there was no documented evidence with regard to when exactly the first stars began to form.

About 400 Million years after the Big Bang, our Universe emerged out of darkness. This period in our Universe's evolution is called the age of "Reionization" in which period <u>clumps of gas consisting of large coulds of all sorts of neutral atoms of many elements produced during the "Recombination Process," collapsed under gravity with internal spinning and swirling to form the very first bright light, which became a star, thereby creating the first star, and followed by more and more stars, which led to building the very first Solar System</u>, and eventually millions of stars along with orbiting planets (Solar Systems). The emitted ultraviolet light from these energetic events cleared out and destroyed most of the surrounding neutral hydrogen gas. The process of reionization plus the clearing of foggy hydrogen gas caused our Universe to become transparent to ultraviolet light for the first time. This dynamic phase of formation of stars and galaxies lasted over 500 million (half a billion) years, and the reionization process lasted about 1 billion years. The first galaxy was formed about 1 billion years after the Big Bang. [27]

## FORMATION OF STARS, GALAXIES, CLUSTERS & SUPER CLUSTERS

The early stars were made up of very simple and light gaseous elements (hydrogen and helium) and so they had very short lifespans of only millions of years. But the nuclear fusion in the cores' of these early stars slowly created all kinds of heavier elements, including the most important carbon and oxygen. When a large star died, it would become a part of a new star in the supernova explosion. In the beginning, these stars were created in small groups and attracted other stars. These stars were grouped in irregular shapes. Then the different shapes merged to form the first galaxies. Then as more and more galaxies formed, they were grouped in galaxy clusters, and then these clusters were contained in super clusters. Today, our scientists know about a force called dark energy. Dark energy acts like an anti-gravity and does the opposite of gravity. Dark energy is currently the cause of the expansion of our Universe. Our Universe is expanding at an accelerating rate today. With the discovery of dark energy, many scientists now believe that our Universe will continue to expand forever and all of the matter in our Universe will eventually decay in about one trillion years. [38]

### <u>How Many Stars Are There in Our Universe?</u> Dr. RK Has Made the Following Calculation:

Our Universe is embedded with 2 trillion galaxies  $= 2 \times 10^{12}$ galaxies.
Our Milky Way Galaxy has 500 billion stars $= (1/2)$ trillion stars $= (1/2) (10^{12})$ stars
Therefore Total Number of Stars $= (2 \times 10^{12}) (1/2) (10^{12}) = 10^{24}$ stars = Trillion Trillion stars.
There are 1,000,000,000,000,000,000,000,000 stars. There are $10^{24}$ stars.
That's a 1 followed by twenty-four zeros.
This is a grossly rough estimate. The exact number of stars is unknown.

# COUNTING STARS IN THE SKY OF OUR UNIVERSE [6, 18]
## METHOD 1

Counting stars in the sky of our Universe is like trying to count the number of sand grains on a beach. We might be able to calculate the surface area of the beach by measuring the length and width of the beach by means of a measuring tape, and we can also measure the depth of the sand grains spread all over the beach by means of a measuring tape, and then we could calculate the volume of the total sand grains on the beach in cubic centimeters ($cm^3$) by using the formula "volume of the total sand grains a beach = length x width x depth". Supposing that each sand grain is a spherical particle, and by measuring the radius of a grain in centimeters, we can calculate the volume of each sand grain in cubic centimeters ($cm^3$) by using the formula $(4/3) \pi r^3$ where r is the radius of the sand grain (a spherical particle). If we divide the volume of the total sand grains of the beach by the volume of each sand grain, we obtain the total number of sand grains in that beach by simple math. This is just a simple example that can be understood by any person with a high school background. Our astronomers in the past used to apply this kind of simple technique in determining the number of stars in our Universe by visual observation using a telescope. The more experience an astronomer has, the more accurate the star-count could be. [6]

Counting stars in the sky of our Universe is always a grossly rough estimate (Even the NASA does not know total stars) as it is impossible to count the stars accurately. Over time, the space research progressed a lot. On space, astronomers wouldn't try to count stars individually, instead they measure integrated quantities like the number and luminosity of galaxies. ESA's infrared space observatory Herschel has made an important contribution by 'counting' galaxies in the infrared, and measuring their luminosity in this range. From these experiments, they found the number of galaxies in our Universe. By multiplying the number of galaxies in our Universe by the number stars in each galaxy, they were able to determine the total number of stars. [6]

For Example, A ESA's Astronomer Has Made The Following Calculations: [6]
Suppose that our Universe has $10^{11}$ to $10^{12}$ Galaxies.
Each Galaxy has has $10^{11}$ to $10^{12}$ Stars.
Total number of Stars in our Universe (grossly rough estimate) = $10^{22}$ to $10^{24}$ Stars.

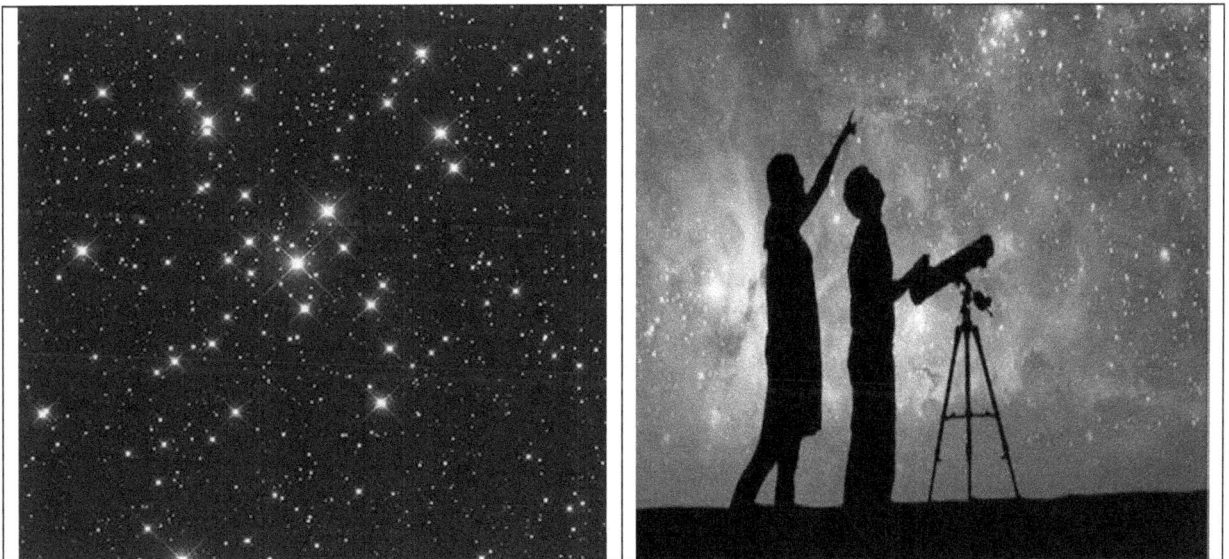

Figure 1.7 Counting stars in the sky of our Universe.
Counting stars in the sky by visual observation by our astronomers is believed to be an art.

## METHOD 2

The primary way astronomers estimate stars in a galaxy is by determining the galaxy's mass. The mass is estimated by looking at how the galaxy rotates, as well as its spectrum using spectroscopy. Once a galaxy's mass is determined, the other tricky thing is figuring out how much of that mass is made of stars. Most of the mass will be made up of dark matter, a type of matter that emits no light but which is believed to make up most of the mass of our Universe. You have to model the galaxy and see if you can understand what percentage of that mass of stars would be. If we can determine mass of the galaxy and the mass of the interstellar space, we can calculate the total mass occupied by stars. By supposing an average mass for each star (Of course, not all stars have equal mass), we can approximately compute the total number of stars in a galaxy. In a typical galaxy, if you measure its mass by looking at the rotation curve, about 90 percent of that is dark matter. [18]

Much of the remaining "stuff" in the galaxy is made up of diffused gas and dust. A scientist estimated that about 3 percent of the galaxy's mass will be made up of stars, but that could vary. Further, the size of the stars itself can greatly vary from something that is the size of our sun, to something dozens of times smaller or bigger. So is there any way to figure out how many stars are for sure? In the end, it comes down to a rough estimate only. In one calculation, the Milky Way has a mass of about 100 billion solar masses, so it is easiest to translate that to 100 billion stars (In general a galaxy is believed to have one trillion stars). This accounts for the stars that would be bigger or smaller than our Sun, and averages them out. However, the mass is tough to calculate. More sophisticated instruments are being manufactured to determine the mass of a galaxy. By multiplying the number of galaxies discovered by the number of stars in each galaxy, our scientists determine the rough estimate of number of stars in our Universe. [18]

## Stars Manufacture Heavier Elements Like Factories Do! [39, 40, 41]

**RECAP:** The nuclei of the primordial elements "hydrogen and helium" were created 3 minutes after the Big Bang. Nearly 380,000 years after the Big Bang, when the first light appeared, the nuclei of the light elements attracted electrons, and formed neutral atoms. Which means the actual stable atoms of the light elements "hydrogen, helium, lithium & beryllium" were created at the time of recombination in a process called nucleosynthesis well before the stars formation. Nearly 400 million years after the Big Bang, the primitive (first) stars formed as clumps of gas (mostly hydrogen) collapsed enough under gravity to form the very first bright light, which became a star, thereby creating the first star, followed by more and more stars, and eventually millions of stars, billions of stars, and even trilions of stars. Hydrogen is the primordial element created 380,000 years after the Big Bang, and is used as the burning fuel in the stars. Hydrogen is never created or produced in stars. But all the other heavier elements are produced in the burning cores of stars 400 million years after the Big Bang. [39]

## • Stellar Nucleosynthesis: When a gigantic interstellar cloud of space dust and primordial gas (mostly hydrogen) is collapsed due to gravity, a protostar forms and proceeds to compact further. The protostar becomes a disk and starts rotating, spinning and swirling under gravity. The rotation of the protostar (the disk) helps preventing further collapse, but internal spinning and swirling continues within the cloud, forming much stronger protostar. The continuing gravitational compaction causes the protostar to heat up more and more until its core reaches a critical temperature of about 15,700,000 °C. At this extremely high temperature, hydrogen atoms are disassociated into protons and electrons, as they no longer bound together. When the temperature in the burning star rises to 15 million to 100 million degrees Celsius, the dissociated protons and electrons are brought back together by a fundamental force called "strong nuclear force", thereby creating a much heavier element called helium. This process in which a heavier element is created in the burning cores of stars is called nuclear fusion or stellar nucleosynthesis. Then the helium star lights up and shines again. [40]

# Stellar Nucleosynthesis (Continued)

Stellar Nucleosynthesis is a process in which heavier elements are created within a star by combining the protons and neutrons together from the nuclei of lighter elements at extremely high temperatures (millions of degrees) when stars run out of fuel, extinguish or die, and then explode into supernovae.

**Supernova explosion** occurs in a galaxy when a huge star runs out of nuclear fuel (hydrogen or helium), collapses and explodes while manufacturing, dumping and scattering all kinds of heavier elements into the interstellar medium, from a gigantic cloud of which a typical Solar System is created.

Primitive stars were massive, short-lived, collapsed under gravity, and exploded into supernovae while manufacturing all kinds of heavier elements. Hydrogen was the primary element from which all heavier elements were created in the following manner: [41]

- **Hydrogen** was first fused to produce helium in the burning core of a star or stars.
- Helium in turn was fused to produce lithium.
- Lithium plus helium in turn was fused to produce beryllium.
- Beryllium plus helium in turn was fused to produce **carbon** (very important element).
- Carbon plus helium was fused to produce **nitrogen** (very important element).
- Carbon/Nitrogen plus helium was fused to produce **oxygen** ( very important element).
- Oxygen plus helium was fused to produce neon.
- Neon plus helium was fused to produce magnesium.
- Magnesium plus helium was fused produce silicon.
- Silicon plus helium was fused to produce **sulfur** (very important element).
- Sulfur plus helium was fused produced argon.
   Sulfur was also produced from silicon via an alpha process.
- **Phosphorus** was produced via neutron capture onto isotopes of silicon (very important).
- Argon plus helium was fused to produce calcium.
- Calcium plus helium was fused to produce titanium.
- Titanium plus helium was fused to produce chromium.
- Chromium plus helium was fused to produce iron.

Similarly all those 117 heavier elements of our periodic table were manufactured in the burning cores of stars.

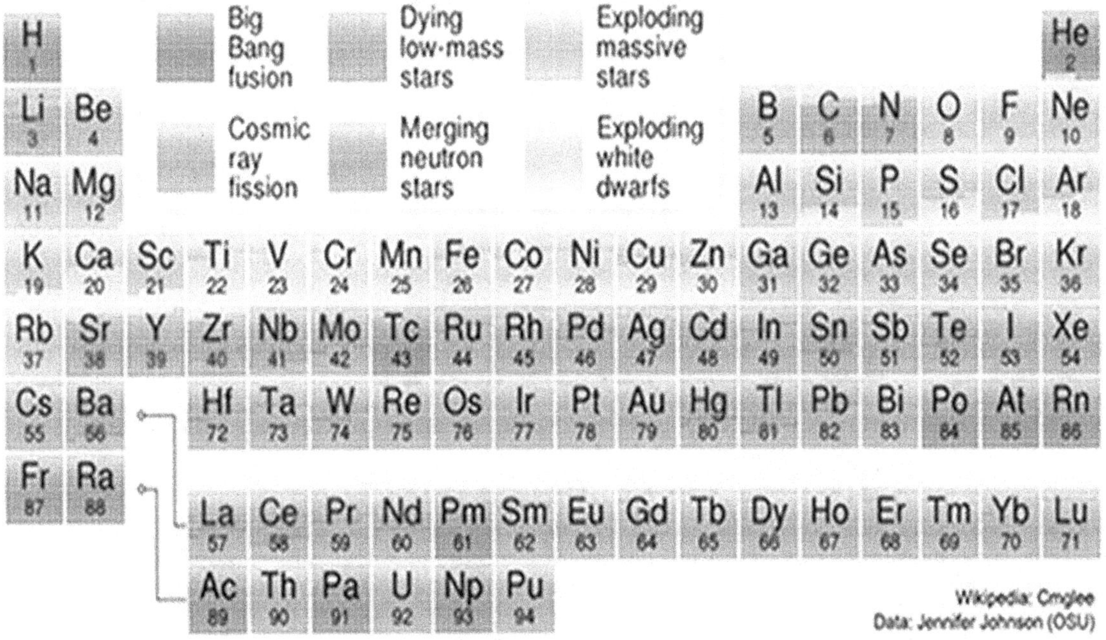

Courtesy of Nasa Science (Nasa.gov) and Wikipedia: Cmglee

Figure 1.8  Periodic Table (All these heavier elements were manufactured in the burning cores of stars).

◉ In the stellar nucleosynthesis, many different reactions take place in many different ways in the interiors of collapsing stars. It is called the triple-alpha process in which helium-4 nuclei (alpha particles) are transformed to produce the next heavier element. Each heavier element is produced when a star reaches a distinct core temperature (sometimes, tens of millions of degrees), heat and radiation. Sometimes the catalytic chemical reaction also takes place.

◉ Early stars were massive, short-lived and exploded into supernovae while manufacturing, dumping and scattering all those 117 heavier elements (except hydrogen) of our periodic table into the interstellar space from a gigantic cloud of which our Solar System was created!

◉ Did you know? When our solar system began its formation 6 billion years ago from a gigantic cloud of space dust and interstellar gas, that gigantic cloud was already enriched with all those 117 elements, and that is how our planet Earth possessed all those 117 heavier elements.

**IMPORTANT NOTE:** NASA's scientists, astronomers & space researchers studied extensively the possibility of the formation and existence of life in the other planets of our Solar Sytem, and always adopted that "Life requires 6 essential elements such as CHNOPS: carbon, hydrogen, nitrogen, oxygen, phosphorus and sulfur." [42, 43]

## WHEN YOU LOOK UP AT NIGHT, YOU ARE SEEING FACTORIES CALLED STARS

When you look up at night, you are seeing factories called stars equipped with nuclear-fusion reactors, working round the clock, without which the constituents for our entire natural world would not exist, including all those 117 heavier elements of our periodic table desperately needed for the formation and survival of every human being, animal & plant. [40]

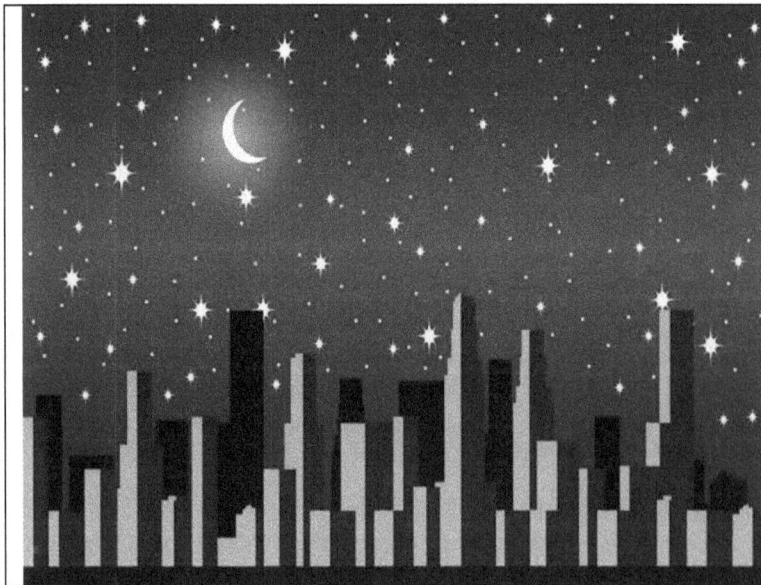

Astronomer Dr. Carl Sagan in his book "Cosmos" wrote: The nitrogen in our DNA, the calcium in our teeth, the iron in our blood, the carbon in our apple pies were all made in the interiors of collapsing stars. We are all made of starstuff. [44]

Almost 99% of the mass of the human body is made up of SIX elements "carbon, hydrogen, nitrogen, oxygen, phosphorus and sulfur." And the remaining 1% is made up of other elements. All organic matter containing carbon was produced originally in the stars. [45]

Figure 1.9  When you look up at night, you are seeing factories called stars.

### The Process of Stars Creation Continued Until Today!

The process of stars creation continued, as our Universe has begun creating millions of stars along with orbiting planets and galaxies, and then billions of stars along with orbiting planets and galaxies, and then even trillions of stars along with orbiting planets and galaxies that are visible today!

### The Current Temperature of Our Universe in the Year 2020

The current temperature of our Universe in 2020 = −270.42 °Celsius = 2.73 °Kelvin. [36]

# FORMATION OF OUR MILKY WAY GALAXY

In general our Universe has 3 types of galaxies (there are 2 trillion galaxies): [46]
(i) Spiral-shaped galaxy
(ii) Elliptical-shaped galaxy
(iii) Irregular-shaped galaxy

● **Milky Way Galaxy:** Please see Figure 1.2. We live on a planet called "Earth" that is a very small part of our solar system, manufactured by our Sun. But our solar system itself is a tiny portion of our Milky Way Galaxy, which is again a tiny portion of our unimaginably humongous Universe that has been expanding unlimitedly for 13. 8 billion years. A galaxy is a huge collection of gas, dust, and of billions or trillions of stars and their solar systems. A galaxy is held together by gravity.

● Our Milky Way Galaxy is spiral-shaped upon which we all live, and our solar system (our Sun, our Earth & other 7 planets, our Moon) formed on one of the spiral arms as shown in the figure below. Astronomers now believe that our Milky Way Galaxy is approximately 13.6 billion years old. [11]

● Just like our planet Earth goes around the Sun, the Sun goes around the center of the Milky Way Galaxy. It takes one year or 365 days for our planet Earth to go around our Sun, and it takes 250 million years for our Sun and our entire solar system to go all the way around the center of our Milky Way Galaxy. [19]

● Our Milky Way Galaxy has 100 billion stars (solar systems) on the lower end and 400 billion stars (solar systems) on the upper end, totaling 500 billion solar systems. Our solar system (our Sun, our planet Earth, 7 other planets and our Moon) is one of them. Inside the Milky Way Galaxy, most stars have at least one planet orbiting the solar system. However, there are many stars without planets orbiting.

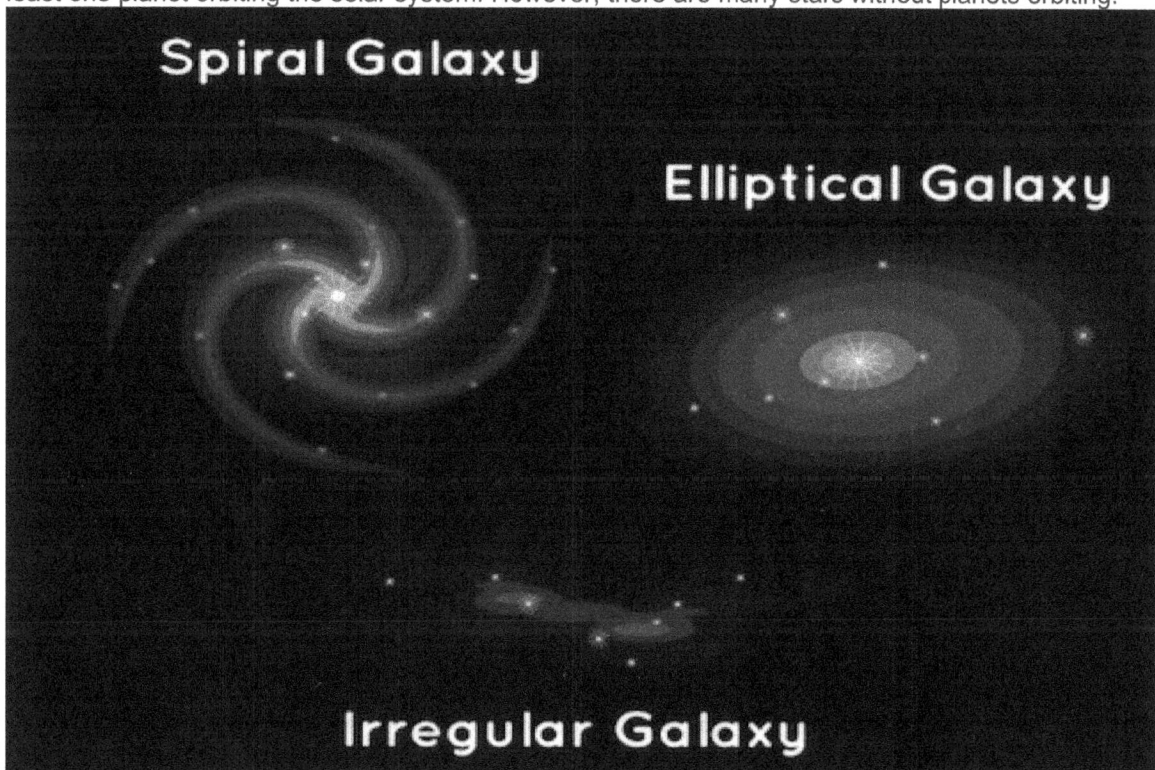

Courtesy of Nasa.gov

Figure 1.10 Galaxies are spiral-shaped, elliptical-shaped, oval-shaped or irregular-shaped. [46]
Milky Way Galaxy is spiral-shaped upon which we all live. Please see Figure 1.2.

⦁ **BLACK HOLE:** Our Milky Way Galaxy has a supermassive black hole, filled with dark energy, in the middle of it. [46] A black hole is a region of space exhibiting extremely strong gravitational acceleration. In black holes, no particles or even electromagnetic radiation such as light can pass through or escape from. The strong gravity occurs because matter has been compressed into a tiny space. This compression can take place at the end of a star's life when it runs out of fuel. Some black holes are a result of dying stars.

⦁ **Why Was It Called Milky Way Galaxy?** At first the Greeks and then the Romans called it "Milky Way" because if you look upward, either with your naked eye or by means of a telescope, on a clear night from the Earth's darkest regions, you could glimpse a broad stripe of stars, cloaked in clouds of dust and gas, arching across sky, and it would make you feel that you are witnessing a **milky patch**. The Milky Way Galaxy was found to glow in the night sky over the Chile's La Silla Observatory, La Higuera, Coquimbo Region, Chile, South America. [47, 48]

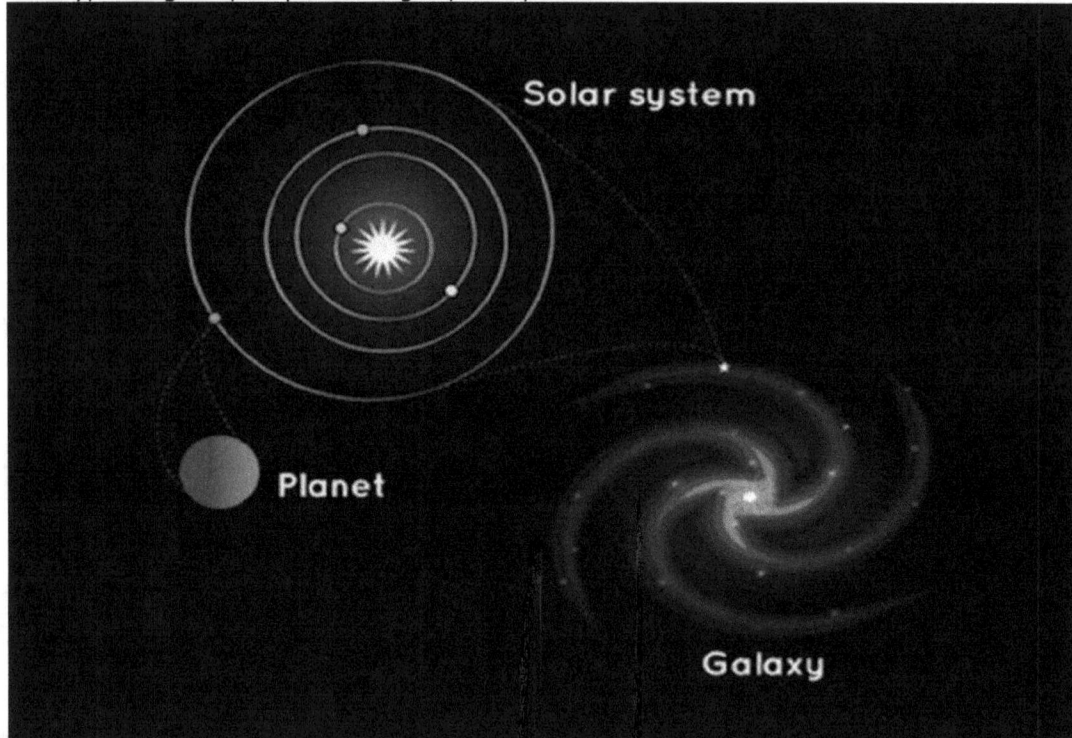
Courtesy of Nasa.gov

Figure 1.11  Our Milky Way Galaxy is spiral-shaped, and our Solar System formed on one of the spiral arms. [46]

## LIGHT-YEAR | NEAREST STAR | NEAREST GALAXY

**LIGHT-YEAR:** A light-year is not time, but a light-year is a unit of distance. It is the distance that light can travel in one year. Light travels at a speed of 186,000 miles per second or 300,000 km per second. So in one year, light can travel about 10 trillion km. More precisely, one light-year is equal to 9,500,000,000,000 kilometers. The distance between stars in our galaxy and in our Universe is so vast that astronomers and scientists cannot indicate it in kilometers or miles, but rather express it in light-years.
⦁ Our Milky Way Galaxy is about 150,000 light-years across.
**NEAREST STAR:** Alpha Centauri is nearest star, much larger star than our Sun. It is 4.3 light-years away. Our scientists believe that for humans to travel to the nearest star, it would take at least 70,000 years.
**NEAREST GALAXY:** Andromeda Galaxy is the nearest spiral galaxy, much larger than our Milky Way Galaxy, and is approximately 2.5 million light-years away. Our Milky Way Galaxy as a whole is moving through space at a rate of approximately 600 km per second and our scientists believe that it will collide with the Andromeda Galaxy in about 4 billion years. By that time our Sun could be exhausted, running out of fuel, extinguishing and about to collapse and explode into supernova. [12]

# FORMATION OF OUR SOLAR SYSTEM [55, 56, 57, 58, 59, 60]
OUR SUN, OUR PLANET EARTH, 7 OTHER PLANETS, OUR MOON, ASTEROIDS, COMETS, Etc.
## Did You Know Our Sun Manufactured Our Solar System?

Astronomers, space researchers and scientists figured out that a Solar System, consisting of a star and several planets that orbit the star, is created from the supernova explosion of a deceased star.

**WHAT IS A SUPERNOVA?**  Supernova explosion occurs in a galaxy when an enormously large star (10 to 20 times larger than our Sun) runs out of nuclear fuel (hydrogen and/or helium), and when some of its mass flows into its core, and the core collapses as it cannot withstand its own gravitational force. Supernovae have been observed by our astronomers as monster explosions in galaxies. Larger stars have shortened lifespan as they need more fuel to burn whereas relatively smaller stars have longer lifespan as they need less fuel to burn. When a massive star runs out of nuclear fuel, it will be collapsed as it cannot withstand its own gravitational force, and explodes into a supernova while manufacturing, dumping and scattering heavier elements into the interstellar space from a gigantic cloud of which, a Solar System is created.

**WHAT IS A SOLAR NEBULA?** [55, 56]
⊕ A gigantic interstellar cloud known as "solar nebula" of space dust (cosmic dust) and space gas that was squeezed by a supernova explosion gave birth to our solar system. A nebula is nothing but a huge cloud of interstellar gas and space dust mixed and coalesced with the leftovers of a previous star upon death. Each cloud of an extinguished or deceased previous star is capable of generating dozens of stars in a galaxy, though some stars are larger than the others.

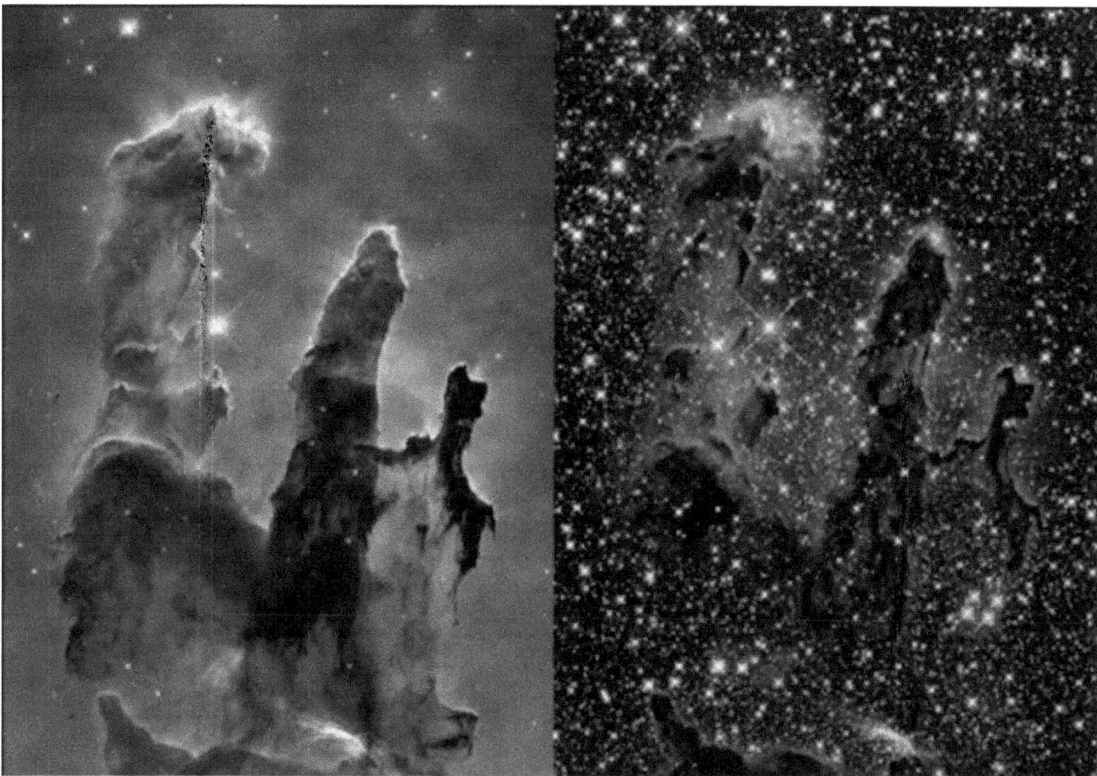

Courtesy of Nasa.gov          **Pillars of Creation**
Figure 1.12  A solar nebula is a gigantic cloud of space dust & gas of a deceased star.

• According to the Big Bang theory, our solar system began its formation some 6 billion years ago. By that time, the stardust in the space and interstellar gas were already enriched abundantly with all kinds of elements. There are 118 all kinds of elements listed in our periodic table such as hydrogen, helium, lithium, carbon, oxygen, nitrogen, calcium, iron, phosphorous, iodine, magnesium, zinc, selenium, copper, manganese, chromium, molybdenum, chloride, and many other components. All these elements (except hydrogen) were manufactured in the burning cores of earlier stars.

• **Please Refer to Figure 1.13:** A gigantic interstellar cloud known as "solar nebula" of space dust and primordial gas that was squeezed by a supernova explosion gave birth to our solar system. A nebula is nothing but a huge cloud of interstellar gas and space dust that was already enriched with all kinds of heavier elements, mixed, coalesced and squeezed together with the leftovers of a previous star upon death. The giant interstellar cloud collapsed under gravity and began rotating, compacting, spinning and swirling for 100s of millions of years or even billions of years, until our solar system formed! Our solar system began its formation some 6 billion years ago. Our scientists estimated that the age of our Earth and therefore the age of our solar system is 4.54 billion years, which means it took some one and half billion years to complete our solar system formation.

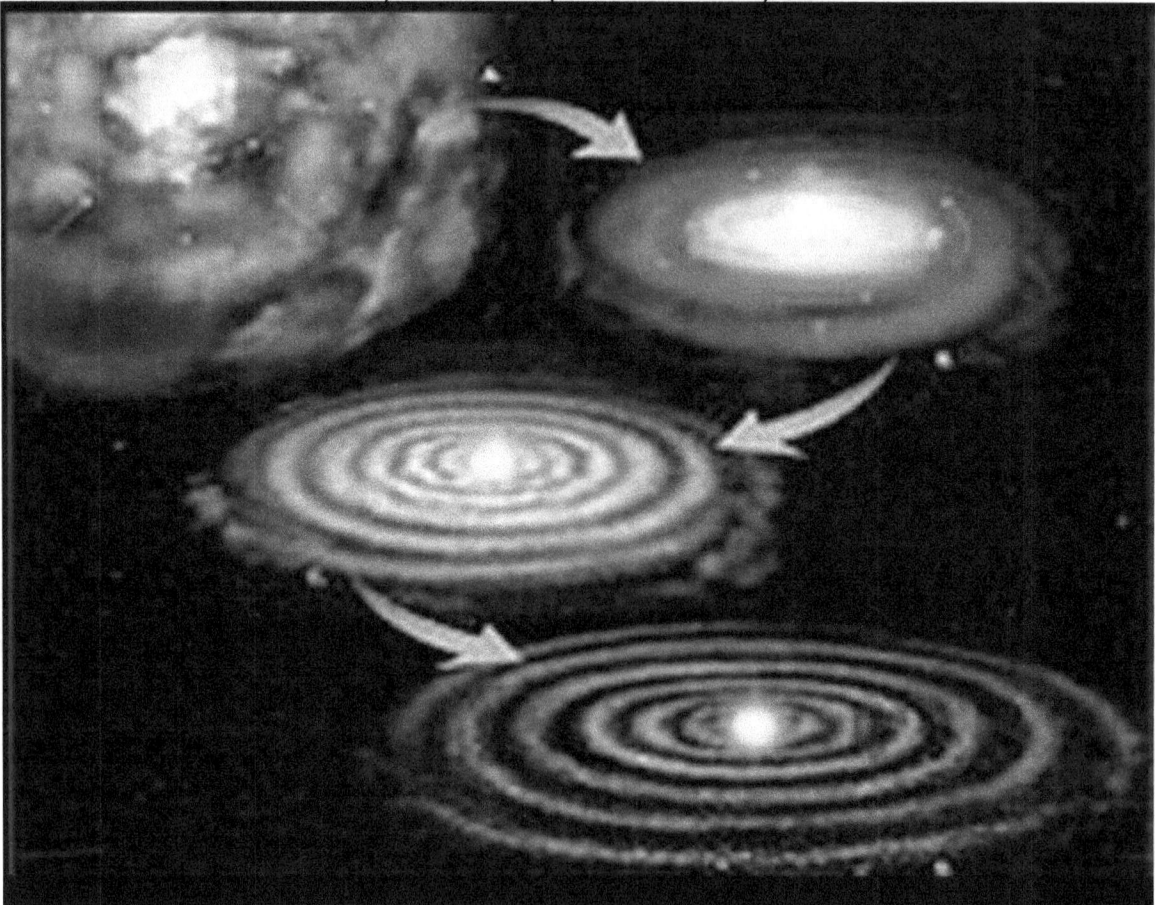

Figure 1.13 Our Solar System was being formed from a solar nebula.
A nebula is nothing but a gigantic cloud of interstellar gas and space dust.

• Experts believe that more than 99% of the gigantic interstellar cloud of the space dust and the interstellar gas, from which our solar system was being developed, becomes the Sun, and the remaining portion (less than 1%) becomes the planets that orbit the Sun for 100s of millions of years, or even billions of years before the solar system is completed its formation.

⦾ **Please Refer to Figure 1.14:** Upon the collapse of the gigantic cloud of space dust and primordial gas (mostly hydrogen), a protostar formed and proceeded to compact further. The protostar became a disk and started rotating under gravity. The rotation of the protostar (the disk) helped preventing further collapse, but internal spinning and swirling continued within the cloud, forming much stronger protostar. The central core reached a balance between the gravitational force and the internal pressure, aka as hydrostatic equilibrium, after 100s of millions of years. The rotation of the disk helped preventing further collapse of the disk, but internal spinning and swirling continued within the cloud, forming the protoplanetary disk.

⦾ Just like a dancer that spins faster as she pulls in her arms, the cloud began to spin as it collapsed. Eventually, the cloud grew hotter and denser in the center, with a disk of gas and dust surrounding it that was hot in the center but cool at the edges. As the disk got thinner and thinner, particles began to stick together and form clumps. Some clumps got bigger, as particles and small clumps stuck to them, eventually forming 8 planets, their moons, asteroids, comets, meteorites, near-earth objects, etc.[60]

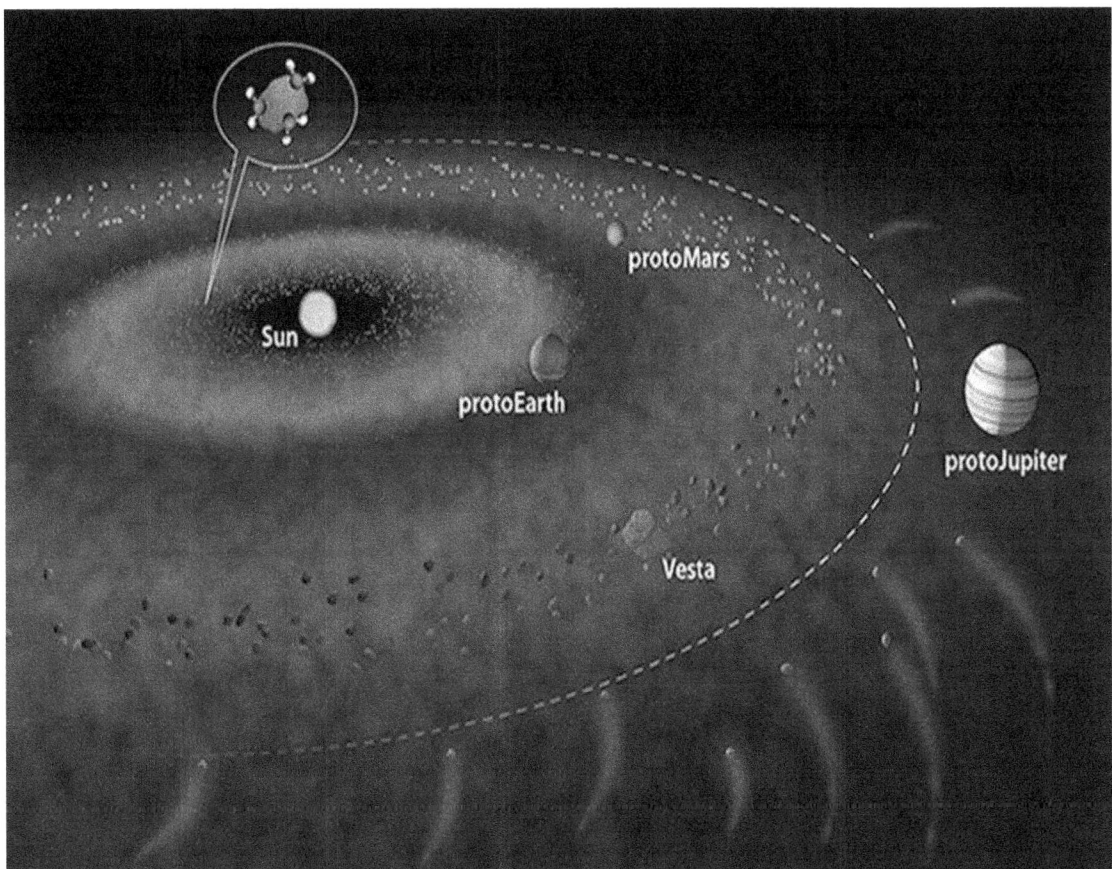

Courtesy of Jack Cook, Woods Hole Oceanographic Institution.
Figure 1.14  Our Solar System formation (Protoplanetary disks).
ProtoEarth, ProtoMars, ProtoJupiter = The planets that are at an early stage of development.
The Protostar (our Sun) was actually being orbited by 8 Protoplanets (some of them were not yet formed).
A protostar is a very young star that is still gathering mass from its parent molecular cloud. A protoplanetary disk or a protoplanet is a rotating circumstellar disk of dense gas and dust surrounding a young newly formed star.

**SUMMARY:** A gigantic cloud of space dust and interstellar gas of the supernova explosion of a massive, collapsing, exploding, spinning and swirling deceased star gave birth to our Solar System. That gigantic cloud was already enriched with all those minerals that we use today to remineralize and alkalize the purified water. That gigantic cloud was also already filled with liquid water. And that is how our planet Earth possessed that much liquid water that we drink to survive today.

# FORMATION OF OUR PLANET EARTH [57, 58, 59, 60]

◉ This process of spinning, swirling and the accretion in the solar system continued for 100s of million of years, or even billions of years, until the larger solid balls of accretion completed, and gave birth to 8 planets, including our planet Earth. It took more than a billion years for the formation of our solar system including all 8 planets, their moons, asteroids, comets, near-earth objects, etc.

**Please Refer to Figure 1.15:** Near the center of the burning Sun where only rocky material could stand the great heat, the four terrestrial or inner planets "**Mercury, Venus, Earth and Mars**" formed. And away from the centre of the burning Sun or farther to the burning Sun, icy and gassy matter settled in the outer regions of the disk, where the other four giant or jovian outer planets "**Jupiter, Saturn, Uranus and Neptune**" formed as shown in the figure below.

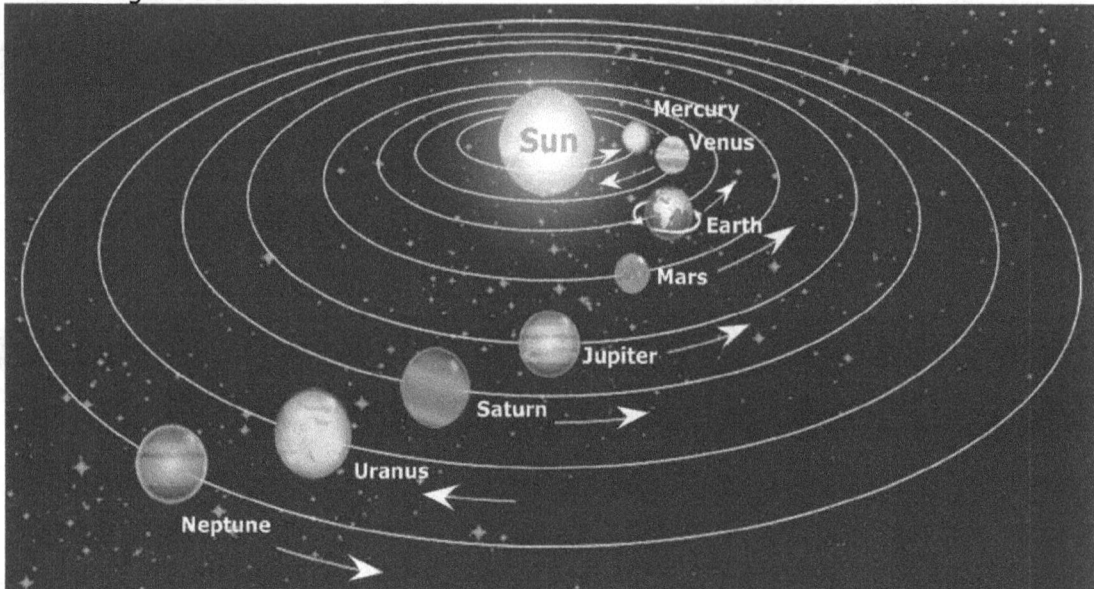

Figure 1.15  Formation of our solar system along with 8 planets, including the Earth.

◉ Our Sun manufactured our solar system, including our planet Earth, as the process of spinning and swirling of a gigantic cloud of the space dust and the interstellar gas continued for one and half billion years! Our Sun is now being orbited by 8 planets named "Mercury, Venus, Earth, Mars, Jupiter, Saturn, Uranus and Neptune". Our solar system began its formation 6 billion years, and completed its formation 4.54 billion years ago. In the next half a billion years, our planet Earth is going to be accompanied by our Moon (read below).

◉ **The Size of our Sun is Enormous:** Our Sun is 864,400 miles (1,391,000 kilometers) across, 109 times the Earth's diameter, weighs about 333,000 times more than Earth, 93 million miles (149.5 million km) away from Earth, [61b, 61c] and our Sun is so humongous that even 1,300,000 Earths could fit inside of it. [61]

◉ **How Long Our Sun Lasts?** Our Sun has a lifespan of 9 to 10 billion years. Which means our Sun will run out of nuclear fuel, extinguish or die after 4 to 5 billion years. When our Sun dies, our planet Earth, our Moon and 7 other planets will be engulfed with it and possibly vaporized. Afterwards our Sun either will become a White Dwarf or will explode into a supernova in which case a new star will born out of the debris. [62]

# FORMATION OF OUR MOON [63, 64]

๏ Our solar system began its formation some 6 billion years ago. The formation of our planet Earth and other 7 planets completed 4.54 billion years ago. After our terrestrial planet Earth was solidifying from its lava, softer elements moved to the surface and harder elements moved to the center of the core of our Earth. Some 4 Billion years ago, suddenly a large object (a meteorite) of the size of the mars smashed on to the surface of our Earth, creating a huge blast. Our planet Earth swallowed up much of the object's particles, ejecting a huge beam of dust and particles on to its atmosphere. These particles of debris gathered together and formed a much smaller planet-like object called Moon. Thus our Moon was formed. The formation of our Moon was an incredibly important event in the history of our Earth, especially in the development of life.

๏ The size of our Moon (equivalent to the size of Mars) perfectly suited our planet Earth, and gave stability to the development of our planet Earth and to the Earth's axis. Our Moon's gravitational force and at the same time its attachment to our planet Earth protected our planet Earth from wabbling while rotating on its own axis and orbiting around our Sun. Our Moon also helped our Earth's rotation by slowing down a little thereby establishing smooth rotation. Our planet Earth, at the time of its birth, was actually rotating so fast that it took only 6 hours to complete one rotation per day. After the formation of our Moon, our Earth's rotation stabilized and started completing one rotation in 24 hours, thereby creating the day-and-night cycle for us.

๏ Our Moon also provided our Earth the very important seasons "spring, summer, autumn and winter" in sequence, which are very important for the plants to grow and life to occur and to survive on our planet Earth.

๏ Our Moon and the presence of the plenty of liquid water in our planet Earth were both greatly responsible for the formation and development of life on our planet Earth.

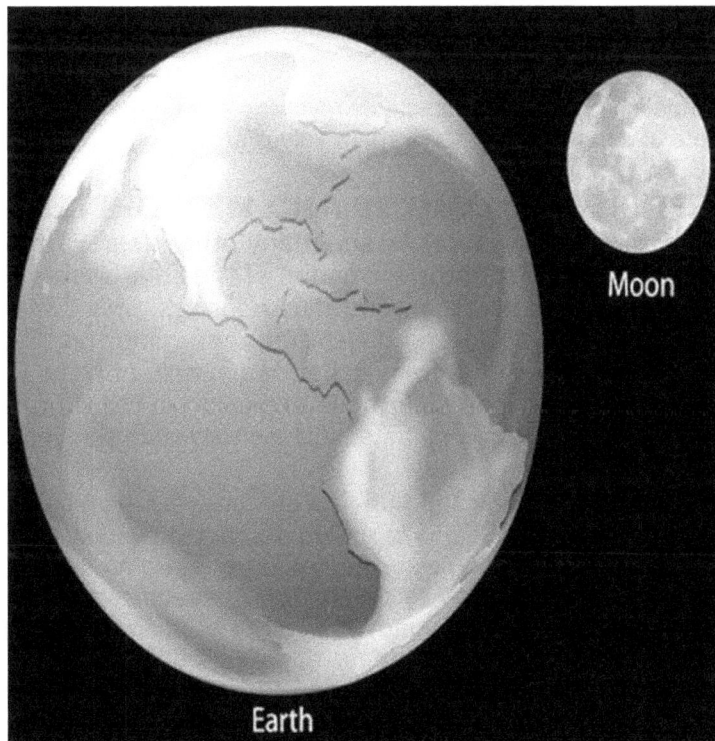

Figure 1.16 Formation of our Moon occurred 4 billion years ago, and gave stability to our Earth's rotation.

# FORMATION OF OUR PLANET EARTH & MOON (Continued)

Our Earth at the time of its birth was rotating so fast to complete one rotation per day. After the attachment of our Moon, Earth's rotation slowed down, stabilized, and started completing one rotation in exactly 24 hours. We now know that the Earth, by rotating around its own axis and by orbiting (revolving) around the Sun, creates day and night. It now takes 24 hours for our Earth to complete one rotation around its own axis (12 hours for the day and 12 hours for the night). It takes precisely 365 ¼ days (1 year) for our Earth to orbit, revolve or circle around the Sun.

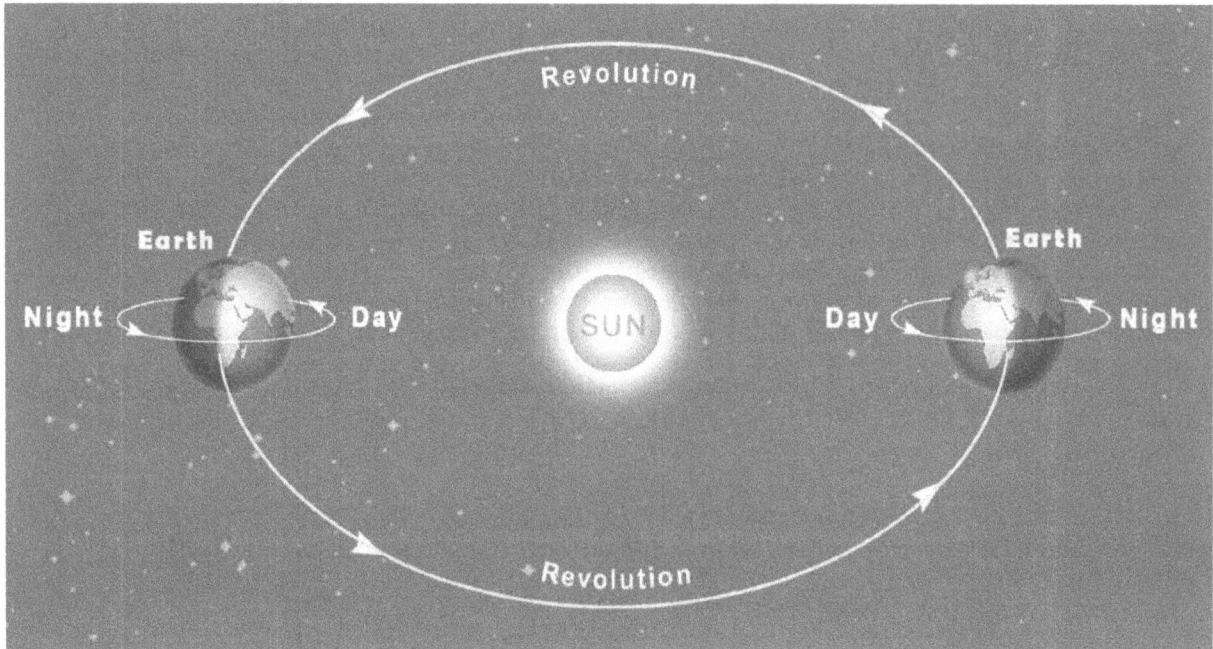

Figure 1.17 Our Earth, by rotating on its own axis and by revolving around the Sun, creates day & night. It takes 24 hours to complete one rotation, and our Earth revolves around our Sun in 365 ¼ days (1 year).

# FORMATION OF ASTEROIDS, COMETS AND METEORITES

Asteroids, comets, moons, meteors, meteorites and many other near-Earth objects are now understood to be the leftover debris from the formation of the solar system. Astronomers and scientists around the world currently think that our solar system's 8 planets (Mercury, Venus, Earth, Mars, Jupiter, Saturn, Uranus and Neptune) and minor bodies, including asteroids, comets, moons, meteorites and many other near-Earth objects all formed from the same cloud of stardust and gas of the supernova explosion of a collapsing massive star. Asteroids & comets cannot be considered as planets because they are relatively small in size.

**Asteroids** are rocky fragments that orbit the Sun in a belt between Mars and Jupiter. Scientists think that there are probably millions of asteroids, ranging widely in size from less than one kilometer wide to hundreds of kilometers across. The asteroid belt is located between Mars and Jupiter. Scientists believe that stray asteroids or fragments from earlier collisions have slammed into our planet Earth in the past, and played a major role in the evolution of our planet Earth. Researchers also determined that ice-bearing asteroids brought water, life-forming substances and other useful elements to the Earth during the period of their bombardment in the early stages of the formation of our planet Earth. Which means our planet Earth by the time of its formation already possessed liquid water. Researchers now have scientific evidence that our planet Earth attained 50% of its water from the bombardment of Asteroids.

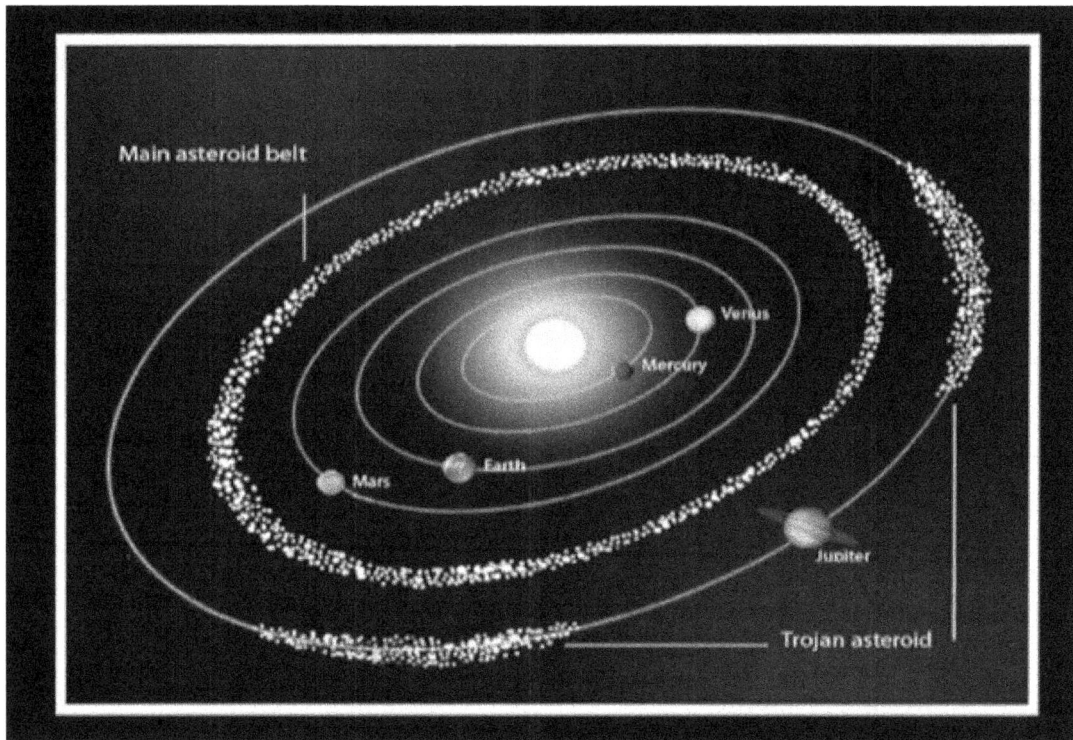

Figure 1.18 The asteroid belt is between Mars and Jupiter.

## AGE OF OUR UNIVERSE & OUR MILKY WAY GALAXY [1, 2, 3, 4, 5, 11, 12, 13]

The Hubble Space Telescope, launched in 1990, has helped our astronomers tremendously to measure the age of our Universe. Our astronomers have figured out several ways of observing and determining the age of our Universe.

(i) By measuring the speeds and distances of galaxies, our astronomers determined the age of our Universe. Because all of the galaxies in our Universe are generally moving apart, we infer that they must all have been much closer together sometime in the past (since our Universe has been created, it has been expanding all the time). Knowing the current speeds and distances to galaxies, coupled with the rate at which our Universe is being accelerated, it became possible to calculate how long it took for them to reach their current locations. The answer was about 13 to 14 billion years repeatedly.

(ii) The second method involves measuring the ages of the oldest star clusters. Globular star clusters orbiting our Milky Way are the oldest objects our astronomers found and a detailed analysis of those stars revealed that they formed about 13 to 14 billion years ago. The good agreement between the above-mentioned two very different methods is an encouraging sign that our space scientists are in the right track.

(iii) The Wilkinson Microwave Anisotropy Probe (WMAP), originally known as the Microwave Anisotropy Probe (MAP), is a NASA Explorer mission that launched in June 2001 to make fundamental measurements of cosmology, the study of the properties of our Universe as a whole. Headed by Professor Charles L. Bennett of Johns Hopkins University, the mission was developed in a joint partnership between the NASA Goddard Space Flight Center and Princeton University. WMAP has been stunningly successful, producing our new Standard Model of Cosmology. WMAP's data stream has ended. In 2012, NASA's Wilkinson Microwave Anisotropy Probe (WMAP), after collecting a vast amount of data for over a period of 9 years, estimated the age of our Universe to be 13.772 billion years, with an uncertainty of plus or minus 59 million years. Therefore,

**The age of our Universe = 13.8 Billion Years.**     **Please see Figure 1.1.**

Some astronomers and scientists believe that first stars appeared after 200 million years, and others believe after 400 billion years. So the Milky Way began its formation 200 to 400 million years after the Big Bang. Therefore,

**The age of our Milky Way Galaxy = 13.4 to 13.6 Billion years. Please see Figure 1.2.**

# AGE OF OUR PLANET EARTH BY RADIOMETRIC DATING [65-71]

⬤ The age of our planet Earth was determined by radiometric dating, which is the most accurate and reliable method to date old rocks. The nuclei of radioactive elements decay or spontaneously break down at predictable rates. For example, half of a given batch of uranium will decay into lead every 710 million to 4.47 billion years, depending on the isotope used (this number is termed the element's "half-life"). That uranium, which was created during a supernova that occurred long before our solar system existed, lingers in trace amounts within the Earth. When a rock is formed in the bowels of the planet, uranium atoms are trapped within it. These atoms will decay as the rock ages, and by measuring the ratio of radioactive isotopes within the rock, scientists can figure out how long it has been around. [66]

⬤ The oldest rocks on Earth, found to date, are the Acasta Gneiss in northwestern Canada near the Great Slave Lake, which are 4.03 billion years old. But rocks older than 3.5 billion years can be found on all continents. Greenland boasts the Isua supracrustal rocks (3.7 to 3.8 billion years old), while rocks in Swaziland are 3.4 billion to 3.5 billion years. Samples in Western Australia run 3.4 billion to 3.6 billion years old. The age of a zircon crystal from Australia was found to be 4.4 billion years, and is the oldest piece of Earth yet found (after our scientists believed the rock of Acasta Gneiss in northwestern Canada is the oldest). Our scientists have collected and calculated the ages of some 70 meteorites that have fallen from sky on to the Earth by using the radiometric dating technique. The oldest of these rocks are reported to be between 4.4 billion and 4.5 billion years old. [67]

⬤ An age of 4.55 ± 0.07 billion years, very close to today's accepted age, was determined by Clair Cameron Patterson using uranium-lead isotope dating (specifically lead-lead dating) on several meteorites including the Canyon Diablo meteorite and published in 1956. [70]

⬤ In 1972, Apollo 17 mission brought back the oldest Moon rocks of our solar system ever collected and archived thus far have the radiometric dates of up to 4.54 billion years. [68]

▷ The age of our planet Earth, our Sun & our Solar System is therefore 4.54 Billion years.

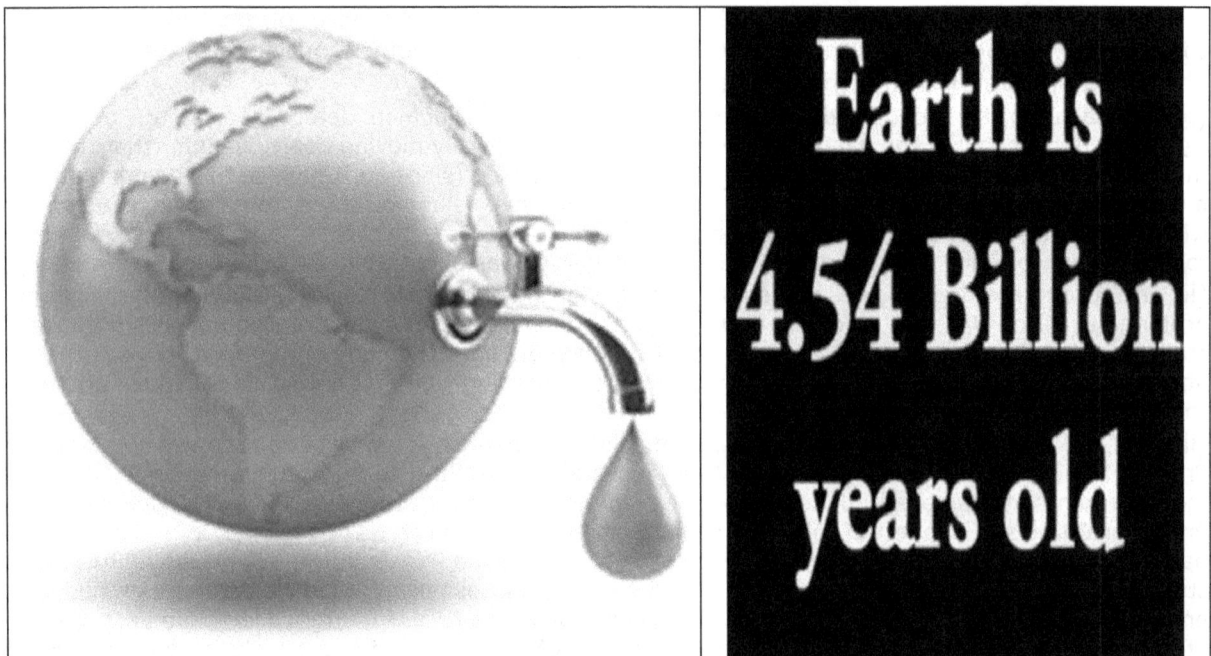

Figure 1.19  Our Planet Earth was manufactured by our Sun 4.54 billion years ago, and was getting ready to harbor life. Our planet Earth, our Sun and our Solar System were all formed at the same time, 4.54 billion years ago.

## Age of Our Planet Earth and Our Sun

● Based on the aforementioned scientific evidence on age determination of diverse ancient rocks by radiometric dating technique of our Earth and Moon, our scientists have confirmed that the age of our planet Earth (and therefore our Sun and all items in our Solar System) as 4.54 billion years. This most updated estimate is being endorsed by the NASA (National Aeronautics and Space Administration), Washington D.C., USA, and many other space agencies around the world.
● Our Sun has a total lifespan of 9 to 10 billion years. Our Sun will extinguish or die after 4 to 5 billion years. When our Sun dies, our planet Earth and other 7 planets will be engulfed with it.

## About Our Planet Earth [72-75]

● Our planet Earth is the third rotating and revolving planet from the Sun, and is the only astronomical object known to harbor life. Based on the radiometric dating and other sources of evidence, astronomers and scientists confirmed and verified that our planet Earth is 4.54 billion years old. So far it is the most accurate measurement or calculation of our Earth's age by highly experienced scientists. This age has been endorsed by NASA and other space agencies around the world.
● Our planet Earth has a surface area of approximately 510 million square kilometers or 196.9 million square miles. [72, 73]
● Our planet Earth as a matter of fact is the only green planet in our Solar System, besides its blue color from the space because of its dominant oceans. Our planet Earth has life or biosphere, possessing vast lengths of free land, oceans, plenty of water, and stable atmosphere to breathe in and breathe out oxygen.
● Our planet Earth's natural resources include air, water, soil, minerals, fuels, plants and animals. Our planet Earth has become the homeland to all forms of life such as humans, animals, plants, vegetation, fishes, birds, microbes, many forms of organisms, and so on.
● Our planet Earth is naturally equipped to recycle all the matter within it, as is highly capable to turn the waste into treasure and makes itself habitable instantly, no matter how much garbage the people throw in it. Much of what is considered a waste is reused in a closed system where matter is always locked in.
● By the year 2017, our planet Earth has become the homeland for more than 7.6 billion human beings.[74]

## Water On Our Planet Earth [74, 75]

● Liquid water, in addition to oxygen, is the principal ingredient necessary for the formation of life and for human body survival on our planet Earth. Without water, we wouldn't have been here on the planet Earth!
● Liquid water is a universal solvent and a mediator of life's chemical reactions, and is the most essential ingredient for the kind of delicate chemistry that helps the formation of life. Water is beneficial and vital to the life of every human being, animal and plant. Did you know more than 99% of an adult body's molecules are water molecules, and 55% to 60% of the adult human body weight is water?
● Liquid water on our planet Earth is very abundant. About 71 percent of our Earth's surface is covered by liquid water. According to NASA's report, there are more than 326 million trillion gallons of liquid water on our Earth. [76]
● Our Earth's oceans contain about 96.5 percent of all the planet's liquid water. Less than 3 percent of all liquid water on our Earth is freshwater, easily accessible and usable for drinking. More than two-thirds of our Earth's freshwater is locked up in ice caps and glaciers. [75, 76]

## Population On Our Planet Earth [74]

● The world population was 7.6 billion in 2017, and is expected to reach 8.6 billion in 2030, 9.8 billion in 2050 and a staggering 11.2 billion in 2100, according to a new United Nations report. Our planet Earth is capable to accommodate all kinds of life forms, no matter how high the world's population growth is (unless a catastrophic incident or incidents may occur).

# WATER FORMATION ON OUR PLANET EARTH (5 THEORIES)? [80-166]

The puzzling question on everyone's mind is: "**How did the Earth possess that much water (more than 326 million trillion gallons)?**" Astronomers, space researchers, scientists and very many academic researchers have been struggling to find out the truth throughout the human history, but were unable to come up with a definitive answer thus far. However all those scientific research findings can be summarized into the following 5 theories. These 5 theories are discussed in detail along with journal publications in Chapter 20.

| THEORIES OF WATER FORMATION ON OUR EARTH | CONCLUSION |
|---|---|
| **1. COMETS COULD HAVE BROUGHT WATER TO EARTH**<br>⊕ Our Solar System (Our Sun, Our Earth and other 7 Planets) began its formation 6 billion years ago, and completed its formation 4.54 billion years ago.<br>Our ancestors believed that ice-bearing comets probably bombarded our Earth 4 to 3.8 billion years ago, and brought water to Earth. This theory is now believed to be wrong because (D/H Ratio) of the water from comets is much higher than that of ocean water. Our ancestors' belief that comets brought water to our planet Earth was however proved by our most recent scientists to be a myth. | MYTH! |
| **2. ASTEROIDS (METEORITES /CARBONACEOUS CHONDRITES) COULD HAVE BROUGHT WATER TO EARTH**<br>⊕ Water-rich asteroids (meteorites / carbonaceous chondrites) impacted the infant Earth about 4 to 3.8 billion years ago, distributing water across the planet by brute force. As a result, our oceans formed. This theory is more accurate because D/H Ratio of the water from asteroids matched well with that of ocean water. Research proved that our planet Earth attained up to 50% of its water from the asteroids during the early stages after the formation of our Solar System. | TRUE! |
| **3. EARTH INHERITED ITS WATER FROM THE INTERSTELLAR MEDIUM**<br>⊕ Water is known to form in the clouds of gas and dust of the interstellar medium (ISM). Our Solar System was created 6 billion years ago from a gigantic cloud of interstellar gas and stardust. That cloud collapsed and formed a solar nebula—a spinning, swirling disk of material under gravity. Scientists found that the primordial water of the interstellar medium survived within the particles of the stardust, and carried forward all the way until and after the formation our Earth. Researchers concluded, from an extensive experimental study and mathematical modelling, that our planet Earth inherited up to 50% of its water from the interstellar medium even before our Solar System was created. Our Solar System completed its formation 4.54 billion years ago.<br>However the water we drink today is at least 4.54 billion years old. | TRUE! |
| **4. EARTH'S DEEP MANTLE HAS THE PRIMORDIAL WATER FROM THE INTERSTELLAR MEDIUM**<br>⊕ The researchers collected samples of primitive rocks from the Baffin Island, Nunavut Territory, Canada back in 1985. Water analysis revealed that these rocks have lower amount of deuterium, and lower D/H Ratio, indicating that the Earth's deep mantle attained the primordial water from the interstellar medium.<br>Which means the water we drink today is at least 4.54 billion years old. | TRUE! |
| **5. THICK HYDROGEN LAYER COULD HAVE REACTED WITH OXYGEN**<br>⊕ Hydrogen could have reacted with oxygen available from the oxides of Earth's mantle, and could have formed water molecules after our Solar System formed. This water from the mantle could have been later transported to the Earth's surface, forming oceans. [ $2 H_2 + O_2 = 2 H_2O$ ]<br>This theory does not have much supporting evidence and so disregarded. | FALSE! |

# THE ORIGIN OF THE EARTH'S WATER REVEALED!

🌐 Astronomers, space scientists and academic researchers have known for decades that there is plenty of water in the interstellar medium. There is sufficient scientific research evidence along with journal publications supporting the fact that our planet Earth inherited up to 50% of its water (it is called primordial water) from the interstellar medium even before before our Solar System was created some 6 billion years ago, and the remaining water was believed and proved to have obtained from the bombardment of asteroids (meteorites/ carbonaceous chondrites) during and after the early stages of the formation of our planet Earth in our Solar System.

🌐 The water samples taken from our Earth's deep mantle (rocks found in 1985 from the Baffin Island, Nunavut Territory, Canada) were analysed and proved to contain primordial water formed in the interstellar medium. This discovery has given the strong supporting evidence that the water we drink today is at least 4.54 billion years old, older than our Solar System.

## How Did the Water Get Into The Interstellar Medium?

🌐 Nearly 380,000 years after the Big Bang, the primary element "hydrogen" was first created, and thereafter it was abundantly available throughout our Universe. Nearly 400 million years after the Big Bang, stars formation commenced using hydrogen as the burning fuel. The massive pressure build-up of the fiery inferno within the stars was so great that hydrogen atoms fused together to form heavier element helium, and helium atoms in turn fused together to form much heavier elements such as lithium, beryllium, carbon, nitrogen, oxygen, and others in a process known as "**stellar nucleosynthesis**." The early stars were massive and short-lived. When the massive stars finished burning their hydrogen or helium fuel, they eventually extinguished, collapsed as they could not withstand their own gravitational force, and exploded into supernovae while manufacturing, dumping and scattering all kinds of heavier elements such as "carbon, nitrogen, oxygen, phosphorus and sulfur and many other elements" across the interstellar medium of our Milky Way Galaxy, and perhaps across the other galaxies our Universe.

🌐 More than 6 billion years ago, even before our Solar System and our Earth were created, during the supernova explosions in our Milky Way Galaxy, those newly formed heavier elements, including the very important oxygen, commingled together and formed all kinds of newer elements that we see in our periodic table today (there are 117 heavier elements). Space scientists discovered that during the time when newer elements were being formed, the abundantly available hydrogen and oxygen commingled together in the star-forming clouds under the appropriate climate conditions, and formed ice-cold water molecules by the chemical reaction ( $2 H_2 + O_2 = 2 H_2O$ ). Those ice-cold water molecules then entered into the space dust (also known as stardust) and interstellar gas in the interstellar medium, from a gigantic cloud of which our Solar System (our Sun, our planet Earth & 7 other planets) was created 6 billion years ago. The formation of our Solar System completed 4.54 billion years ago. And that is how our planet Earth inherited liquid water even before it was born. Our planet Earth was thus born with water.

🌐 **The intriguing idea** is that the ices from the interstellar medium were incorporated with a lot of organic material in them, which could have helped kick-start the life on our planet Earth.

**CONCLUSION:** The Water We Drink Today Is At Least 4.54 Billion Years Old, Older Than Our Planet Earth, Older Than Our Sun, and Older Than Our Solar System! Our planet Earth inherited up to 50% of its water from the interstellar medium even before it was born, and the remaining water came to our planet Earth by the bombardment of Asteroids (not Comets) during and after the early stages of our Solar System formation.

**Please refer to APPENDIX-A (Chapter 20)** for the detailed scientific studies and complete evidence, including journal publications, on water formation on our planet Earth.
**Please Note:** Drinking Water Guide-II does not come with Chapter 20.

# DRINKING WATER STATISTICS AT A GLANCE [77]

Please take a hard look at the following jaw-dropping statistics, posted by the World Health Organization (WHO) in 2018, and avoid becoming another statistic:

● Globally, at least 2 billion people use a drinking water source contaminated with faeces.
● Contaminated water can transmit water-borne diseases such as diarrhea, cholera, malaria, dysentery, typhoid, polio and other illnesses.
● Toxic chemicals arsenic, lead, chromium, beryllium or nickel could cause kidney damage, cancer, birth defects, and other illnesses if you drink contaminated tap water.
● Contaminated drinking water is estimated to cause 502,000 diarrhea deaths each year.
● By the year 2025, half of the world's population will be living in water stressed areas.
● In low and middle-income countries, 38% of health care facilities lack any water source, 19% do not have improved sanitation, and 35% lack water and soap for hand washing.
● It is being reported on the TV channels and in newspapers in USA and in many other countries that many children in schools are being exposed to lead-poison after drinking contaminated tap water in the campuses of schools. This is an alarming news to us because many schools fail to exercise appropriate caution in providing clean and purified water to children.

# LIVE LIKE AN ADVANCED HUMAN BEING (RECOMMENDATIONS by Dr. RK)

● Please do not drink tap water, well water, or bottled water of any kind directly without knowing how pure it is. Please always drink purified water (RO water, distilled water, zero water, or other).

● Learn how to monitor water pH by using pH testing drops, and urine pH by using pH paper.
● Also learn how to monitor TDS level of water by using a TDS meter. The TDS level of purified water (RO water) should be under 5 ppm. The TDS level of distilled water should be zero.
● Also learn how to test for chlorine and fluoride in your drinking water using test strips every now and then. The allowable chlorine level in drinking water is up to 5 ppm or mg/L.
The allowable fluoride level in drinking water is 1.5 for children and 2.4 ppm or mg/L for adults.

● World Health Organization (WHO) reported that drinking water with no minerals is potentially harmful to human health. So learn how to remineralize the purified water by adding Himalayan pink salt, Celtic sea salt, or ConcenTrace mineral drops to purified water. Learn how to remineralize the purified water up to a TDS (Total Dissolved Solids) level of 200 ppm.
● Or purchase a reliable pitcher that purifies tap water, adds minerals, and raises pH. Make sure that the pitcher is working perfectly by testing the water with a TDS meter and a pH meter.
● Get your drinking water tested by a certified laboratory in your area frequently, and make sure that the water you drink is one hundred percent free of contaminants.
● Consume one whole lemon a day including the pulp to neutralize your body's urine. Learn how to raise the pH of purified water by adding a tiny bit of baking soda or by adding ConcenTrace mineral drops. Make sure that the pH of your drinking water is 7, or between 7 and 7.25. Please do not drink the water that is acidic (If the water pH is below 7, that is acidic). Learn how to neutralize or slightly alkalize the purified water before drinking.
● There were many reported health benefits of alkaline ionized water, Kangen water, hydrogen water, and alkaline RO water. Learn how to make your own alkaline water, and start drinking alkaline water periodically (not every day), and get you blood pH tested routinely. Normal blood pH should be between 7.35 and 7.45. By trial and error, find out how much alkaline water would suit your body and help feel healthy. Adjust your drinking water pH until it suits your body.

● Drinking Water Guide teaches you everything you need on how to remineralize and alkalize the purified water at the comfort of your home without purchasing expensive purification systems.
● The RECOMMENDATIONS provided by the author at the end of each chapter would guide you on what exactly you need to do to protect your health.
● You are about to discover very many extremely useful drinking water strategies in this book, so please proceed to the next chapter and the following chapters.

# REFERENCES

**AMAZING FACTS ABOUT OUR UNIVERSE, OUR STARS, OUR MILKY WAY GALAXY, OUR SOLAR SYSTEM, OUR SUN & OUR EARTH!**

**AGE OF OUR UNIVERSE**
1. How Old is the Universe? by NASA (The National Aeronautics and Space Administration), NASA posted that we can estimate the age of the universe to be about 13.77 ± 0.059 billion years! Posted on Dec 21, 2012.
https://wmap.gsfc.nasa.gov/universe/uni_age.html

2. Age of the Universe, Wilkinson Microwave Anisotropy Probe, From Wikipedia, the free encyclopedia, Last edited Feb 21, 2019. NASA's Wilkinson Microwave Anisotropy Probe (WMAP) estimated in 2012 the age of the universe to be 13.772 billion years, with an uncertainty of plus or minus 59 million years. The current measurement of the age of the universe is approximately 13.8 billion years.
https://en.wikipedia.org/wiki/Age_of_the_universe
https://en.wikipedia.org/wiki/Wilkinson_Microwave_Anisotropy_Probe

3. How Old Is The Universe?, Frequently Asked Questions by Hubblesite.org.
The universe is approximately 13.8 billion years old.
https://hubblesite.org/quick-facts/science-quick-facts
https://hubblesite.org/quick-facts/mission-quick-facts

4. How old are galaxies? by NASA Space Place. Our universe is about 13.8 billion years old, and our own Milky Way galaxy is approximately 13.6 billion years old. Article last updated on, Jan 24, 2019, Posted on March 12, 2019, Last updated on Sept 16, 2020.
https://spaceplace.nasa.gov/galaxies-age/en/

5. How Old is the Universe? "In 2012, WMAP estimated the age of the universe to be 13.772 billion years, with an uncertainty of 59 million years" by Nola Taylor Redd, Posted on June 08, 2017, Science & Astronomy, Space.com.
https://www.space.com/24054-how-old-is-the-universe.html

**HOW MANY STARS ARE THERE IN OUR UNIVERSE?**
6. How many stars are there in the Universe? by European Space Agency. There are $10^{11}$ to $10^{12}$ stars in our Galaxy, and there are perhaps something like $10^{11}$ or $10^{12}$ galaxies. Simple calculation gives you $10^{22}$ to $10^{24}$ stars in the Universe.
https://www.esa.int/Our_Activities/Space_Science/Herschel/How_many_stars_are_there_In_the_Universe
https://www.esa.int/Science_Exploration/Space_Science/Herschel/How_many_stars_are_there_in_the_Universe

7. How many Stars in the Universe? by Fraser Cain, Posted on January 03, 2013.
If you multiply the number of stars in our galaxy by the number of galaxies in the Universe, you get approximately $10^{24}$ stars (That's a 1 followed by twenty-four zeros).
https://www.universetoday.com/102630/how-many-stars-are-there-in-the-universe/

**HOW MANY GALAXIES ARE THERE IN OUR UNIVERSE?**
8. Galaxy, From Wikipedia, the free encyclopedia, Number of galaxies in the observable universe has been changed from a previous estimate of 200 billion ($2\times10^{11}$) to a suggested current estimate of 2 trillion ($2\times10^{12}$) or more, Posted on March 7, 2017. https://en.wikipedia.org/wiki/Galaxy

9. Hubble Reveals "Observable Universe Contains 10 Times More Galaxies Than Previously Thought," by Editor Karl Hille, Nasa.gov, Posted on Oct 13, 2016, Updated on Aug 6, 2017. https://www.nasa.gov/feature/goddard/2016/hubble-reveals-observable-universe-contains-10-times-more-galaxies-than-previously-thought

10. This Is How We Know There Are Two Trillion Galaxies In The Universe by Ethan Siegel, PhD, Senior Contributor, Science, Posted on Forbes.com. https://www.forbes.com/sites/startswithabang/2018/10/18/this-is-how-we-know-there-are-two-trillion-galaxies-in-the-universe/#79bb52055a67

## HOW OLD IS OUR MILKY WAY GALAXY?

11. How old are galaxies? "Milky Way galaxy is approximately 13.6 billion years old." Posted by NASA Space Place, Article last updated on March 12, 2019. https://spaceplace.nasa.gov/galaxies-age/en/

12. Milky Way Facts by The Planets. The oldest star in the Galaxy is HD 140283, also known as the "Methuselah Star," and it is at least 13.6 billion years old. https://theplanets.org/milky-way/

13. Milky Way's Age Narrowed Down (The study puts its age at 13.6 billion years, give or take 800 million years) by Robert Roy Britt, Space.com, Posted on August 17, 2004. https://www.space.com/263-milky-age-narrowed.html

## HOW MANY SOLAR SYSTEMS ARE IN OUR MILKY WAY GALAXY?

14. How Many Stars in the Milky Way? by Maggie Masetti, Posted on July 22, 2015. There are 100 billion stars in the Milky Way on the low-end and 400 billion on the high end. https://asd.gsfc.nasa.gov/blueshift/index.php/2015/07/22/how-many-stars-in-the-milky-way/

15. Astronomy Course "Exploring the Universe" Being Offered at eDynamic Learning by Edgenuity.com. Our Sun is just one of approximately 500 billion stars in our galaxy, meaning that there could possibly be up to 500 billion solar systems. https://www.edgenuity.com/Syllabi/edynamics/EDL028-Syllabus_Astronomy.pdf

16. ASTRONOMY Course Being Offered at the National University Virtual High School, Chula Vista, CA 91910-5200, USA, Posted in April 2016. Our Sun is just one of approximately 500 billion stars in our galaxy, meaning that there could possibly be up to 500 billion solar systems. https://www.nuvhs.org/assets/resources/courseResources/Syllabus_Astronomy1.pdf

17. Milky Way, From Wikipedia, the free encyclopedia, March 9, 2019. Milky Way Galaxy is estimated to contain 100–400 billion stars and as many as 100-400 billion planets. https://en.wikipedia.org/wiki/Milky_Way

18. How Many Stars Are in the Milky Way? by Elizabeth Howell, Space.com, Posted on March 30, 2018. Talks about counting stars by determining the galaxy's mass, dark energy, etc. The estimate of the total stars in our Milky Way Galaxy at 100 billion (based on solar mass). https://www.space.com/25959-how-many-stars-are-in-the-milky-way.html

19. The Milky Way Galaxy, Imagine the Universe by NASA.gov, Goddard Space Flight Center. Milky Way is made up of approximately 100 billion stars (This information is outdated). It takes 250 million years for our Sun and our entire solar system to go all the way around the center of our Milky Way Galaxy. https://imagine.gsfc.nasa.gov/science/objects/milkyway1.html

20. How many solar systems are in our galaxy? Sun is one of about 200 billion stars (or perhaps more) just in the Milky Way galaxy alone, Posted by Spacespace of Nasa. https://spaceplace.nasa.gov/review/dr-marc-space/solar-systems-in-galaxy.html

21. The Reference # 21 is not assigned and not being used.

## FORMATION OF OUR UNIVERSE: BIG BANG THEORY

22. Discovery of the Cosmic Microwave Background (CMB), Our Universe, WMAP's Universe by NASA.gov, Posted and Updated on Sept 05, 2016. https://wmap.gsfc.nasa.gov/universe/bb_tests_cmb.html

23. The Universe: Big Bang to Now in 10 Easy Steps by Denise Chow, Science & Astronomy, Posted on October 19, 2011. https://www.space.com/13320-big-bang-universe-10-steps-explainer.html

24. Origin of Universe and Big Bang Theory, Published on Slideshare by Salim Lakade, Student at Latthe Polytechnic, Sangli, Maharashtra State, India, Published on Sep 8, 2017. https://www.slideshare.net/salimlakade/origin-of-universe-big-bang-theory

25. Step by Step of The Big Bang Theory by jonval21, Steemit Social Media Network. https://steemit.com/universe/@jonval21/step-by-step-of-the-big-bang-theory

26. The SIX Things you may not know about the afterglow of the Big Bang by Physics.org. http://www.physics.org/featuredetail.asp?id=45

27. Our Expanding Universe: Age, History & Other Facts by Charles Q. Choi, Space.com Contributor, Posted on June 17, 2017. https://www.space.com/52-the-expanding-universe-from-the-big-bang-to-today.html

28. The Early Universe by Las Cumbres Observatory, 6740 Cortona Drive, Suite 102, Goleta, CA 93117, USA, 2019. https://lco.global/spacebook/early-universe/ https://lco.global/spacebook/cosmology/early-universe/

29. Timeline of the Big Bang by The Physics of the Universe, 2019. https://www.physicsoftheuniverse.com/topics_bigbang_timeline.html

## PRIMORDIAL SOUP CONDITION RECREATED BY CERN, SWITZERLAND

30. Big Bang 'soup recipe' confirmed by Rolf Haugaard Nielse, Posted on June 13, 2003. https://www.newscientist.com/article/dn3821-big-bang-soup-recipe-confirmed/

31. Scientists at CERN Catch a Glimpse of the Universe's Primordial Soup by Todd Jaquith, Posted on Feb 10, 2016. https://futurism.com/scientists-at-cern-catch-a-glimpse-of-the-universes-primordial-soup

32. LHC (Large Hadron Collider) Produces 'Primordial Soup' of The Universe Using Less Particles Than Thought Possible by Bec Crew, Posted on Sep 7, 2015. https://www.sciencealert.com/lhc-produces-primordial-soup-of-the-universe-using-less-particles-than-thought-possible

33. The Universe's Primordial Soup Flowing at CERN by You Zhou & Jens Jørgen Gaardhøje, Niels Bohr Institute, University of Copenhagen, Denmark, Posted on February 9, 2016.
https://phys.org/news/2016-02-universe-primordial-soup-cern.html
https://www.nbi.ku.dk/english/news/news16/the-universes-primordial-soup-flowing-at-cern/

## FORMATION OF OUR UNIVERSE: BIG BANG THEORY (Continued)
34. General Astronomy, The First 3 Minutes by Wikibooks, Posted on Oct 16, 2018.
https://en.wikibooks.org/wiki/General_Astronomy/The_First_Three_Minutes

35. Abundance of the chemical elements, From Wikipedia, the free encyclopedia, Last updated March 27, 2019.
https://en.wikipedia.org/wiki/Abundance_of_the_chemical_elements

36. Chronology of the Universe, From Wikipedia, the free encyclopedia, Updated on March 27, 2019.
https://en.wikipedia.org/wiki/Chronology_of_the_universe
37. First Light & Reionization by NASA.gov.
https://jwst.nasa.gov/firstlight.html

38. YouTube Video, The Big Bang Theory Explained The Simple Way by gphhawkins, Published on Sep 22, 2011.
https://www.youtube.com/watch?v=wt4TmZVS0Do

## STELLAR NUCLEOSYNTHESIS
39. Is my body really made up of star stuff? by StarChild Authors (Phil Newman and Others) of NASA.
https://starchild.gsfc.nasa.gov/docs/StarChild/questions/question57.html

40. Stars: Element Factories, Stellar fusion creates most elements in the Universe; "When you look up at night, you are seeing factories called stars" by Kent Fairfield, Lifelong Amateur Astronomer, The Bulletin, Posted on Oct 29, 2014.
https://www.bendbulletin.com/outdoors/2523761-151/stars-element-factories

41. Stellar Nuceosynthesis, How elements from helium and hydrogen are created by Andrew Zimmerman Jones, Updated on December 07, 2018.
https://www.thoughtco.com/stellar-nucleosynthesis-2699311

42. NASA Finds a "Weird" Kind of Life on Earth. Life requires the six elements CHNOPS (carbon, hydrogen, nitrogen, oxygen, phosphorus and sulfur), Posted by Nancy Atkinson, Universe Today, Space and Astronomy News, December 2, 2010.
http://www.universetoday.com/81106/nasa-finds-a-weird-kind-of-life-on-earth/

43. What are the Ingredients of Life? Posted by Natalie Wolchover, February 02, 2011.
All organisms are built from the same six essential elemental ingredients: carbon, hydrogen, nitrogen, oxygen, phosphorus and sulfur (CHNOPS).
https://www.livescience.com/32983-what-are-ingredients-life.html#:~:text=Nonetheless%2C%20all%20organisms%20are%20built,Why%20those%20elements%3F

44. Dr. Carl Sagan, "Cosmos," Paperback, Ann Druyan (Introduction), Neil deGrasse Tyson (Foreword), ISBN number 978-0345539434, Amazon.com, December 10, 2013.

45. Composition of the human body, From Wikipedia, the free encyclopedia.
https://en.wikipedia.org/wiki/Composition_of_the_human_body#:~:text=Almost%2099%25%20of%20the%20mass,11%20are%20necessary%20for%20life

## FORMATION OF OUR MILKY WAY GALAXY

46. What is a galaxy (galaxy pictures posted)? by Space Place of Nasa.gov.
https://spaceplace.nasa.gov/galaxy/en/

47. Why Do We Call Our Galaxy the Milky Way? by Deanna Kerley, Posted on November 13, 2013.
http://mentalfloss.com/article/53589/why-do-we-call-our-galaxy-milky-way

48. How Did the Milky Way Get Its Name? by Mindy Weisberger, Senior Writer, Posted on November 7, 2016.
https://www.livescience.com/56756-milky-way-name-origin.html

References from 49 to 54 are not assigned and not being used.

## FORMATION OF OUR SOLAR SYSTEM

55. Mysteries of the Universe (The picture of a nebula posted) by Nasa.gov. Pillars of Creation, Eagle Nebula, a cloud of gas and dust created by an exploding star from which new stars and planets are forming.
https://www.nasa.gov/specials/60counting/universe.html
https://www.nasa.gov/image-feature/the-pillars-of-creation
https://www.nasa.gov/image-feature/eagle-nebula-s-pillars-of-creation-in-infrared

56. How to build a solar system (The picture of a nebula posted) by Karla Panchuk, Department of Geological Sciences, University of Saskatchewan, Canada.
https://opentextbc.ca/geology/chapter/22-3-how-to-build-a-solar-system/

## FORMATION OF OUR PLANET EARTH

57. How Planets Are Born, Story by Alison Takemura, Posted on June 16, 2016.
https://nasaviz.gsfc.nasa.gov/12278

58. Our Sun Came Late to the Milky Way's Star-Birth Party by Donna Weaver, Editor: Lynn Jenner, Space Telescope Science Institute, Baltimore, Maryland, Posted & Updated on Aug. 6, 2017.
https://www.nasa.gov/content/goddard/our-sun-came-late-to-the-milky-way-s-star-birth-party

59. Did a Supernova Give Birth to Our Solar System? by Charles Q. Choi, Space.com Contributor, Posted on December 28, 2016.
https://www.space.com/35151-supernova-trigger-solar-system-formation.html

60. Solar System Formation, Windows to the Universe, Brought to you by the National Earth Science Teachers Association, 2012.
https://www.windows2Universe.org/our_solar_system/formation.html

## THE SIZE OF OUR SUN & LIFESPAN OF OUR SUN

61. How large is the Sun compared to Earth? Posted by Cool Cosmos.
https://coolcosmos.ipac.caltech.edu/ask/5-How-large-is-the-Sun-compared-to-Earth-

61b. How Hot Is the Sun? by Tim Sharp, Reference Editor, Posted on October 18, 2017.
The sun is about 93 million miles (149.5 million km) from Earth.
https://www.space.com/17137-how-hot-is-the-sun.html

61c. How do scientists know the distance between the planets? by the Spaceplace of NASA.
The Sun is about 93 million miles from Earth.
https://spaceplace.nasa.gov/review/dr-marc-solar-system/planet-distances.html

62. How old is the Sun?, NASA Space Place, Posted on March 12, 2019. Our Sun is 4.54 billion years old. Stars like our Sun burn for about 9 or 10 billion years. So our Sun is about halfway through its life.
https://spaceplace.nasa.gov/sun-age/en/

## FORMATION OF OUR MOON
63. YouTube Title: Whole Story from the Big Bang to the Present Day - Full Documentary (History of the World in 2 Hours) by Perfect Toys, Published on Apr 24, 2016. Narrators: Alex Filippenko (Astrophysicist), Peter Ward (Paleontologist), Clifford V. Johnson (Physicist, University of Southern California), and others.
https://www.youtube.com/watch?v=_ITHx8SKD5g        (This vodeo is unavailable now!)

64. History of the World in 2 Hours by Alex Filippenko (Astrophysicist), Peter Ward (Paleontologist), and others, DVD, ASIN: B006ENHGLS, Available on Amazon.com.

## AGE OF OUR PLANET EARTH BY RADIOMATRIC DATING
65. The Earth is 18 Galactic Years Old, Astronomy, Earth Facts, Posted on January 16, 2018. The age of the Earth is approximately 4.54 billion years.
https://ourplnt.com/Earth-18-galactic-years-old/

66. Dear Science: How do we know how old the Earth is? by Sarah Kaplan March 6, 2017. Researchers used uranium-lead techniques to date the meteorite back 4.54 billion years, give or take about 70 million — the best age for our planet so far, according to the U.S. Geological Survey.
https://www.washingtonpost.com/news/speaking-of-science/wp/2017/03/06/dear-science-how-do-we-know-how-old-the-earth-is/?noredirect=on&utm_term=.c0d5c099c3a5

67. How Old Is Earth? by Nola Taylor Redd, Science & Astronomy, Space.com, February 07, 2019.
https://www.space.com/24854-how-old-is-earth.html

68. Age of the Earth – Timeline by Science Learning Hub, Updated on April 22, 2014. Chronological order of scientific discoveries of the measurement of the age of the Earth.
https://www.sciencelearn.org.nz/resources/1553-age-of-the-earth-timeline

69. How old is the Earth?, Posted by NASA.gov. Earth's age: About 4.5 billion years based on radioactive dating using uranium and thorium isotopes.
https://image.gsfc.nasa.gov/poetry/ask/a10597.html

70. Age of the Earth, From Wikipedia, the free encyclopedia, Last edited on March 11, 2019. The age of the Earth is 4.54 ± 0.05 billion years (4.54 × 109 years ± 1%)
https://en.wikipedia.org/wiki/Age_of_the_Earth

71. How is Earth's Age Calculated? by Jeanna Bryner, Live Science Managing Editor, Posted on November 29, 2012.
https://www.livescience.com/32321-how-is-earths-age-calculated.html

## ABOUT OUR PLANET EARTH
72. Space and Astronomy News, Universe Today, Posted on Feb 10, 2017. Our planet Earth has a surface area of approximately 510 million square kilometers or 196.9 million square miles.
https://www.universetoday.com/25756/surface-area-of-the-earth/

73. Our Sun by the Numbers, Solar System Exploration by NASA.gov. Our planet Earth has a surface area of approximately 510 million square kilometers or 196.9 million square miles.
https://solarsystem.nasa.gov/solar-system/sun/by-the-numbers/

74. World population projected to reach 9.8 billion in 2050, and 11.2 billion in 2100, by United Nations, Dept of Economics and Social Affairs, Posted in 2017.
https://www.un.org/development/desa/en/news/population/world-population-prospects-2017.html

75. How much water is there on, in, and above the Earth? by US Geological Survey (USGS) Water Science School, Posted on Dec 2, 2016.
https://water.usgs.gov/edu/earthhowmuch.html

## WATER FORMATION ON OUR PLANET EARTH
76. Oceans Worlds, Water in the Solar System and Beyond by NASA. According to NASA's report, there are more than 326 million trillion gallons of liquid water on our Earth.
https://www.nasa.gov/specials/ocean-worlds/

77. Drinking Water Statistics by World Health Organization (WHO), Posted on Feb 07, 2018.
http://www.who.int/news-room/fact-sheets/detail/drinking-water
http://www.who.int/en/news-room/fact-sheets/detail/drinking-water

# FORMATION OF OUR UNIVERSE: SUMMARY

🕑 Our Universe is about 13.8 billion years old. The NASA's Wilkinson Microwave Anisotropy Probe (WMAP) mission precisely determined the age of our Universe.

🕑 Our Universe was born 13.8 billion years ago with the Big Bang as an unbelievably and unimaginably hot and dense point of singularity, which was at infinite temperature and infinite density. When our Universe was just $10^{-34}$ of a second young — that is, when it was a hundredth of a billionth of a trillionth of a trillionth of a second young — it underwent an incredible burst of expansion known as inflation, in which period the space itself expanded like a magical balloon faster than the speed of light, and doubled its size at least 90 consecutive times. At that very beginning stage of formation, our Universe existed in the form of quark-gluon plasma, also called the primordial soup. No stable atoms were created yet.

🕑 Nearly one second after the Big Bang, the temperature of our Universe dropped to 1 billion degrees or $10^9$ degrees Kelvin, and as a result, the most fundamental particles such as quarks, electrons, photons and neutrinos just formed, but not yet bound together.
Nearly 3 minutes after the Big Bang, our Universe underwent a cooling process in which the quarks coalesced and bound into hadrons such as protons and neutrons. It was called hadrons era. The protons and neutrons in turn combined to form nuclei of light elements such as hydrogen and helium (no neutral atoms were created yet). This is one of the most important events of the history of the Big Bang because our visible Universe today is composed of 90% hydrogen, 8% helium, and 2% everything else.

🕑 Nearly 380,000 years after the Big Bang, the primary element "hydrogen" was created, and thereafter hydrogen was abundantly available throughput our Universe. The nuclei of the light elements such as hydrogen, helium, lithium and beryllium attracted electrons, and formed neutral atoms (stable atoms formed) in a process known as "stellar nucleosynthesis". This is one of the most important events of the history of the Big Bang because our visible Universe today is composed of 90% hydrogen, 8% helium, and 2% everything else.

🕑 Our Universe kept expanding unstoppably and unimaginably without boundaries, and the temperature kept dropping exponentially. Our Universe then entered into an era of dark ages for 100s of millions of years because there were no stars.

🕑 Nearly 400 million years after the Big Bang, stars formation commenced, as clumps of gas collapsed enough under gravity while spinning and swirling took place to form the very first bright light, which became a star, thereby creating the first star, and followed by more and more stars, and eventually millions of stars along with the orbiting planets.

🕑 The early stars were massive and made up of very simple and light gaseous elements (hydrogen and helium) and so they had very short lifespans of only millions of years. But the fiery inferno and nuclear fusion in the cores of these early stars slowly created all kinds of heavier elements (there are 117 heavier elements in our periodic table), including the most important Carbon, Nitrogen, Oxygen, Phosphorus and Sulfur. When a large star died, it would become a part of a new star in the supernova explosion. In the beginning, these stars were created in small groups and attracted other stars. These stars were grouped in both regular and irregular shapes. Then the different shapes merged to form the first galaxies. Then as more and more galaxies formed, they became grouped in galaxy clusters, and then these clusters were contained in super clusters.

🕑 Likewise, our Universe has been creating millions of stars along with orbiting planets and galaxies, and then billions of stars along with orbiting planets and galaxies, and then even trillions of stars along with orbiting planets and galaxies that are visible today!

---

### In CHAPTER 1, You Have Learned All About The Origin of the Earth's Water

The Big Bang Theory explained in Chapter 1 of this book "Drinking Water Guide-II" is the most relevant, most essential, and most important part. This book teaches that all those heavier elements of our periodic table, including all those minerals that we use today to remineralize and alkalize the purified water, were originally manufactured in the burning cores of collapsing stars by a process known as "stellar nucleosynthesis," even before our Solar System and our planet Earth were created. Stars are responsible for all the constituents of our planet Earth (Carbon, Hydrogen, Nitrogen, Oxygen, Phosphorus and Sulfur are the most important elements) that are needed for the formation and survival of every human being, animal and plant.

In the Remaining Part of This Book, You Will Learn
Water Statistics, Types of Drinking Water, Importance of Drinking Water, and How to Drink Only Purified Water
That is Properly Remineralized and Slightly Alkalized.

*Purified water (zero water) that is either neutralized (pH=7) or slightly alkalized (pH= 7 to 7.5), and remineralized up to a TDS level of 200 ppm is the healthy drinking water.*

---

## CHAPTER 2  DRINKING WATER FACTS & STATISTICS

## TABLE OF CONTENTS

# Facts and Statistics Posted by Water For People [1]

- 2.1 billion people around the world don't have access to safe water.
- 4.5 billion lack access to adequate sanitation.
- Women and children spend more than 4 hours walking for water each day.
- More than 840,000 people die each year from water-related diseases.

The aforementioned numbers are based off the following data:
- UNC Water Institute Study
- World Health Organization (WHO)
- National Center for Biotechnology Information (NCBI)

# Facts and Statistics Posted by Water Aid [2]

- About 844 million people don't have clean water (WHO Report 2017).
  WHO = World Health Organization.

- About 2.3 billion people don't have a decent toilet (WHO Report 2017).

- About 31% of schools don't have clean water (UNICEF Report 2015).
  UNICEF = United Nations Children's Fund
          (formerly, United Nations International Children's Emergency Fund).

- About 443 million school days are lost every year because of water-related illnesses.

- Every minute a newborn dies from infection caused by lack of safe water and an unclean environment. (WHO Report 2015).

- Diarrhea (also spelled diarrhoea), caused by dirty water and poor toilets kills a child under 5 every 2 minutes. (WASHWatch.org Report).

- Every $1 invested in water and toilets returns an average of $4 in increased productivity.

- The World Bank says promoting good hygiene is one of the most cost effective health interventions.

- If everyone, everywhere had clean water, the one-third of the number of diarrhoeal (relating to diarrhea) deaths would be prevented.

# Drinking Water Statistics Posted by WHO in 2018 [3]

● About 844 million people lack even a basic drinking-water service, including 159 million people who are dependent on surface water.

● Globally, at least 2 billion people use a drinking water contaminated with faeces. Contaminated water can transmit water-borne diseases such as "diarrhea (also spelled diarrhoea), cholera, polio, typhoid, and dysentery". Contaminated drinking water is estimated to cause 502,000 diarrhea deaths each year.

● By 2025, half of the world's population will be living in water-stressed areas. In low and middle income countries, 38% of health care facilities lack an improved water source, 19% do not have improved sanitation, and 35% lack water and soap for handwashing.

● In 2015, 5.2 billion people used safely managed drinking-water services. The remaining 2.1 billion people without safely managed services in 2015 included:

 ⇛ 1.3 billion people with basic services, meaning an improved water source located within a round trip of 30 minutes.

 ⇛ 263 million people with limited services, or an improved water source requiring more than 30 minutes to collect water.

 ⇛ 423 million people taking water from unprotected wells and springs.

 ⇛ 159 million people collecting untreated surface water from lakes, ponds, rivers and streams. Sharp geographic, sociocultural and economic inequalities persist, not only between rural and urban areas but also in towns and cities where people living in low-income, informal, or illegal settlements usually have less access to improved sources of drinking-water than other residents.

● In 2013 to 2014, water-borne diseases caused 289 cases of illnesses, 108 hospitalizations, and 17 deaths in the United States alone. As many as 63 million people from rural central California to the boroughs of New York City were exposed to potentially unsafe water more than once during the past decade. Industrial dumping, farming pollution, and pipe deterioration are the main causes of the contaminated water. In some instances it took nearly two years for the issues causing the contaminated water to be resolved.

# Drinking Water Statistics Posted by New York Times [4, 5]

● 35 years after the U.S. Congress passed the Safe Drinking Water Act, some regulators and environmentalists state the law is now so obsolete that it fails to protect people from the most obvious threats.

● In the USA, the NY Times reported on violations of the Clean Water Act, a federal law which governs water pollution, and has shown household water that is contaminated with lead, nickel, and other heavy metals. Some extreme side-effects of this contamination have resulted in skin burns, rashes, and eroded tooth enamel.

● The Times interviewed more than 250 state and federal regulators, water-system managers, environmental advocates and scientists. That research showed that an estimated 1 in 10 Americans have been exposed to drinking water that contains dangerous chemicals or fails to meet a federal health benchmark in other ways.

● An estimated 19.5 million Americans fall ill each year from drinking water contaminated with parasites, bacteria or viruses, according to a study published last year in the scientific journal Reviews of Environmental Contamination and Toxicology. That figure does not include illnesses caused by other chemicals and toxins.

● The NY Times has compiled a database of violations of the Safe Drinking Water Act, finding 40% of the nation's community water systems in violation at least once, exposing millions to potentially harmful chemicals, toxins, and heavy metals. More than 23 million people received drinking water from municipal systems that violated a health-based standard. State officials noted that they had cited more than 4,200 water pollution violations at mine sites around the state since 2000.

● Chemical factories, manufacturing plants and other workplaces have violated water pollution laws more than half a million times in the past 5 years. The violations range from failing to report emissions to dumping toxins at concentrations regulators say might contribute to cancer, birth defects and other illnesses.

● In the nation's largest dairy states, like Wisconsin and California, farmers have sprayed liquefied animal feces onto fields, where it has seeped into wells, causing severe infections. Tap water in parts of the Farm Belt, including cities in Illinois, Kansas, Missouri and Indiana, has contained pesticides at concentrations that some scientists have linked to birth defects and fertility problems.

● In parts of New York, Rhode Island, Ohio, California and other states where sewer systems cannot accommodate heavy rains, untreated human waste has flowed into rivers and washed onto beaches. Drinking water in parts of New Jersey, New York, Arizona and Massachusetts shows some of the highest concentrations of tetrachloroethylene, a dry cleaning solvent that has been linked to kidney damage and cancer.

● Records analyzed by The Times indicate that the Clean Water Act has been violated more than 506,000 times since 2004, by more than 23,000 companies and other facilities, according to reports submitted by polluters themselves. Companies sometimes test what they are dumping only once a quarter, so the actual number of days when they broke the law is often far higher. And some companies illegally avoid reporting their emissions.

● In 46 states of USA, local regulators have primary responsibility for crucial aspects of the Clean Water Act. Though the number of regulated facilities has more than doubled in the last 10 years, many state enforcement budgets have remained essentially flat when adjusted for inflation. In New York, for example, the number of regulated polluters has almost doubled to 19,000 in the last decade, but the number of inspections each year has remained about the same.

● Three coal companies — Loadout, Remington Coal and Pine Ridge, a subsidiary of Peabody Energy, one of the largest coal companies in the world — reported to state officials that 93% of the waste they injected near this community had illegal concentrations of chemicals including arsenic, lead, chromium, beryllium or nickel.

◉ More than 350 other companies and facilities in West Virginia have also violated the Clean Water Act in recent years, records show. Those infractions include releasing illegal concentrations of iron, manganese, aluminum and other chemicals into lakes and rivers.

◉ Department officials say they continue to improve the agency's procedures, and note that regulators have assessed $14.7 million in state fines against more than 70 mining companies since 2006.

## Water-Borne Diseases [6, 7]

Water-borne diseases are developed due to contaminated water and lack of sanitation. Water-borne diseases are the leading cause of death around the world, and it's almost inexcusable on the part of local governments and municipalities. The following are the most common water-borne diseases being faced around the world:

**a. Diarrhea** (also spelled diarrhoea): Diarrhea is a symptom of infection caused by a host of bacterial, viral and parasitic organisms most of which can be spread by contaminated water. It is more common when there is a shortage of clean water for drinking, cooking and cleaning and basic hygiene is important in prevention. Water contaminated with human faeces for example from municipal sewage, septic tanks and latrines is of special concern. Animal faeces also contain microorganisms that can cause diarrhoea. Diarrhoea can also spread from person to person, aggravated by poor personal hygiene. Food is another major cause of diarrhoea when it is prepared or stored in unhygienic conditions. Water can contaminate food during irrigation, and fish and seafood from polluted water may also contribute to the disease.

**b. Malaria:** When you think of malaria you probably think of mosquitos, but malaria is also a water-borne disease. Malaria is a life threatening illness that causes high fever, chills, vomiting, and even the state of coma.

**c. Cholera:** Cholera is an infection of the small intestine or bowels that, if left untreated, can be fatal. Cholera typically can be contracted from infected water supplies and causing severe vomiting, diarrhea and often death. Diarrhea may seem harmless enough, but believe it or not, in developing countries without access to modern medicine and clean drinking water, cholera kills about 2.2 million people per year, usually due to severe dehydration.

**d. Polio (short for Poliomyelitis):** Polio is a serious infectious water-borne disease that can cause permanent paralysis (being unable to move the or body body parts).

**e. Typhoid:** Typhoid is an infectious bacterial fever with an eruption of red spots on the chest and abdomen and severe intestinal irritation. Contaminated water is blamed to cause this disease.

**e. Dysentery:** Dysentery is an infection of the intestines resulting in severe diarrhea with the presence of blood and mucus in the feces.

Keeping our water safe and clean to prevent the spread of disease should be a high priority. It's very important to clean the water that has been contaminated and keep the safe environment. Point-of-use water and sanitation technologies reduce the number of deaths caused by water-borne diseases.

# Water and Sanitation [8, 9, 10]

Water sanitation is the key factor in preventing the water-borne diseases and keeping the adequate conditions for safe water supply. Water sanitation measures at any given public water supply facility include the development, application and maintenance of sanitary measures for the sake of cleanliness, protecting health, etc. Major attention should be given to maintaining clean toilets, urinary devices, sinks, showers in bathrooms, maintaining clean swimming pools, piped water to the house or yard, public taps or standpipes, boreholes, protected dug wells, protected springs and rainwater collection tanks, etc. It is very important to take responsibility is installing the systems for taking and recycling the dirty water and other waste products away from buildings in order to protect people's health. Lack of sanitation is the world's biggest cause of infection. Hand washing reduces the risk of disease by 50%. (The Global Public-Private, globalhandwashing.org, Health Impact).

The water and sanitation crisis claims more lives through disease than any war claims through guns. (United Nations Development Programme (UNDP), Human Development Report 2006, Beyond Scarcity: Power, Poverty, and the Global Water Crisis, UNDP, 2006).

At any given time, half of the world's hospital beds are occupied by patients suffering from a water-related disease. (UNICEF/WHO, Progress on Drinking Water and Sanitation: Special Focus on Sanitation, UNICEF/WHO, 2008).

# Contaminants Found in Drinking Water [11, 12]

Drinking water supplies in the United States are among the safest in the world. However, according to Centers for Disease Control and Prevention (CDC), even in the USA, drinking water sources can become contaminated. In particular, people on well water in rural areas could have a higher risk of health impacts from contaminants in their tap water, making regular testing important. In developing countries, water contamination is a more serious problem.

## Contaminants can be classifies into several categories:
a. Organics,
b. Inorganics,
c. Heavy Metals,
d. Fecal Matter (Cysts), and
e. Legionella.

**Organics:** The word organic refers to carbon-based chemicals including solvents, pesticides, and insecticides that make their way into our water through cropland runoff and factory discharge.

**Inorganics:** Inorganics are compounds lacking a carbon atom in their molecular structure. There are very many chemical contaminants in drinking water called inorganics. Examples include chlorine, boron, and cyanide.

**Heavy Metals:** Lead, Aluminum, Arsenic are the leading contaminants in drinking water. The lead particles leached out of old pipes in cities like Flint, MI and Sacramento, CA, and caused serious contamination problems.

**Fecal Matter/Cysts:** Microbial cysts from both human and animal fecal matter, the resting or dormant state of microorganisms, can be lurking in your drinking water. Examples would be cryptosporidium and/or giardia lambia (generally found in rural wells). They also cause gastrointestinal illnesses and cramps from long-term exposure. In 1993 there was a huge outbreak of cryptosporidium in Milwaukee Wisconsin in which 1.6 million residents became ill, and 104 people died as a result.

**Legionella:** The legionella bacteria are actually a naturally occurring contaminant in water, which can lead to Legionnaires' disease (a type of serious lung infection). While it's normally spread through tiny water droplets in the air, usually in buildings with larger plumbing systems, it can make it's way into your body by aspiration of drinking water if the water passes through wrong pipelines. The legionella bacteria very often affects seniors, smokers, or those with a chronic lung condition or weakened immune system.

# REFERENCES

1. Safe Water and Sanitation for Generations by Water for People.
https://www.waterforpeople.org/

2. Facts and Statistics by Water Aid.
https://www.wateraid.org/facts-and-statistics

3. Drinking Water Statistics by World Health Organization (WHO), Posted on Feb 07, 2018.
http://www.who.int/news-room/fact-sheets/detail/drinking-water
http://www.who.int/en/news-room/fact-sheets/detail/drinking-water

4. Clean Water Laws Are Neglected, at a Cost in Suffering by Charles Duhiggsept by Charles Duhigg, New York Times, Posted on Sept 12, 2009.
http://www.nytimes.com/2009/09/13/us/13water.html?_r=2&pagewanted=all

5. Find Water Polluters Near You, Toxic Water, New York Times by Charles Duhigg, Posted on May 16, 2012.
http://projects.nytimes.com/toxic-waters/polluters
https://www.nytimes.com/interactive/projects/toxic-waters/polluters/index.html
https://www.nytimes.com/2009/09/13/us/13water.html

6. Water Sanitation Hygiene, Water-related Diseases, WHO Report.
http://www.who.int/water_sanitation_health/diseases-risks/diseases/diarrhoea/en/

7. Critical Facts About Water-borne Diseases In The United States and Abroad, by John Hawthorne, Posted on Feb 15, 2018.
https://businessconnectworld.com/2018/02/15/critical-facts-water-borne-diseases-us/

8. Global Water Poverty Facts by Watering Malawi.
http://wateringmalawi.org/global-water-poverty-facts/

9. Water, Sanitation and Hygiene, Global Health Observatory Data (GHO).
http://www.who.int/gho/phe/water_sanitation/en/

10. Water, Sanitation and Hygiene by UNICEF.
https://www.unicef.org/wash/

11. How to Distill Water by Pure Water, Posted on May 04, 2017
https://mypurewater.com/blog/2017/05/04/how-to-distill-water/

12. Common Contaminants Found in Drinking Water by Jeff Hayward, Posted on November 14, 2016.
https://www.activebeat.co/your-health/7-common-contaminants-found-in-drinking-water/?streamview=all

# CHAPTER 3  IMPORTANCE OF DRINKING WATER

# TABLE OF CONTENTS

# AMAZING FACTS ABOUT WATER AND DRINKING WATER

## Water On Our Planet Earth [1, 2, 3]

⚫ Our beautiful and wonderful planet Earth is the third rotating and revolving planet from the Sun, and is the only astronomical object known to harbor life in our Solar System. Based on the radiometric dating and other sources of evidence, astronomers and scientists confirmed that our planet Earth is 4.54 billion years old. [1] Our planet Earth has a surface area of approximately 510 million square kilometers or 196.9 million square miles. [2]

⚫ Water on our planet Earth is very abundant. About 71 percent of Earth's surface is covered by water. According to NASA's report, there are more than 326 million trillion gallons of water on Earth. [3]

⚫ The oceans of our planet Earth contain about 96.5 percent of all the planet's water. Less than 3 percent of all water on Earth is freshwater (usable for drinking). More than two-thirds of Earth's freshwater is locked up in ice caps and glaciers. [3]

## Human Body Is Made Up Of Water and Needs Water [4, 5, 6, 7, 8]

⚫ Water is the primary molecule required and the most important ingredient necessary for the formation of life on the planet Earth. The average human adult male is approximately 60% water (by weight) and the average adult female is approximately 55% (by weight). [4]

### ⚫ 99% of Your Body's Molecules Are Water Molecules: [5a, 5b]

Scientists have determined that a typical teenager's body with 57 Kg (127 Pounds) of body weight has the following composition: 61 % water, 16 % fat, 16 % protein, 6% minerals, and 1% carbohydrate. Scientists also estimated that the same body consists of $1.2 \times 10^{25}$ molecules, and more than 99% of them are water molecules. [5a, 5b]

⚫ Every part of your body from your skin to your brain relies on ample hydration to function. Up to 60% of the adult human body weight is made up of water. Women have less water in their bodies compared to men. Infants bodies have 78% to 93% water, and by the age one, the water content drops to 65%. Some organisms and plants contain up to 90% of water. Up to 85% of the brain is submerged in the water that helps feed and cushion it. A scientist H.H. Mitchell reported in the Journal of Biological Chemistry that the brain and heart are composed of 73% water, and the lungs are about 83% water, the skin contains 64% water, muscles and kidneys are 79% water, and the bones are 31% water. Even the fat contains up to 20% of water. [6]

⚫ The amazing human body is composed of roughly 206 bones, 600 muscles, 10,000 nerve fibers, 2 million optic nerve fibers, 100 billion nerve cells, 30 trillion blood cells, 62,000 miles in total length of blood vessels, capillaries and arteries, and so on. All body parts, which work together round the clock, 24 hours a day and 7 days a week, possess large sums of water and need fresh and pure water every single day to survive. Every cell, tissue and organ in your body possesses water and needs fresh and pure water every single day to function correctly. [7a, 7b]

⚫ Water is beneficial and vital to the life of every human being, animal and plant. To feel fit and healthy, the human body should stay hydrated all the time. When you water your plants, you watch them grow taller and greener. Exactly like that, when you drink water, water acts on your body to grow and keeps you active and healthy. [8]

• Water transports nutrients throughout the entire body, especially to the brain. Water circulates throughout the human body by transporting, dissolving, replenishing nutrients and organic matter, and at the same time by carrying away waste material. Water also is needed to regulate the activities of fluids, tissues, cells, lymph, blood and glandular secretions. The shortage of water intake overtime could result in the deficiency in cell activity and thereby chronic dehydration. [8]

• Water is essentially required in your stomach, small intestine and colon for the digestion, transportation and distribution of nutrients in and out of the body's cells, lubrication, temperature regulation, removal of wastes, etc. Water regulates body temperature precisely and aids digestion process. Large amount of water is needed to transport and digest solid foods. When you eat solid foods, you should drink a lot of water. Water is lost from your body when you urinate, sweat and even when you breath out. You should immediately replace lost water by drinking more and more water throughout the day. Just listen to your body, and whenever your body demands, you must drink water. [8]

• Every part of your body relies on ample hydration to function properly. Water lifts you up, opens your senses and makes you feel refreshed and ready to take on any activity, including even sleeping. [8]

• Water lubricates and cushions your body's bones and joints. Water helps heal quickly the joint damages. Water helps maintain muscle tone as muscles are composed primarily of water. [8]

• Water helps your kidneys and liver function properly and helps reduce the fat deposits. The kidneys need plenty of water to remove salt from the blood and to remove toxins and waste. Water lubricates all your organs so that they function at their best. Water also helps the blood from thickening. [8]

## DEHYDRATION & ITS SYMPTOMS
### Human Body Dehydrates and Dies Within A Few Days Without Water: [9, 10, 11, 12]
• Humans need food and water to survive. The water content by weight of the human body ranges between 42% and 75%, depending on age, health, weight and gender. The average human adult male is approximately 60% water. And 99% of your molecules are water.
A human can go without food for about three weeks. Mahatma Gandhi survived 21 days of complete starvation when he went on hunger strike. But a human would typically last only three to four days without water. The maximum time an individual can go without water seems to be a week, though it depends in individual body condition.

• If we expose ourselves to a hot environment and/or vigorous exercise, the body temperature rises. The only physiological mechanism humans have to keep from overheating is sweating. Evaporation of sweat cools blood in vessels in the skin, which helps to cool the entire body. Under extreme conditions of hot environment and vigorous exercise, an adult can lose between 1 and 1.5 liters of sweat per hour. If that lost water is not replaced, the total volume of the body fluid can fall quickly and, most dangerously, blood volume may drop. If this happens, two potentially life-threatening problems arise: (i) blood pressure decreases because of the low blood volume, and (ii) sweating stops and body temperature can soar even higher. Under such conditions, death occurs quickly. Children are more susceptible to rapid overheating and dehydration because of their relatively larger skin surface-to-volume ratio. A child left in a hot car unattended or an athlete exercising hard in hot weather without drinking water can dehydrate, overheat and die in a a few hours.

⊛ Your body uses water to maintain its temperature, remove waste, and lubricate joints. Your body need water is to maintain good health. Water makes up more than half of your body weight. Your body loses water each day when you go to the bathroom, sweat, and even when you breathe out. You lose water even faster when it is really hot outside, when you walk and exercise, even if if you have fever, and even illnesses such as vomiting and diarrhea can also lead to rapid water loss. If you don't replace the water you lose throughout the day, you can become dehydrated.

## The Symptoms of Dehydration Are: [12]
- ⊛ Little or no urine
- ⊛ Urine that is darker than usual
- ⊛ Dry mouth
- ⊛ Sleepiness or fatigue
- ⊛ Extreme thirst, Headache, Confusion
- ⊛ Dizziness or lightheaded feeling
- ⊛ No tears when crying

⊛ Even the mild dehydration can negatively affect your physical performance, leading to reduced endurance. A study reported that fluid loss of 1.36% after exercise, when water is not consumed, did impair both mood and concentration, while increasing the frequency of headaches. Another study reported that mild dehydration caused by exercise or heat can negatively affect many other aspects of brain function.

# How Much Water A Person Should Drink? [13, 14, 15, 16, 17]
(i) An Adult Must Drink At least 8 Cups of Water Per Day.
It is very important that you must replace water you have been losing throughout the day, by drinking a glass of water every now and then, even when you are not eating, and even when you are not thirsty. Health experts recommend that an adult must drink 8 cups or 2 liters of water per day.

1 Cup = 1 Glass = 8 Ounces = 250 mL = 1/4 Liter

⊛ According to several studies, drinking 2 cups (500 mL) of water can temporarily boost metabolism by 24-30%. Some researchers estimated that drinking 8 cups (2 liters) of water in one day can increase energy expenditure by about 96 calories per day. Drinking cold water is also recommended because your body works hard and burns calories to heat the cold water to your body temperature.

⊛ Drinking water about a half hour before meals can also reduce the amount of calories people end up consuming, especially in older individuals. One study showed that dieters who drank 500 ml of water before meals lost 44% more weight over a period of 12 weeks, compared to those who did not drink water before meals.

## (ii) RESEARCH STUDY: How Much Water A Person Should Drink?
According to the research study conducted by National Academies of Sciences, Engineering and Medicine, healthy sedentary men need about 15.5 cups of fluid and women need 11.5 cups of fluid each day, and they get only about 20 percent of that fluid from daily food consumption (all natural foods contain water). [17]

## (iii) Did You Know "Extreme Weight Loss Contestants" Drink 16 cups (4 Liters) of Water Per Day to Achieve Their Weight-Loss Goals?
⊛ After started drinking 16 cups of purified water (RO water) per day, the author of this book (Dr. RK) lost weight fast, and achieved his weight-loss goal.

# HOW DRINKING WATER SPEEDS UP WEIGHT LOSS?

### Drinking Water May Speed Up Weight Loss [18]

● Researchers in Germany found that drinking lots of water may speed up weight loss. Metabolic rate increases slightly with an increase in water consumption. After drinking approximately 17 ounces (2 cups) of water, the subjects' metabolic rates increased by 30% for both men and women.

### How Does Water Flush Fat Out of Your System? [19]

● Drinking water before you eat may help you eat less. A 2010 study published on Obesity investigated the effects of drinking 2 cups of water before meals on weight loss among a group of people following a low-calorie diet. The study found that the water-drinking group lost more weight than the control group. Drinking water before you eat helps fill you up so you eat less, which may help you lose weight.

### Does Water Flush Out Fat? (Discussion Forum) [20]

● Water flushes out fat cells and ketones. Hydration is extremely important for this and it also keeps our bowels working correctly. Water also flushes out water weight. It sounds stupid and does not make sense, but some of our weight is in water and by drinking water we flush out that old water weight that is sticking onto us and you actually may lose a few pounds after drinking water.

● Whether you are dieting or not, water consumption is essential for good health. You're not flushing out fat cells, but rather flushing out the waste products your body makes. Water retention becomes a serious problem and the body tends to hold onto water if there isn't enough coming into your body.

## Water: How 8 Glasses A Day Keep Fat Away? [21]

● Drinking Enough Water is the Best Treatment for Fluid Retention. Water is needed in great quantities for fat metabolism and for the disposal of waste generated once fats are metabolized. When a person is obese or overweight, he/she needs more water than he/she would require with normal body weight. Water flushes away the waste. When a person loses weight (losing weight means burning fat), the body becomes very busy getting rid of a lot of waste generated due to fat metabolism.

● When water retention becomes a serious problem, you need to cut salt consumption. When you consume excess salt, your body retains more and more water to dilute the sodium. If you want to get rid of excess sodium in your system, drink plenty of water. As water is forced through the kidneys, it will remove the excess sodium.

● When you drink limited quantity of water, the body perceives that there is scarcity of water for future survival, and begins to store water in the extracellular spaces, outside the cell walls. This kind of water storage could cause swollen feet, swollen legs and swollen hands. Doctors then prescribe diuretics to their patients to force out the stored water from the extracellular spaces. But if you drink plenty of water (at least 8 glasses per day), you would not encounter such situations. Drinking plenty of water also helps constipation.

### IF YOU DRINK LOTS OF WATER, YOU MUST REMINERALIZE WATER

● Drinking too much water in an attempt to lose weight could lead to dangerously low levels of sodium in your blood. Therefore when you drink more than 8 cups of purified water per day, you should learn how to remineralize and slightly alkalize the purified water at home. This book teaches "How to Remineralize and Alkalize the Purified Water at Home!" in Chapter 14, Chapter 17 & Chapter 18.

# The Water Report: [22]
# How 8 Glasses of Water Per Day Fights Weight Gain!

◉ Pure and clean water such as distilled water or RO water may be the only true Magic Potion for permanent weight loss! If you stop drinking enough water, your body fluids will again be thrown out of balance. So never stop drinking water.

## DRINKING ICE-COLD WATER BURNS MORE CALORIES

◉ Cold water is absorbed more quickly into the system than warm water. Evidence suggests that by drinking ice-cold water a person can actually burn more calories. In order to raise the ice-cold water temperature to your normal body temperature (normal body temperature is 37°C/98.6°F), your body has to work harder and burn more calories. When your body burn more calories, you lose weight and you feel good.

◉ When the body gets enough water to function optimally, all the body system fluids will achieve perfect balance. As a result, the endocrine gland function improves, fluid retention is alleviated as stored water is lost, more fat can be used as fuel because the liver is free to metabolize stored fat, natural thirst to drink water returns, and there is a loss of hunger almost overnight.

## DRINKING LOTS OF WATER REDUCES FAT DEPOSITS

◉ Kidneys cannot function properly without drinking enough water. When the kidneys do not function, the liver takes responsibility to do the kidney's job. But the liver's primary function is to metabolize stored fat into usable energy for the body. But if the liver has to do some of the kidney's work, it cannot work at full throttle. So you must drink lots of water to help your body.

## DRINK ONLY PURIFIED WATER ALL THE TIME (Recommendations by Dr.RK)

◉ Environmental Protection Agency (EPA) began enforcing the water purification and treatment standards for municipal water systems long ago. But there continues to be incidents of contamination, which could be harmful to your health. So you cannot trust tap water even if your local municipality says that the tap water is being purified. You must take your own measures to make sure that the water you drink is indeed purified.

**OPTION 1:** Installing a reliable and high-quality faucet-filtration system to your kitchen sink at home is one option. And get your filtered water tested by a certified lab.
**OPTION 2:** Purchasing RO water or distilled water from supermarkets or local vendors is the much easier alternative option. RO water is much cheaper than distilled water.

◉ However, you should test the purified water every now and then and make sure that the water you drink is indeed purified, and not contaminated. You can do the following:

(i) Use a TDS meter to monitor the TDS (Total Dissolved Solids) level of purified water. The TDS level of purified water should be below 5 ppm, and the TDS level of distilled water should be precisely zero.
(ii) Use pH drops or pH meter, chlorine test kits and fluoride test kits every now and then.
(iii) Get your drinking water tested by a certified laboratory in your area at least once or twice a year.
(iv) Please also learn how to neutralize your body by consuming a lemon a day (Chapter 18).
(v) Please also learn how to neutralize or slightly alkalize, and remineralize the purified water up to a TDS level of 200 ppm. Please refer to Chapter 14, Chapter 17, Chapter 18 & Chapter 19. There are more than 10 experiments conducted at home.

◉ These healthy water-drinking habits would protect your health, keep you out of trouble, and save your own life and lives of all your family members.

# What 8 Cups of Purified Water Per Day Would Do To Your Body?
## How Drinking Water Would Help Improve Your Overall Health!

- Increases metabolism (cold water).
- Makes you feel full (warm water).
- Helps you lose weight.
- Flushes out toxins.
- Gets you healthier skin.
- Reduces risk of certain cancers.
- Helps digestion and constipation.
- Relieves fatigue and energizes.
- Improves overall health.

▷ All of the above for ZERO calories.

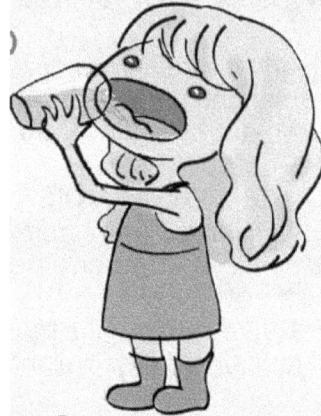

- Did you know more than 99% of your amazing body's molecules are water molecules, and 55% to 60% of your body weight is water? You therefore should make sure that the water in your body is clean, healthy and nutritious, and more importantly one 100% free of contaminants.

- So please do not drink tap water, well water, or bottled water of any kind without knowing how pure it is. Please always drink AT LEAST 8 CUPS OF PURIFIED WATER (RO water, distilled water, or zero water). And learn how to remineralize and slightly alkalize the purified water at home!

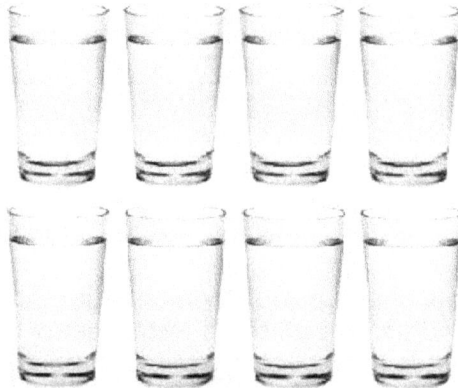

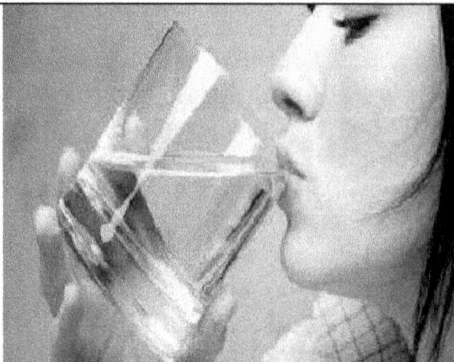

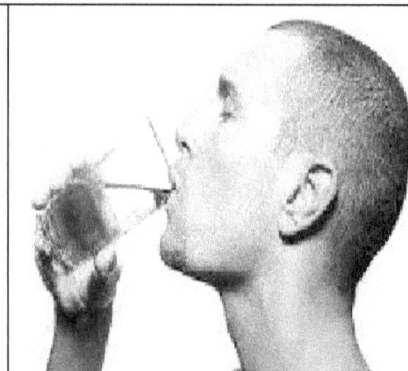

Figure 3.1  How drinking water would help improve your overall health!

# REFERENCES

1. Earth, from Wikipedia, the free encyclopedia.
https://en.wikipedia.org/wiki/Earth

2. Space and Astronomy News, Universe Today, Posted on Feb 10, 2017.
https://www.universetoday.com/25756/surface-area-of-the-earth/

3. Oceans Worlds, Water in the Solar System and Beyond by NASA.
https://www.nasa.gov/specials/ocean-worlds/

4. Body water from Wikipedia, the free encyclopedia.
https://en.wikipedia.org/wiki/Body_water

5a. 99% of Your Molecules are Water by Malaga Bay, Posted on March 15, 2014.
https://malagabay.wordpress.com/2014/03/15/99-of-your-molecules-are-water/

5b. How many molecules are in the human body? by Ernest Z, Posted on June 18, 2016.
https://socratic.org/questions/how-many-molecules-are-in-the-human-body

6. The Water in You by the USGS (The United States Geological Survey) Water Science School, Contact: Howard Perlman, Posted on Dec o2, 2016.
https://water.usgs.gov/edu/propertyyou.html

7a. Permanent Diabetes Control (Book), Authored by Rao Konduru, MS, PhD, Reviewed and Endorsed by Dr. Marshal Dahl, MD, PhD., Page 31.

7b. The Amazingly Complex Human Body by Cloversites.com.
http://storage.cloversites.com/makinglifecountministriesinc/documents/Amazing%20Human%20Body_3.pdf

8. Benefits of Water, Posted by Brita.ca.
https://brita.ca/water-wellness/benefits/

9. Here's how many days a person can survive without water by Dina Spector, Posted on March 8, 2018.
http://www.businessinsider.com/how-many-days-can-you-survive-without-water-2014-5

10. How Long Can a Person Survive Without Water? by Rafi Letzter, Staff Writer, Posted on November 29, 2017.
https://www.livescience.com/32320-how-long-can-a-person-survive-without-water.html

11. How Long Can the Average Person Survive Without Water? by Randall K. Packer, a professor of biology at George Washington University, Scientific American.
https://www.scientificamerican.com/article/how-long-can-the-average/

12. Hydration: Why It Is Important by FamilyDoctor.Org.
https://familydoctor.org/hydration-why-its-so-important/

13. How much water should you drink per day? By Southwest Family Medicine Associates, Dallas, Texas, USA.
https://www.southwestfamilymed.com/blog/how-much-water-should-you-drink-per-day

14. How Much Water Does Your Body Need To Prevent Health Problems?, Posted by Gayatri Friday, May 01, 2020.
https://www.nyoooz.com/features/health/how-much-water-does-your-body-need-to-prevent-health-problems.html/3538/

15. Should You Drink 3 Liters of Water per Day? Written by Rachael Link, Healthline, Updated and Posted on June 10, 2020.
https://www.healthline.com/health/3-liters-of-water

16. Water consumption increases weight loss during a hypocaloric diet intervention in middle-aged and older adults, Randamized Study, by Elizabeth A Dennis 1, Ana Laura Dengo, Dana L Comber, Kyle D Flack, Jyoti Savla, Kevin P Davy, Brenda M Davy, Obesity (Silver Spring), 2010 Feb;18(2):300-7. doi: 10.1038/oby.2009.235. Epub 2009 Aug 6.
https://pubmed.ncbi.nlm.nih.gov/19661958/
https://www.ncbi.nlm.nih.gov/pmc/articles/PMC2859815/

17. Is alkaline water really better for you? by Christy Brissette, Posted on August 28, 2019.
https://www.washingtonpost.com/lifestyle/wellness/is-alkaline-water-really-better-for-you/2019/08/27/8c646d26-c462-11e9-b72f-b31dfaa77212_story.html

18. Drinking Water May Speed Weight Loss by WebMD.com.
http://www.webmd.com/diet/news/20040105/drinking-water-may-speed-weight-loss

19. How Does Water Flush Fat Out of Your System? by JILL CORLEONE, RDN, LD Last Updated: Jun 17, 2015.
http://www.livestrong.com/article/545311-how-does-water-flush-fat-out-of-your-system/

20. Does Water Flush Out Fat? (Discussion Forum).
http://forum.lowcarber.org/archive/index.php/t-336946.html

21. Water: How 8 Glasses A Day Keep Fat Away by Angelfire.com.
http://www.angelfire.com/ca2/LowcarbingDream/water.html

22. The Water Report: How 8 Glasses of Water per Day Fights Weight Gain! by Colon Therapists Network.
http://www.colonhealth.net/healtharticles/8-glasses-water-per-day-fights-weight-gain.html

# CHAPTER 4:  TYPES OF DRINKING WATER
## A QUICK REVIEW

## TABLE OF CONTENTS

Table 4.1  Types of drinking water available for human consumption.

| TYPES OF DRINKING WATER | |
|---|---|
| Tap Water, Well Water, Even Boiled Tap Water, Bottled Water & Spring Water Are Unpurified Waters. So You Should Avoid Drinking Them. | |
| **I. Tap Water**<br>**CHAPTER 5** | Tap water is untrustworthy although almost all local Government municipalities encourage you to drink it. You never know what contaminants are lurking in your tap water that endanger your health. Do not become another statistic! Install a high-quality faucet filter, and replace it once every 3 months or whenever the lifespan of the filter cartridge exhausts. Get your filtered water from tap tested at least once every 6 months, and make sure it is free of contaminants. Consider drinking purified water instead!<br>As an example, read the tap water disaster story that took place recently in Flint, Michigan, USA (Chapter 5), and learn your lesson. |
| **II. Boiled Water**<br>**CHAPTER 6** | Boiled tap water kills most of the pathogens (all kinds of bacteria, viruses, fungi, parasites), microorganisms and E. coli instantly, preventing diseases. But the harmful heavy metal and mineral contaminants such as lead, arsenic, aluminum, etc. may still remain in tap water even if it is boiled. |
| **III. Bottled Water**<br>**(Including Vitamin Water**<br>**and Mineral Water)**<br>**CHAPTER 7** | Bottled water is made from tap water by adding artificial vitamins, minerals, artificial flavors, and additives. It is untrustworthy and unreliable. Testing revealed (there are many reports) that it could contain harmful chemicals, microplastics, pesticides and very many dangerous contaminants. Natural Resources Defense Council (NRDC) found that the harmful contaminants in bottled water outweigh the benefits of the filtered water. Also, bottled water is horrific for the environment and ecosystems surrounding you. Approximately only 1 in 5 plastic bottles are recycled, and those un-recycled bottles remain in the environment and it can take some 400 to 1000 years for those plastics to decompose. |
| **IV. Spring Water**<br>**CHAPTER 8** | Spring water is bottled water. Spring water is the natural water possessing trace minerals in it, but it is not purified water. Even though it contains trace minerals, you never know what contaminants are present in it so it is untrustworthy. However, many people still like and drink spring water because of its taste and mineral composition. |
| **V. Well Water**<br>**CHAPTER 9** | Well water is the groundwater that is reached by drilling, and then pumped to the surface.  Well water in rural areas is highly contaminated. Boiled well water may minimize the risk but it still may contain dangerous heavy metal contaminants, pesticides, both human and animal feces. Get your well water tested at least once every 6 months, and filter the water with a reliable filter, and boil it before drinking. |

# PURIFIED WATER

**Distilled Water, RO Water, Demineralized Water or Deionized Water, Desalinated Water Are Most Commonly Used Purified Waters.**

Test your purified water with a TDS meter, and pH drops or digital pH meter. Make sure it is what it says on their labels. Do not be illuded by empty promises. Make sure their promises are true by testing the water. When Dr. RK tested Santevia water pitcher, it failed miserably. The pH and TDS value of filtered water were found to be unchanged from tap water. The company manager, when questioned, was found suspicious, and refused to provide any further information.

| | |
|---|---|
| **VI. Demineralized Water/Deionized Water CHAPTER 10** | Both demineralization and deionization processes use "ion exchange" as the basic principle to produce purified water. This kind of water has no minerals in it. WHO warned that drinking demineralized water is harmful to your health. So you should consume well-balanced diet by eating leafy vegetables & fruits, and supplement your diet with high-quality multivitamins and minerals (magnesium, calcium, potassium, and others of your choice). |
| **VII. Reverse Osmosis Water/RO Water CHAPTER 11** ◉ Purchase RO water from local vendors, or in supermarkets at Refill Yourself Stations. | It is the best "purified water" after distilled water. It is the most economical purified water available to consumers in supermarkets (a lot cheaper than buying distilled water in pharmacies). The process removes chlorine, mineral content and all other contaminants of water by forcing the water through a semi permeable membrane. This process filters out 95% to 99% of the "total dissolved solids (salts & minerals)" present in tap water. So you should consume a well-balanced diet by eating leafy vegetables & fruits, and supplement your diet with high-quality multivitamins and minerals (magnesium, calcium, potassium, and others of your choice). Please consider remineralizing the RO water with a tiny bit of Himalayan pink salt, Celtic sea salt, or ConcenTrace mineral drops in order to remineralize it (See Chapter 17). |
| **VIII. Desalinated Water CHAPTER 12** | It is the same as RO water without any minerals or trace minerals. Consider remineralizing this water, and consume balanced meals, and take supplements (vitamins and minerals). |
| **IX. Distilled Water CHAPTER 13** ◉ Purchase a counter-top home distiller that makes 1 gallon of distilled water in 5.5 hours. | Distilled water is the purest form of water. This process removes one 100% of the total dissolved solids (salts and minerals). WHO reported that the distilled water lacks nutritional value (minerals) to the human health, and it could suck the minerals out of your body, if consumed for long time, causing diseases and disorders. However there is no solid scientific proof of these claims. Many people still drink the distilled water. Some people remineralize the distilled water before drinking. You will be fine if you consume a well-balanced diet and supplement with high-quality multivitamins and minerals. Please consider neutralizing your body by eating one lemon a day, and/or slightly alkalizing you body by adding a tiny pinch of baking soda to distilled water you drink. |
| **X. ZeroWater, Brita and Pur Filtration Systems CHAPTER 14** | If genuine RO water and distilled water are not available in the market, this book suggests that a consumer must switch to zero water. Make your own purified water using a ZeroWater pitcher. |

| | And learn how to remineralize and slightly alkalize the zero water at home. Everything is explained clearly in Chapter 14. |
|---|---|
| **XI. Remineralized Water**<br>**CHAPTER 17**<br>( A Very Important Chapter) | Purified and remineralized water, made at home, is the healthy & nutritious mineral water. Remineralized water can be obtained by adding a tiny bit of Himalayan pink salt, Celtic sea salt, or ConcenTrace mineral drops to the purified water (RO water, distilled water, or zero water) up to a TDS level of 200 ppm. Please see Chapter 17 for the experiments conducted at home, and to learn how to do it correctly.<br><br>Whenever you remineralize the purified water for the first time, test it by using a TDS meter, and do not exceed the TDS level over 200 ppm. It is the best way to make and drink your own mineral water at home instead of purchasing that overpriced and dangerous "bottled mineral water ". |

## XII. ALKALINE WATER: CHAPTER 18
### ( A Very Important Chapter)

**Alkaline Water Can Be Obtained by 10 Methods As Listed Below:**
Purchase pH testing drops or a reliable digital pH meter to test the water pH, and learn how to neutralize, slightly alkalize and fully alkalize the purified water by adding a tiny bit of baking soda or a few ConcenTrace mineral drops.
Drinking alkaline water will help your body neutralize the acidity that it gains from different foods, juices and beverages as well as stress. Most alkaline substances become carbon dioxide and water once they are oxidized. Your body spends less energy neutralizing overly acidic substances if you drink alkaline water, and they can easily be excreted by the kidneys.
On the other hand, drinking too much alkaline water for a long term is harmful to your body as your stomach needs acidity for the digestion process and to kill bacteria. So you need to optimize the quantity of alkaline water consumption by drinking it periodically.

| | |
|---|---|
| **1. Add Lemon Juice** to purified water. Lemon does not alkalize the water. The urine pH does not rise above 7 (pH < 7). | The best natural method to live healthy. Upon drinking lemon water, urine pH rises to 7 only. Lemon slightly neutralizes your body & does not alkalize. More importantly you cannot make alkaline water by adding lemon juice. |
| **2. Add a Pinch of Baking Soda** to purified water. It is perfectly alkaline water. Drinking water pH can be increased up to 8.5. | Upon adding it to purified water and drinking it, urine pH rises up to 8.5. This method has side effects (gastrointestinal distress) so make sure it suits your body. |
| **3. Add ConcenTrace mineral drops** to purified water. Drinking water can be easily alkalized. | It is very easy to remineralize and alkalize the purified water by adding only 2 drops of ConcenTrace mineral drops. Highly recommended. |
| **4. Purchase Alkaline Water from Local vendors.** | Research in your area, and find out the addresses of local vendors who sell both purified water (RO water) and alkaline water. These vendors routinely test the water and make sure that the unit is working perfectly. Therefore the water you purchase is reliable and trustworthy. |

| | |
|---|---|
| **5. Purchase pH booster drops**, and add to purified water. It is perfectly alkaline water. pH can be adjusted up to 9, 10, or more. | pH drops are unreliable unless the company provides the report of analysis. Drops may contain contaminants or toxins. So get your drinking water tested before you start drinking this kind of alkaline water. |
| **6.** Purchase an **Alkaline Water Pitcher** that adds minerals to tap water or purified water and raises water pH, making it alkaline. | Pitchers filter tap water and add minerals such as calcium, magnesium, potassium, sodium and iron. Do not believe their labels and verbal promises. Test it before using it and make sure it works by using a TDS meter and a digital pH meter. It is not reliable until you test the final product. |
| **7. Purchase a Water Ionizer** that purifies and turns your tap water to alkaline water at the touch of a button. | pH can be adjusted (8 to 11 or more). However, maintaining this kind of unit at home is tedious. You need to test drinking water every day and make sure it is working. You never know if it is working or broke down. |
| **8. Purchase a Kangen Water Machine** that turns your tap water to alkaline water and acidic water (pH adjustable). | KANGEN WATER MACHINE: Maintaining this kind of unit at home is tedious. You need to test drinking water every day and make sure it is working. You never know if the machine is working or broke down. |
| **9. Purchase a Hydrogen Water Generator**. (Not necessarily alkaline water, it could have neutral pH). | HYDROGEN WATER MACHINE: It produces either alkaline water or non-alkaline water depending on the brand name. Needs to check for H2 concentration in drinking water frequently. Again you need to test final product and make sure it is working. |
| **10. Purchase a Reverse Osmosis System** that purifies tap water, remineralizes and pours alkaline water (pH adjustable) into your jug at the touch of a button. | REVERSE OSMOSIS SYSTEM: Maintaining this kind of unit at home is tedious. You need to test drinking water every day or every now and then and make sure it is working. You never know if the machine is working or broke down. Purchase a TDS meter, and test your water for TDS level. Do not drink water with TDS > 200 ppm. |

# OTHER TYPES OF WATER

| | |
|---|---|
| **XIII. Water From Atmospheric Water Generators CHAPTER 15** | Water from atmospheric air is produced through dehumidification of air. The moisture in air is cooled, captured, condensed into droplets and collected into a receiver or reservoir, which is then filtered and purified to obtain safe drinking water.<br>You should consider remineralizing this purified water in order to comply with the WHO suggestion that drinking water should contain minimal mineral content. Also please consider neutralizing or slightly alkalizing your drinking water before consuming. |

**FINAL MESSAGE:** Please do not drink tap water, well water, or bottled water of any kind without knowing how pure it is. Please always drink purified water that is either neutralized or slightly alkalized, and remineralized up to a TDS (Total Dissolved Solids) level of 200 ppm, which is the healthy drinking water.

Purchasing expensive water purification systems for home use is unnecessary. Learn how to purchase or make your own purified water at home. Please refer to the 2nd Part of this book (Chapter 17, Chapter 18 and Chapter 19), and learn how to remineralize and alkalize the purified water at home.

# CHAPTER 14: ZEROWATER, BRITA AND PUR FILTRATION SYSTEMS TO PRODUCE PURIFIED WATER AT HOME

# TABLE OF CONTENTS

# ZEROWATER'S 5-STAGE ION EXCHAGE FILTRATION IN ACTION [1]

Tap water may look clean, but could pick up hidden contaminants while traveling through pipes. ZeroWater company claims that its 5-stage Ion Exchange filtration removes more dissolved solids than ANY other pour-through filter in the world. By removing 99.6% of all TDS (Total Dissolved Solids), the filter leaves nothing behind but the pure water H2O. ZeroWater filter with its advanced technology is certified to remove virtually all dissolved solids from tap water, including the most commonly found contaminants like lead, chromium, mercury, and PFOA & PFOS.

As tap water passes through five distinct sections vertically, the filter removes the visible solids, inorganic compounds, and contaminants that lurk in our tap water so that we can drink the purest tasting and contaminant-free water worry-free. The 5-stage filtration process removes everything from tap water, leaving behind zero dissolved solids as shown below:

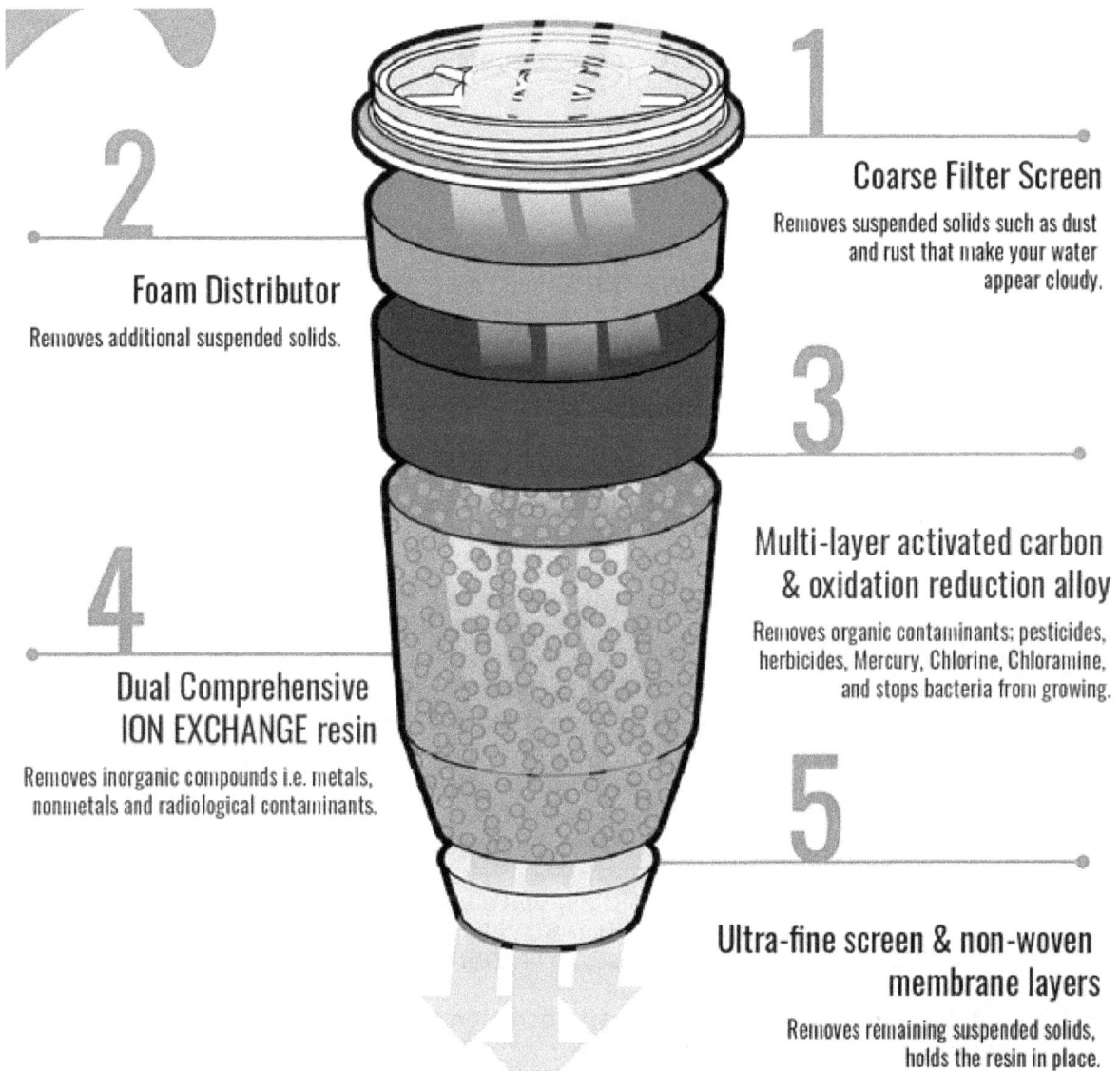

Courtesy of ZEROWATER
Figure 14.1 The 5-stage ZroWater filtration process is explained. [1]

# WHAT ARE PFAS, PFOA & PFOS? [2]

PFAS = polyfluoroalkyl substances
PFOA = perfluorooctanoic acid
PFOS = perfluorooctane sulfonate

PFAS are a group of man-made, large, complex, and ever-expanding group of manufactured chemicals that are widely used to make various types of everyday needful products. These chemicals because of their unique ability to repel oil and water do not degrade over time, but they accumulate within the environment, and could slowly end up in the water we drink. For example, they prevent food from sticking to nonstick cookware, make clothes and carpets resistant to stains (stain repellents), and create firefighting foam that is more effective, waterproof clothing and shoes, fast food wrappers, personal care products, and many other fancy consumer goods. PFAS are vastly used in industries such as aerospace, automotive, construction, electronics, and military.

In general, there are two types of PFAS most commonly produced worldwide:
(i) PFOA (perfluorooctanoic acid) and
(ii) PFOS (perfluorooctane sulfonate)

ZeroWater filter is certified to reduce these most dangerous PFOA & PFOS, thereby making the drinking water safe.

## THE SUPERIORITY OF THE ZEROWATER'S 5-STAGE FILTRATION TECHNIQUE [2, 3]

ZeroWater company (Zero Technologies, LLc) has been designing, manufacturing and marketing many 5-Stage filtration pitchers and dispensers for getting TDS free water at home or in the office. All pitchers remove 99.6% of dissolved solids, including organic and inorganic materials, such as metals, minerals, salts, and ions dissolved in water. TDS can affect the taste and appearance of water but are not harmful to consume. All pitchers and dispensers fit perfectly either on on the counter or in the refrigerator. All pitchers and dispensers come with a ZeroWater® TDS meter so that a customer can easily monitor the TDS level the zero water made using any pitcher.

ZeroWater claims that: Even if all the municipalities with superior technological advancements achieve the removal of 99.6% of total dissolved solids, the water could pick up chemicals, lead and dirt on its way from the treatment plant, through pipelines, to the faucet. Even the minute quantities of the added chlorine by municipalities is harmful to the children. The taste of the tap water may not be appreciated and the quality may not be trustworthy.

ZeroWater's products are internationally certified against NSF/ANSI standards, delivering the purest tasting water of any pour-through water filter. ZeroWater's 5-stage filtration system is far superior to the Brita filtration system in removing the following contaminants: [3]

METALS SUCH AS: ANTIMONY, ARSENIC, BARIUM, BERYLLIUM, CADMIUM, CHROMIUM, COPPER, IRON, LEAD, MANGANESE, MERCURY, SELENIUM, SILVER, THALLIUM, ZINC, and
INORGANIC NON-METALS SUCH AS: CHLORINE, CYANIDE, FLUORIDE, NITRATE, NITRITE.

The results can be seen on a comparison chart shown on the following webpage:
https://zerowater.com/pages/results

# ZEROWATER PRODUCTS (PITCHERS, DISPENSERS & FAUCET FILTERS) [4]

All ZeroWater products are made from BPA-Free hard plastic so that they last longer.

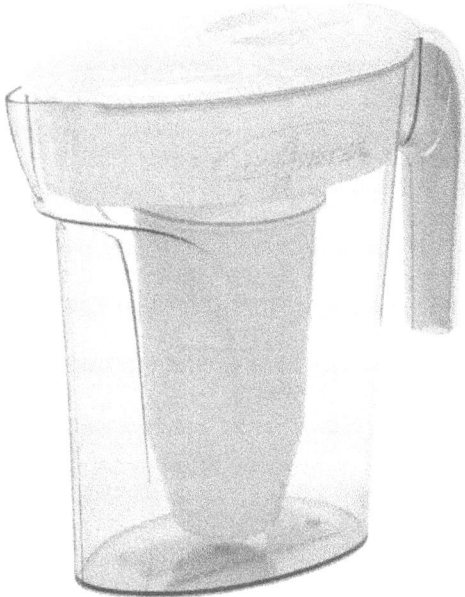

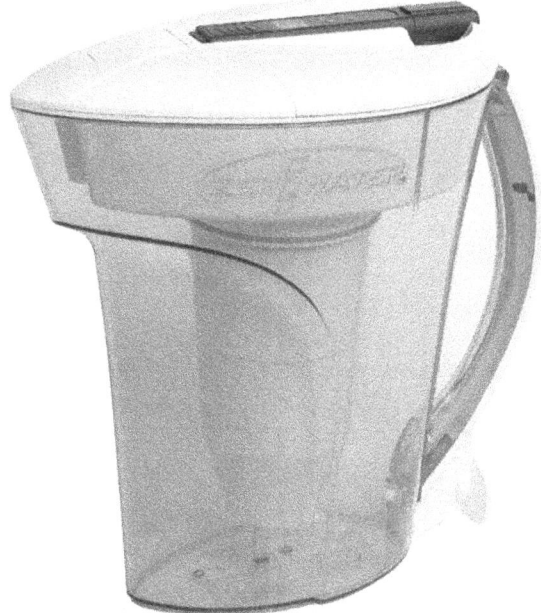

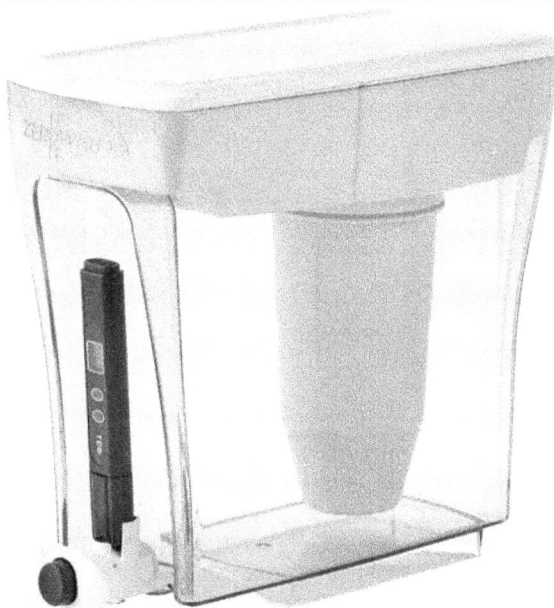

| | |
|---|---|
| ZeroWater 7-Cup Pitcher | ZeroWater 10-Cup Pitcher |
| ZeroWater 20-Cup Pitcher | ZeroWater 40-Cup Pitcher (Glass Container) |

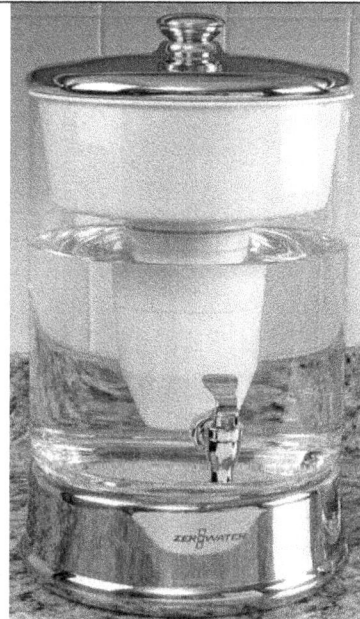

**FAUCET FILTERS** are installed to the tip of kitchen sink faucet to remove contaminants from tap water. Faucet filters do not reduce the TDS level of tap water. The major advantage is that if you install a faucet filter to sink, the ZeroWater filter lasts longer.

Courtesy of ZEROWATER

Figure 14.2 ZeroWater 5-Stage Water Filtration Products to purify water.

# HOW TO REMINERALIZE AND SLIGHTLY ALKALIZE THE ZERO WATER
## (Same Procedure Can Be Used for Any Kind of Purified Water)

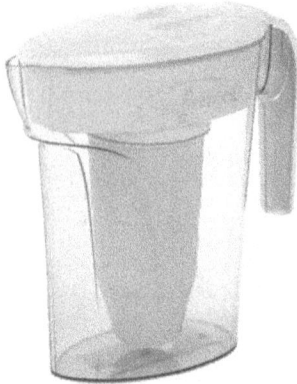

**1.** Purchase a ZeroWater pitcher on Zerowater.com or from any local retail store. It comes with a ZeroWater filter and also a TDS meter.

**2.** Install the filter inside the pitcher, and learn how to make zero water from tap water. After making zero water, monitor the TDS level using the TDS meter. The TDS level of zero water should be precisely 0 ppm.

**3.** The filter lifetime depends on the TDS level of your tap water. In Canada, the TDS level is only 20 ppm and so it lasts long. In USA, the TDS level varies from 100 ppm to 300 ppm so the filter is exhausted in 3 to 4 weeks for a single person if he/she drinks 8 cups of water per day. You can use the filter until TDS=5 ppm.

**4.** Make enough zero water for a week, and store zero water in four 4-liter bottles as show below.

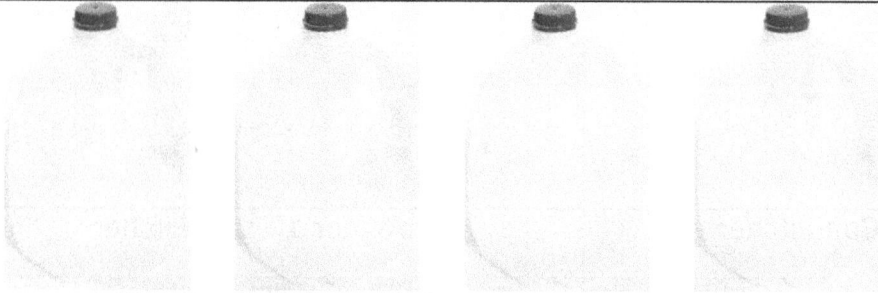

ZeroWater Pitcher

4-Liter Bottles Filled With Zero Water (TDS = 0 ppm)

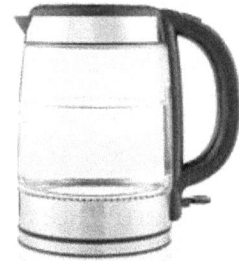

Glass Kettle (1.7 Liters)

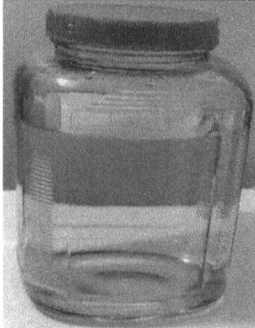

Glass Bottle Filled With 4-Liters of Zero Water

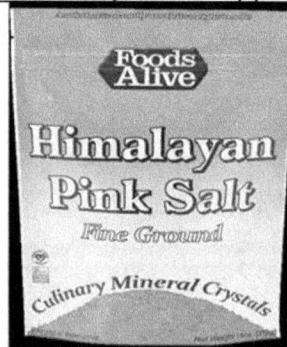

Himalayan pink salt

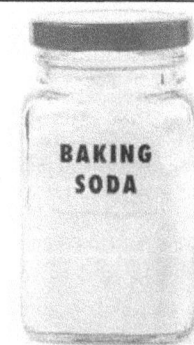

Baking Soda

**5.** Transfer 4 liters of zero water (you have just made) into a glass bottle.

**6.** Add a tiny pinch (only a few kernels) of Himalayan pink salt, and shake the bottle in a circular motion so that all water is remineralized. Monitor TDS level. Make sure that TDS is 20 ppm, 50 ppm, or 100 ppm (your desired TDS level). Add more Himalyan pink salt if the TDS level is below your desired level. Do not exceed TDS=200 ppm.

**7.** Add a tiny pinch of baking soda (only a few kernels), shake the bottle thoroughly and measure the pH. pH should be close to 7 (maximum 7.25).

**8.** Boil this remineralized and slightly alkalized zero water by using a glass kettle, store it in glass bottle until it is cooled, transfer to 4-liter plastic bottles, refrigerate it, and drink it.

**9. IMPORTANT NOTE:** When you use baking soda to increase the pH of the purified water, you must do urine test frequently and make sure that your urine pH is under 8.

*Purified water (zero water) that is either neutralized (pH=7) or slightly alkalized (pH= 7 to 7.5), and remineralized up to a TDS level of 200 ppm is the healthy drinking water.*

Figure 14.3 How to make healthy drinking water from zero water.

# HOW TO USE TWO ZERO WATER FILTERS SIMULTANEOUSLY AND SAVE MONEY?

**1.** ZeroWater company suggests that whenever the TDS level of filtered water reaches 6 ppm, you must dispose the filter, purchase a replacement filter, and use it to produce zero water on an ongoing basis.
**2.** But Drinking Water Guide advises that if you use two filters simultaneously and wisely as explained here, you can save a lot of money in a long run.

**3.** Purchase two ZeroWater pitchers. Start using Pitcher-I until the TDS level reaches 6 ppm. Do not dispose this filter and keep using it. Store this filtered (not drinkable) water at 6 ppm to 10 ppm in 4-liter bottles as shown below.
**4.** Filter this water at 6 ppm in Pitcher-II, which will reduce TDS level from 6 ppm to 0 ppm. Store this filtered (drinkable) water at 0 ppm in different 4-liter bottles as shown below.

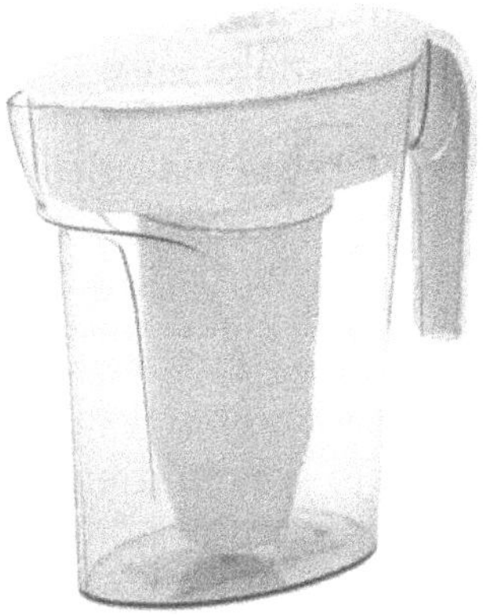

### ZeroWater Pitcher-I
Tap water TDS is reduced from 100 ppm to 6 ppm.
This filter will last 3 to 4 weeks.

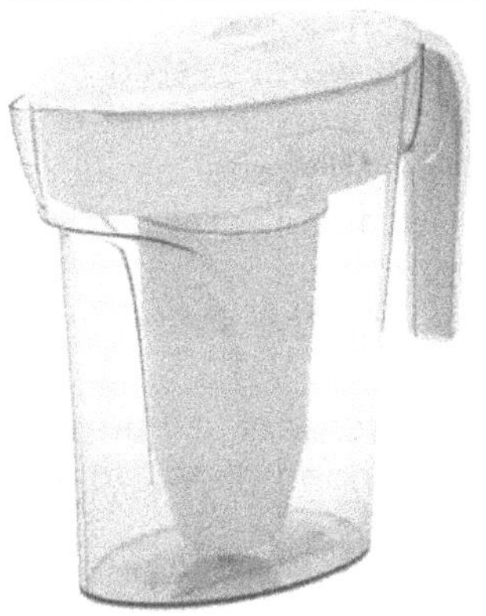

### ZeroWater Pitcher-II
Filtered water TDS is reduced from 6 ppm to 0 ppm.
This filter will last a lot longer than 4 weeks.

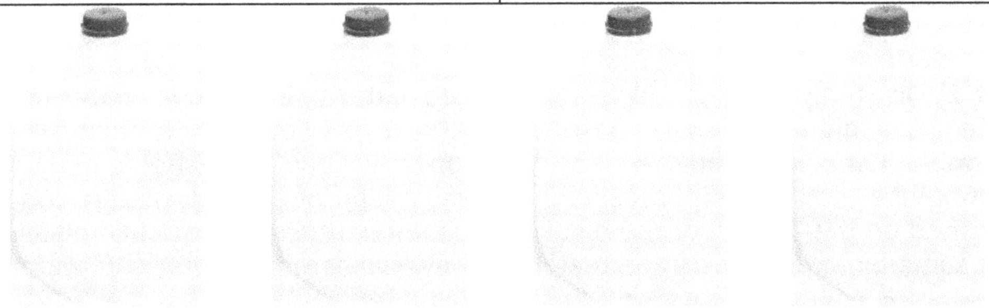

4-Liter Bottles Filled With Filtered Water (TDS = 6 ppm to 10 ppm, not drinkable)

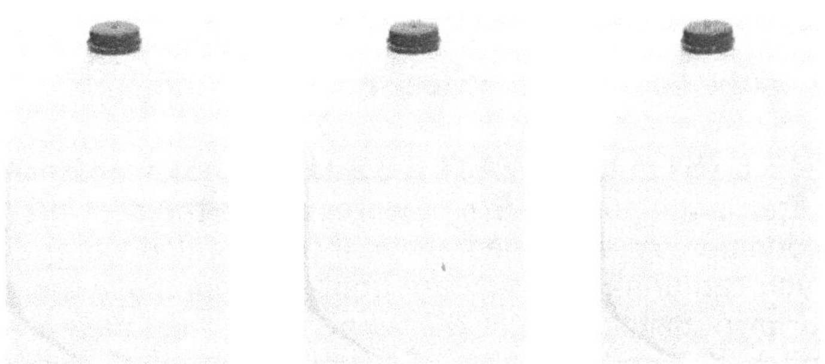

4-Liter Bottles Filled With Zero Water (TDS = 0 ppm, drinkable water)

Figure 14.4 How to use two ZeroWater filters simultaneously and save money.

# WHY IS ZERO WATER PREFERABLE
## COMPARED TO DISTILLED WATER AND RO WATER?

If it is manufactured, distributed and available in pristine condition, if it is genuine and trustworthy, and if it is one 100% free of contaminants, distilled water is the purest form of water (perfectly H2O), and is the best water for human consumption.

However under current day circumstances, the distilled water distribution industry is totally corrupt as it is very difficult to find the genuine distilled water in the market nowadays.

## CHEAP HOME DISTILLERS ARE UNTRUSTWORTHY

◦ When you purchased a home distiller and started making your own distilled water, please get your distilled water tested by a local certified laboratory, and make sure that there are no contaminants present in the distilled water you made.

◦ CAUTION: Cheap home distillers can release contaminants from the materials of construction such as metal and/or plastic. Make sure that the home distiller's steam chamber, upper cover with condensing coil, fan and cap are properly designed and manufactured with the safe materials of construction so that the distilled water is free of contaminants.

◦ A customer purchased a home distiller on Amazon, and got his distilled water tested by a laboratory, and found elevated level of nickel contaminant. There was nothing he could do about it but stopped using that distiller. So please be careful when using home distillers.

## STORE BOUGHT DISTILLED WATER IN BOTTLES IS UNTRUSTWORTHY

An innocent consumer can easily get into a trap by purchasing and drinking distilled water in bottles readily available all over the supermarkets. Bottled water is untrustworthy. Whenever you purchased distilled water or reverse osmosis water in bottles, make sure that it is genuinely purified water by testing it as explained below:

◦ **METHOD 1:** Dr. RK purchased and tested distilled water being sold in 4-liter bottles in Walmart, Real Canadian Superstore, Safeway and Save-On-Foods, in Vancouver area, British Columbia, Canada. He distilled this distilled water again in his home distiller. After the completion of the distillation process, there was a kind of colored, greasy and sticky SCUM deposited on the bottom of the distiller. It is dangerous to drink such distilled water. He had the same experience when he tested the reverse osmosis water (RO water).

◦ **METHOD 2:** He also boiled this distilled water in a stockpot with glass lid on the stove. He left the lid slightly opened so that the vapors would escape out. After all the distilled water is evaporated and escaped out, he found some golden brown colored scars (large scars and small scars) on the bottom of the stock pot. It is dangerous to drink such distilled water.

## IF GENUINE DISTILLED WATER IS UNAVAILABLE, SWITCH TO ZERO WATER

◦ Distilled water is the purest form of water and is the best drinking water if it is available in its pristine condition. As explained above if the distilled water was tested and approved by a laboratory, you can drink it. If you are unable to purchase genuine distilled water or unable to make your own distilled water that is genuine, then please switch to zero water using a ZeroWater pitcher. ZeroWater filter removes 99.6% of dissolved solids from the tap water (everything is removed exactly as in distillation process).

TDS level of distilled water is 0 ppm. TDS level of zero water is also 0 ppm.

◦ When drinking zero water, learn how to remineralize and slightly alkalize zero water.

## LEARN HOW TO REMINERALIZE AND SLIGHTLY ALKALIZE THE ZERO WATER
World Health Organization (WHO) reported that demineralized water (distilled water) leaches minerals from the body's cells, and develop many serious health risks including cancer and heart disease. This topic is discussed extensively in Appendix-13A (see below). Please refer to Chapter 17, Chapter 18 & Chapter 19 and learn how to remineralize and alkalize the purified water at home. There are experiments conducted at home.

# RECOMMENDATIONS (by Dr. RK)
When you remineralize the zero water, please do not add too much Himalayan pink salt. Himalayan pink salt, Celtic sea salt or ConcenTrace mineral drops which contain extremely high quantity of sodium. Beware of that important information regarding the high sodium content. Research showed that many people who overconsumed sodium chloride (NaCl) beyond the RDA developed and suffered from hypertension, osteoporosis, kidney stones, Menierre's Syndrome (ear ringing), insomnia, motion sickness, asthma, and a variety of cancers. So learn how to add only a few kernels of Himalayan pink salt, Celtic sea salt so that the TDS level could be 50 ppm, 100 ppm, or maximum 200 ppm (Never exceed 200 ppm).
When you try to alkalize the zero water, please not add too much baking soda. If you do so, the pH will shoot up to 8.5. It is dangerous to drink water at pH=8.5 every day. Add only a few kernels of baking soda and measure pH. Let the pH be close to 7.
After making the zero water using ZeroWater pitcher, and after remineralizing and slightly alkalizing, boil the zero water using a glass kettle, store it in a glass bottle, and refrigerate it. Zero water because of its high purity should never be stored in metal containers. So make sure that you are not using any metal kettle.
When you boil the water, no matter what kind of water it is, pathogens (all kinds of bacteria, viruses, fungi, parasites), microorganisms and E. coli would be destroyed, and so you can drink the purified water worry-free.
Always drink zero water that is boiled and refrigerated, remineralized (up to a TDS level of 200 ppm, and slightly alkalized (pH=7 to 7.25).
RULE TO BE ADOPTED: Purfied water that is either neutralized (pH=7) or slightly alkalized (pH=7 to 7.25), and remineralized up to a TDS level of 200 ppm is the healthy drinking water.

## Advantages of Zero Water Compared to Distilled Water
It takes 1 hour to make 1 liter of distilled water or 4 hour to make 4 liters of distilled water using a countertop home distiller, where as 1 liter of zero water can be made in 15 to 20 minutes using a Zerowater Pitcher or 4 liters of zero water can be made in 1 hour using a ZeroWater pitcher.
Countertop water distillers don't last long as they break down in a few weeks or few months where as ZeroWater Pitcher lasts long.
Zero water can be self-made at home. You can make your own zero water from tap water at the comfort of your home without depending on supermarkets or local delivery companies or other vendors. You don't have to purchase bottled water, which is untrustworthy.

## DRAWBACKS OF ZEROWATER, BRITA & PUR FILTERS
These filters are not guaranteed to remove all contaminants from the tap water. They are designed to remove only some commonly found contaminants as listed on their websites.
You the consumer need to see your municipality's annual water quality report, and find out what contaminants are actually lurking in your tap water, and research and use an appropriate water purification system that is designed to remove the remaining contaminants (other than those removed by ZeroWater, Brita, or PUR filters).

# BRITA WATER FILTRATION SYSTEM [5]

## MAJOR DIFFERENCE BWTWEEN ZERO WATER FILTER & BRITA FILTER
While ZeroWater filter removes all contaminants from tap water and reduces the TDS level to zero, Brita® claims that their filters are meant to remove most commonly found contaminants (not all) from tap water, and that they are not committed to reduce the TDS level to zero.

Brita® claims that their products are tested and certified by the WQA (Water Quatoty Association) and also tested against NSF/ANSI Standards 42 and 53 for the reduction of the claims specified on the Performance Data Sheet. Brita® claims that their filters remove Lead, Mercury, Cadmium, Benzene, Asbestos, Particulates, Copper, Zinc, Tricholorobenzene, Select pharmaceuticals, pesticides/herbicides, TTHMs, Atrazine, and many other contaminants, making the tap water safe to drink. [5]

The major drawback of Brita® filter is that it is not certified to remove the dangerous contaminants (i) PFOA (perfluorooctanoic acid) and (ii) PFOS (perfluorooctane sulfonate).

Brita® manufactures and distributes a variety of pitchers, dispensers, faucet mounts: [5]
## BRITA PITCHERS & DISPENSERS
(i) Brita® Colour Series Grand Pitcher
(ii) Brita® Marina Water Filtration Pitcher
(iii) Brita® Slim Water Filtration Pitcher

(iv) Brita® Soho Water Filtration Pitcher
(v) Brita® Space Saver Water Filtration Pitcher
(vi) Brita® Ultramax Dispenser with 1 Brita®

## BRITA SINK FAUCET MOUNTS
(i) Brita® Faucet Mount Filtration Basic System - Chrome
(ii) Brita® Faucet Mount Filtration Basic System – White
In addition, Brita also sells "Carry-on Water Bottles" with filter inside.

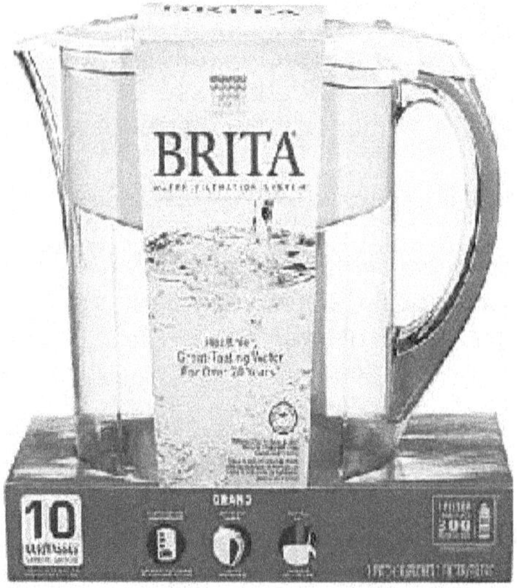

Courtesy of Brita®

Dr. RK personally tested the Brita Water Pitcher. He did the following experiment to test the Brita filtration unit. He purchased the Brita Water Pitcher in the local supermarket, and made purified water from tap water. He monitored the TDS level in the tap water and in the purified water obtained from Brita Water Pitcher. He noted the results of TDS carefully.

• For the tap water (in Burnaby, British Columbia, Canada), TDS = 22 ppm.
• For the purified water obtained from Brita Water Pitcher, TDS = 22 ppm.

**CONCLUSION:** Brita does not reduce TDS level in Canadian tap water. It might reduce TDS level in US tap water, if TDS level is very high, by 20%.

Figure 14.5  A typical Brita water filtration system to purify water.

# PUR WATER FILTRATION SYSTEM [6]

Tap water may look clean, but can pick up potentially harmful contaminants and pollutants while traveling through very many zigzag pipelines before reaching your kitchen sink. So filtering your tap water before drinking is of utmost importance. PUR water pitcher filters are certified to reduce these chemical and physical contaminants, lurking in the tap water.

PUR pitcher filters and faucet filters are certified to reduce more contaminants than Brita's leading water filters, with easy tool-free installation. PUR's superior filtration technology removes 99 percent of lead and over 70 other contaminants, including 96% of Mercury and 92% of certain pesticides. Also reduces chlorine (taste and odour). Each PUR water filter gives you 30 gallons (480 Cups) of clean, healthy, great tasting water with unique Maxion filter technology by using activated carbon and ion exchange to reduce more contaminants than any other brand. The slim design of dispensers allows to fit comfortably in a fridge . [6]

PUR manufactures and distributes a variety of pitchers, dispensers, faucet mounts: [6]

## PUR PITCHERS & DISPENSERS
(i) PUR 7-Cup Pitcher & (ii) PUrRPlus 7-Cup Pitcher
(iii) PUR 11-Cup Pitcher & (iv) PUR Plus 11-Cup Pitcher
(v) PUR 10-Cup Pitcher & (vi) PUR Plus 12-Cup Pitcher
(vii) PUR 18-Cup Dispenser & (viii) PUR 44-Cup Dispenser
(ix) PUR 30-Cup Dispenser & (x) PUR Plus 30-Cup Dispenser

## PUR SINK FAUCET FILTERS
(i) PUR Faucet Filtration System, Vertical
(ii) PUR Faucet Filtration System, Horizontal
(iii) PUR Plus Faucet Filtration System, Horizontal
(iv) PUR Plus Faucet Filtration System, Horizontal with Bluetooth

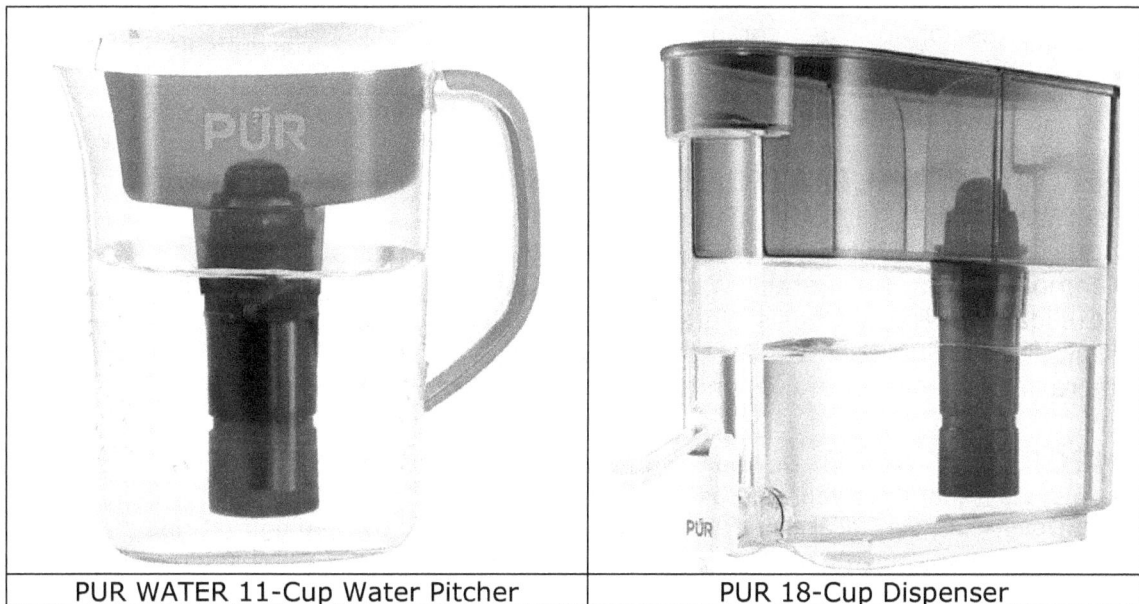

| PUR WATER 11-Cup Water Pitcher | PUR 18-Cup Dispenser |

Figure 14.6  PUR Water filtration systems to purify water (Courtesy of PUR).

# AQUAGEAR WATER FILTRATION SYSTEM [7]

The Aquagear company claims that their filter with its robust filtering technology (proprietary blend of activated carbon and ion exchange media) catches contaminants like a magnet, and removes most dangerous impurities and toxins like PFOA/PFOS (Forever Chemicals), microplastics, lead, mercury, cadmium, copper, chlorine, asbestos, herbicides, pesticides, and trace pharmaceuticals, Volatile Organic Compounds (VOCs), and more.

Aquagear targets contaminants only without removing healthy minerals like calcium and magnesium. The Aquagear filter lasts up to 120 gallons of purified water. That is 3 times longer than competitor filters. Aquagear products are 100% BPA-free, lightweight, vegan, and recyclable.

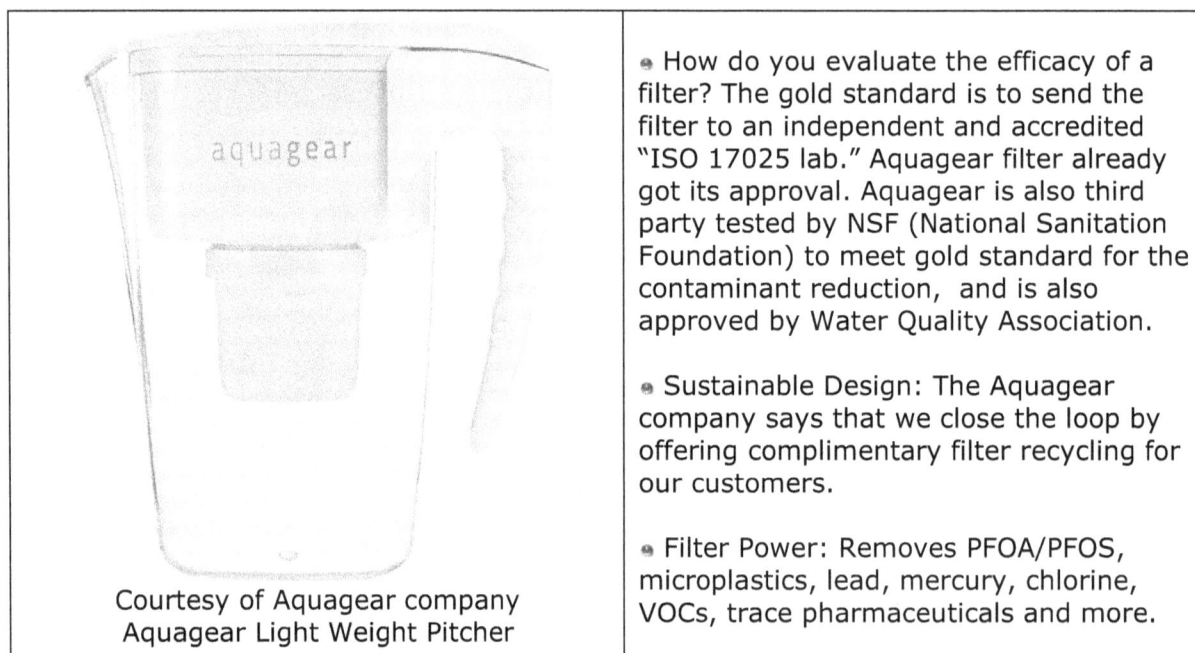

● How do you evaluate the efficacy of a filter? The gold standard is to send the filter to an independent and accredited "ISO 17025 lab." Aquagear filter already got its approval. Aquagear is also third party tested by NSF (National Sanitation Foundation) to meet gold standard for the contaminant reduction, and is also approved by Water Quality Association.

● Sustainable Design: The Aquagear company says that we close the loop by offering complimentary filter recycling for our customers.

● Filter Power: Removes PFOA/PFOS, microplastics, lead, mercury, chlorine, VOCs, trace pharmaceuticals and more.

Courtesy of Aquagear company
Aquagear Light Weight Pitcher

Figure 14.7  Aquagear Water filtration systems to purify water.

## OTHER WATER FILTRATION SYSTEMS
(i) Nakii Water Filter, (ii) LARQ Water Bottles
(iii) Aquasana Water Filters, (iv) Waterdrop Under Sink Filters
(v) Kenmore Filters, (vi) Berkey Water Filters, (vii) Pure Aqua Water Filtration Systems
(viii) Culligan Reverse Osmosis Water Filters, (ix) Soma Water Filters
(x) Frigidaire Refrigerator Water Filtration System
and there are many other brands on tap water filtration.

● **IMPORTANT NOTE:** Do your own research thoroughly, and purchase and use a water filtration system that suits your purpose and interest. Request the "Water Quality Report" from the municipality of your local Government where you live, and by reading that report, learn how many contaminants could be present in the tap water, and find out a suitable filter that removes all or most of the contaminants. In addition, you should consider the fact that municipality water could pick up hidden contaminants while traveling through so many pipes before reaching your sink. In addition, you should consider the fact that plumbers could be working to repair pipes, and accidentally contaminated the water passing through pipelines. However it is important that you should never use tap water as the drinking water before you thoroughly purify it.

# REFERENCES

1. ZeroWater Website.
https://zerowater.com/

2. PFAS (Perfluoroalkyl and Polyfluoroalkyl Substances) by NIH (National Institute of Environmental Health Sciences), Health and Education Section, Last Reviewed on November 17, 2021.
https://www.niehs.nih.gov/health/topics/agents/pfc/index.cfm

3. Performance Laboratiry Test Results (Compared to 2-Stage Filters).
https://zerowater.com/pages/results

4. ZeroWater Products (Pitchers to produce zero water at home).
https://zerowater.com/collections/all-water-filter-products

5. Brita Website
https://www.brita.com/
https://www.brita.com/why-brita/better-water/
https://www.brita.com/why-brita/better-water/

6. PUR website
https://www.pur.com/
https://www.pur.com/shop/pitchers
https://www.pur.com/shop/dispensers
https://www.pur.com/shop/faucet-systems

7. The Aquagear Filter
https://www.goaquagear.com/
https://www.goaquagear.com/pages/filter-performance

# 2nd Part: Drinking Water Guide
# 2nd Part of the Book Begins Here!
2nd Part of the Book Contains Very Important Information!

---

**Remineralization and Alkalization Methods
Are Simplified and Explained Briefly in 2 Pages.**

**By Reading These 2 Pages Only,**
**You Can Remineralize and Alkalize The Purified Water**
**(RO Water, Distilled Water, or Zero Water)**
**Like a Layperson at Home!**

**MAKE YOUR OWN NUTRITIOUS MINERAL WATER!**
**It Is Very Easy to Remineralize and Alkalize!**
[You Don't Have to Read all Scientific Experiments!]

---

# 2nd Part Contains 3 Chapters
# With Scientific Experiments
**These Three Chapters Are Very Important!**
Please Read These 3 Chapters Very Carefully
If You Have Basic Scientific Backgroung!

| | |
|---|---|
| CHAPTER 17 | REMINERALIZATION OF THE PURIFIED WATER<br>▶ How to Remineralize the Purified Water at Home? |
| CHAPTER 18 | ALKALINE WATER<br>▶ How to Alkalize the Purified Water at Home? |
| CHAPTER 19 | DRINKING WATER GUIDE IN A NETSHELL<br>▶ QUICK-REFERENCE & DOI-IT-YOURSELF GUIDELINES |

● However, you should adopt the following concept permanently into your mind: Purified water that is either neutralized (pH=7) or slightly alkalized (pH=7 to 7.25), and remineralized up to a TDS (Total Dissolved Solids) level of 200 ppm is the healthy drinking water!

**"How to Remineralize and Slightly Alkalize
the Purified Water Like A Layperson?"**

**This Topic Is Briefly Explained in the Next 2 Pages!**

**By Reading Through Next 2 Pages Only,**
**YOU CAN MAKE YOUR OWN NUTRITIOUS MINERAL WATER!**
**You Can Remineralize and Alkalize the Purified Water at Home!**
[You Don't Have to Read all Scientific Experiments!]

# HOW TO ALKALIZE AND REMINERALIZE LIKE A LAYPERSON

## HOW TO SLIGHTLY ALKALIZE THE PURIFIED WATER LIKE A LAYPERSON

**1.** Fill up a glass bottle with 4 liters of purified water (RO water, distilled water, or zero water).
**2.** Add a tiny pinch of baking soda (only a few kernels), shake the bottle thoroughly, and measure the pH using one of the following items:
**a.** Enagic pH drops with color chart (you can purchase this at local Enagic store), or
**b.** pH test kit (pH drops) with color chart (you can purchase this in a pet store), or
**c.** Digital pH meter (practice and learn how to use this digital pH meter correctly).

⚬ If you add 3 drops of Enagic pH drops to a cup of slightly alkalized water, the water should turn green color. pH should be close to 7. If you add too much baking soda, pH shoots up to 8.5 (too alkaline). You should never drink such water with pH=8.5.
You should always drink water with pH close to 7 (maximum 7.25).
⚬ By trial and error, and with practice, you will be able to add only a few kernels of baking soda, and will be able to adjust the purified water pH close to 7. It is very easy!
**IMPORTANT NOTE:** When you use baking soda to increase the pH of the purified water, you must do urine test frequently and make sure that your urine pH is under 8.

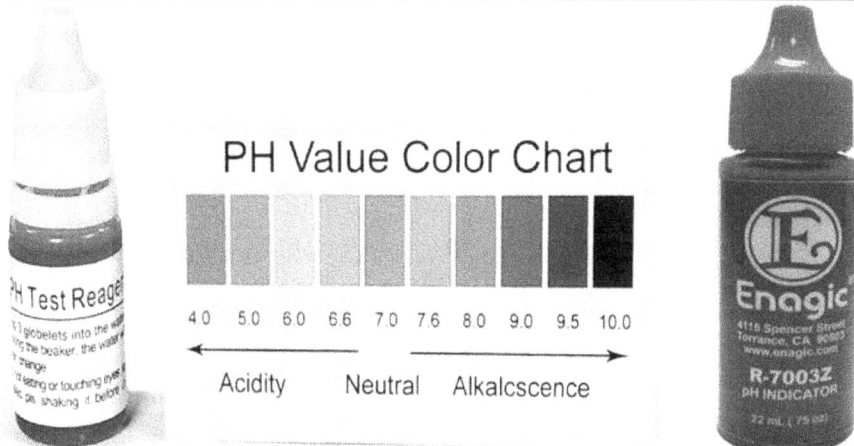

**a.** On the right is the Enagic pH Testing Drops.
**b.** On the Left is pH Testing Reagent Drops with color chart to measure the water pH.

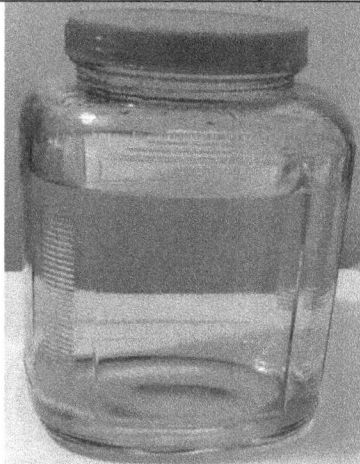

Glass Bottle Filled With 4 Liters of Purified Water.

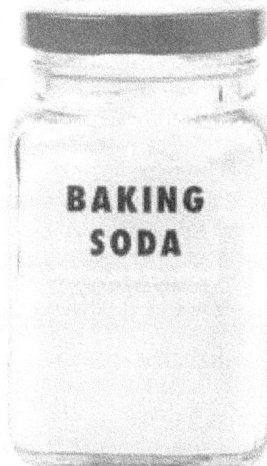

Baking Soda

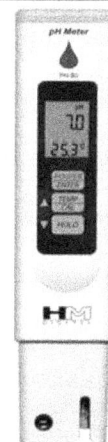

**c.** Digital pH meter Courtesy of H.M. Digital.

Figure 17.1 How to alkalize the purified water like a layperson.

# HOW TO REMINERALIZE THE PURIFIED WATER LIKE A LAYPERSON
## [ Continued from Previous page ]

**1.** You have just alkalized the purified water (RO water, distilled water, or zero water) by adding a tiny pinch of baking soda so that pH is close to 7, as explained in previous page .
**2.** You now remineralize this same water by adding a tiny pinch (only a few kernels) of Himalayan pink salt or Celtic sea salt into the same glass bottle of purified water without using digital kitchen scale, but with your fingers. After adding salt, shake the bottle thoroughly in a circular motion so that all the purified water is remineralized.
**3.** Monitor the TDS level using a TDS meter. Make sure that the TDS level is 20 ppm, 50 ppm, 100 ppm, or 150 ppm (your desired TDS level). Some people like 20 ppm, and some others like 50 ppm or 100 ppm. Add more Himalayan pink salt (only a few kernels) if the TDS level is below your desired level. Do not exceed TDS=200 ppm.

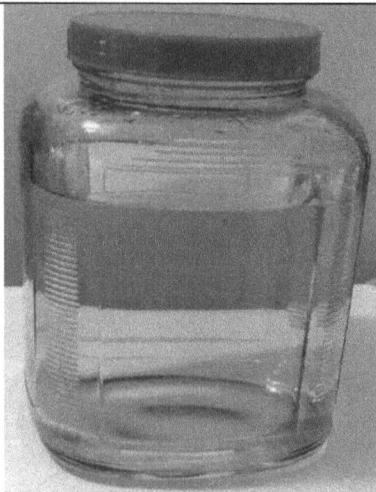
Glass Bottle Filled With 4-Liters of Purified Water.

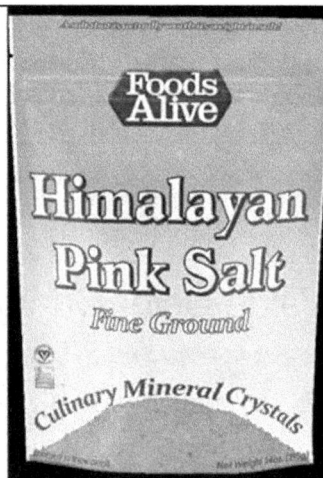
Himalayan pink salt, Or Celtic Sea salt

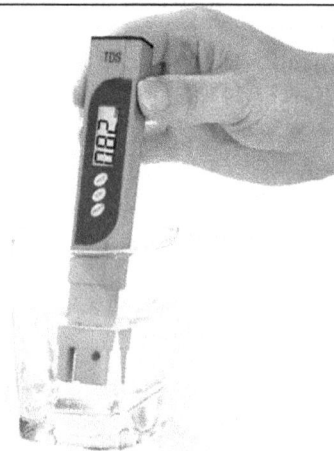
TDS Meter
Courtesy of H. M. Digital

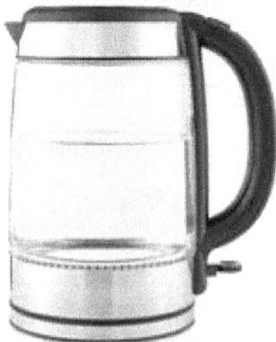
Glass Kettle (1.7 Liters)

**4.** Boil this purified water that is remineralized and slightly alkalized using a glass kettle (do not use metal kettle).
**5.** Store this boiled water in 4-liter glass bottles, and leave them to be cooled to room temperature.
**6.** Then transfer this cold water into a 4-liter plastic bottles (as many bottles as you wish), and refrigerate it before drinking. If you store water in FOUR 4-liter plastic bottles, that would be enough for a week (if you drink 8 cups a day).

● *REMEMBER: Purified water that is either neutralized (pH=7) or slightly alkalized (pH= 7 to 7.5), and remineralized up to a TDS level of 200 ppm is the healthy drinking water.*

Figure 17.2 How to remineralize the purified water like a layperson.

# CHAPTER 17:  REMINERALIZATION OF THE PURIFIED WATER
## [A Very Importannt Chapter]
## TABLE OF CONTENTS

## What is Purified Water?

Purified water is the water that has been mechanically filtered and processed to remove all impurities, bacteria, parasites, viruses, microorganisms, E. coli, organic chemicals, inorganic chemicals, heavy metals, and all other kinds of contaminants (physical contaminants, chemical contaminants, biological contaminants & radiological contaminants) found in tap water, well water, and any other unprocessed water. When attempting to remove all those impurities, such purification process unfortunately also removes valuable minerals that are necessary for human health. The following items can be classified as purified water:

a. Distilled Water.
b. RO Water (Reverse Osmosis Water).
c. Drinking Water obtained by using ZeroWater, Brita or Pur Water filtration units.
d. Demineralized Water or Deionized Water obtained by ion exchange process.
e. Desalinated Water obtained by reverse osmosis process.
f. Purified water obtained by any other process including carbon filtering, microfiltration, ultrafiltration, ultraviolet oxidation, or electrodeionization, atmospheric water generators, or using the combinations of a number of these processes in series.

**RO Water, Distilled Water and Zero Water** are readily available everywhere, and so are most commonly used by many people as purified water.

## WHY SHOULD WE REMINERALIZE THE PURIFIED WATER?

World Health Organization (WHO) reported, based on certain scientific investigations, that drinking water with no minerals, or drinking demineralized water such as distilled water or RO water is potentially harmful to human health. WHO also warned the people that drinking water with a low mineral content, or with low or zero TDS (Total Dissolved Solids) level had a negative effect on functions in the body that control water and mineral metabolism, and so is potentially harmful to human health. [1, 2, 3]

Many studies throughout the world have reported that people drinking water that is low in calcium and magnesium (soft water) is tied to higher incidence of death from cardiovascular disease compared to those drinking regular water. When demineralized water is consumed, our intestines have to add electrolytes to this water first, pulling them from body reserves. This leads to the dilution of electrolytes and insufficient body water redistribution which may compromise the function of vital organs. At the early stages of this condition, symptoms may include fatigue, headaches, weakness, as well as muscle cramps and even heart rate abnormalities. [4]

**It is therefore of utmost importance** that you should learn how to remineralize the purified water by adding the correct amount of Himalayan pink salt, Celtic sea salt, or ConcenTrace mineral drops to purified water in order to maintain a healthy TDS level of up to 200 ppm. This chapter is designed to teach you how to do that.

**WHY NOT SPRING WATER?** Spring water is unpurified natural water with minerals in it. In nature, pure water picks up minerals, other impurities, and dangerous contaminants by flowing through soil, rock and clay. While spring water is the naturally filtered and purified by passing through the porous layers of soil, rock and clay in the mountain valleys, there is no way we can tell scientifically that spring water is indeed purified water. Many people like and drink spring water because of the tradition and belief that the spring water has a wide spectrum of mineral composition and drink it because of its taste and natural occurrence, but there is no guarantee that spring water has no harmful chemicals and impurities in it. That is why, a civilized person would prefer to drink purified and sterilized water, and would remineralize it in order to consume minerals and would enjoy all advantages of spring water but without consuming impurities or contaminants that would jeopardize health and cause strange diseases.

# How to Know If The Water We Drink is Purified Or Not?

By using a TDS meter, and by dipping the TDS meter probe into a cup of water, you can monitor TDS (Total Dissolved Solids) level of any water.

(i) The TDS level of RO water or any other purified water should be below 5 ppm.

(ii) The TDS level of distilled water and zero water should be precisely zero.

## TDS METER [5]

a. Here is a TDS testing meter on Amazon.com/Amazon.ca. HM Digital TDS-4TM Handheld Hydro Tester TDS and Temperature Tester, ASIN # B001RK38LU, Price: Close to $20.

https://www.amazon.ca/HM-Digital-TDS-4TM-Handheld-Temperature/dp/B001RK38LU/ref=sr_1_1?ie=UTF8&qid=1437459250&sr=8-1&keywords=TDS-4+Water+Tester+by+HM+Digital

b. Also purchase several calibration solutions (NaCl solution) so that you can calibrate it and test it.

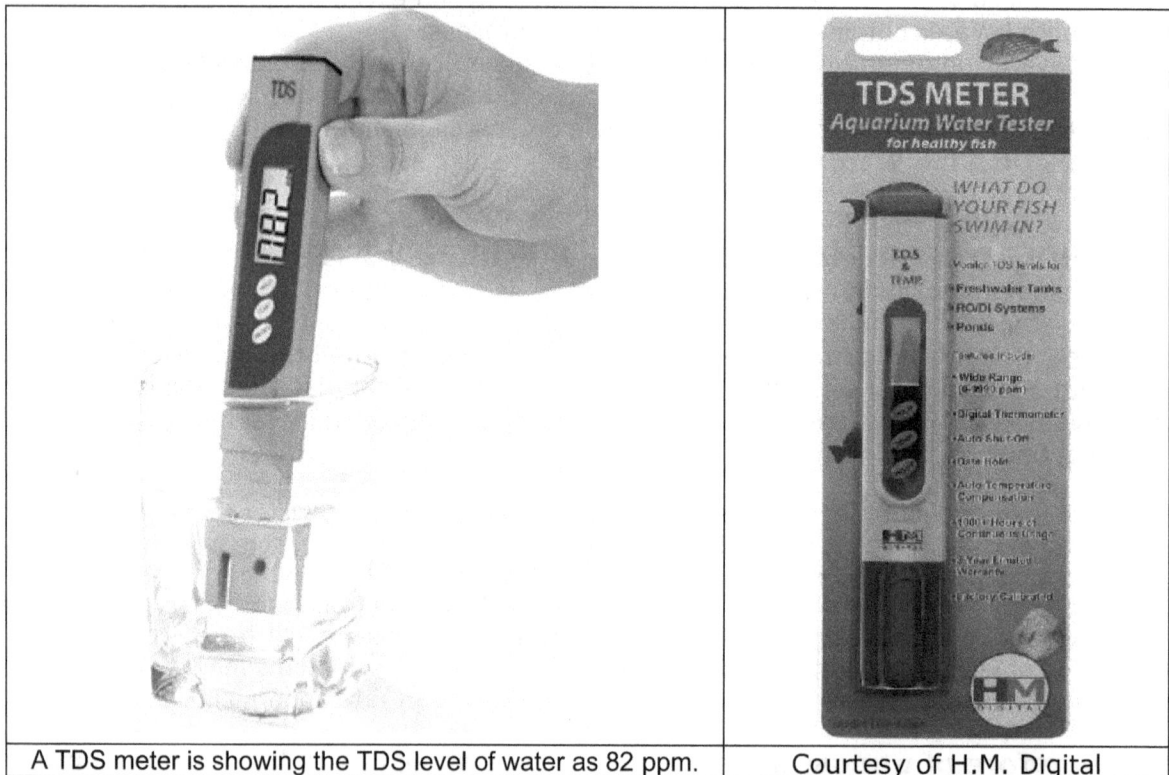

| A TDS meter is showing the TDS level of water as 82 ppm. | Courtesy of H.M. Digital |

Figure 17.3  TDS meter to test the presence of total dissolved solids in water.

**HOW TO USE THE TDS METER?** I have purchased this TDS meter some 10 years ago, and it still works perfectly well. I test it every now and then with distilled water and calibration solutions, and make sure that the meter is working fine, reliable & trustworthy.

It is very easy to use this TDS meter. It has an on-off button. Whenever you want to use it, just turn on by pressing the on-off button, and just dip the probe into a cup of water one inch deep. It immediately shows you the TDS level of the water. After using it, turn it off or it will automatically turn off itself if unused for a long time. Also, clean the probe by dipping it into a cup of  distilled water, wipe the probe with a cloth or paper, and put on the cap.

**TEST IT:** The best way to test it every time you use is by dipping the probe into a cup of distilled water. The TDS level of distilled water is precisely zero so it should read perfectly zero. You can also test it by using the calibration solution manufactured at a specific TDS level.

# ACCEPTABLE TDS LEVEL IN DRINKING WATER [6, 7, 8, 9, 10, 11, 12, 13]

TDS (Total Dissolved Solids) comprise all the inorganic salts and small amounts of organic matter that are dissolved in water. The principal constituents are usually the cations calcium, magnesium, sodium, potassium, phosphorus and the anions carbonate, bicarbonate, chloride, sulphate and  nitrate (particularly in groundwater). TDS is expressed in milligrams per unit volume of water (mg/L), and also referred to as ppm (1 ppm = 1 mg/L). [6, 7]

**Permissible Range of TDS in Drinking Water:** Different governments set different regulations and standards for the TDS level. The United States EPA sets the maximum level for TDS as 500 ppm where as the World Health Organization (WHO) has different prescribed limits, depending on the location and circumstances of water source available to public.

An aesthetic objective (palatability of water) of ≤500 mg/L has been established for total dissolved solids (TDS) in drinking water by WHO. At higher levels, excessive hardness, unpalatability, mineral deposition and corrosion may occur. At low levels, however, TDS contributes to the palatability of water. Most people think of TDS as being an aesthetic factor. In a study by the World Health Organization, a panel of tasters came to the following conclusions about the preferable level of TDS in water:

Table 17.1  TDS Values Established by World Health Organization. [8, 9]

| TDS Level (ppm or mg/L) | Palatability of Water |
|---|---|
| < 300 | Excellent |
| 300 – 600 | Good |
| 600 – 900 | Fair |
| 900 – 1200 | Poor |
| > 1200 | Unacceptable |

The palatability of water only describes the acceptability of the taste of the water. It does not indicate whether the water is healthy or unhealthy to drink. The above-mentioned standards can be considered outdated because WHO set and published these standards in 1996, and has not updated the TDS standards since then.

In Kent's Health Organization, a panel of tasters & health professionals proposed the following standards about the preferable level of TDS in drinking water:

Table 17.2  TDS Values Established by Kent's Health Organization. [10]

| TDS Level (ppm or mg/L) | Rating |
|---|---|
| 50 to 150 | Excellent! |
| 150 to 250 | Good! |
| 250 to 300 | Fair (Bad for kidneys)! |
| 300 to 500 | Poor (very bad for kidneys)! |
| Above 500 | Unacceptable! |

**IMPORTANT:** Under any circumstances, a person should not drink any water that has a TDS level above 500 ppm. A TDS level equal to or beyond 500 ppm in drinking water could have a devastating effect on kidneys at least to some people.

However some health experts believe that the TDS levels for ideal drinking water should be 50 ppm or under 50 ppm. Even the TDS levels of 50 ppm would be too high for older people with health issues. For example, the tap water in Vancouver and surrounding areas, British Columbia, Canada is awesome with a TDS level of only 16 ppm. It regularly ranks among the best in the world, and the City of Vancouver has committed to making it even better by 2020. Therefore health experts in general recommend to drink purified water with lesser TDS level. The RO water has a TDS level of 2 ppm to 4 ppm, and distilled water has a TSD level of zero. Some older people drink purified water (RO water, distilled water, or zero water), knowing that purified water lacks essential minerals within it, but eat balanced meals and take high quality multivitamins and mineral supplements.

It does not mean that this book recommends you to drink tap water. The clean tap water in Vancouver, British Columbia, Canada is an exception. A disaster could happen even in this carefully controlled area. That is why this book recommends that please do not drink tap water, well water and bottled water of any kind without knowing how pure it is. This book also recommends that "drinking distilled water is far better than drinking any water that is not purified".

However remineralizing the purified water (RO water, distilled water, or zero water) is a very important aspect especially for young people. This chapter is designed to help you achieve that goal.

## Sources of TDS [10, 13]
Some dissolved solids come from organic sources such as leaves, silt, plankton, and industrial waste and sewage. Other sources come from runoff from urban areas, road salts used on street during the winter, and fertilizers and pesticides used on lawns and farms. Dissolved solids also come from inorganic materials such as rocks and air that may contain calcium bicarbonate, nitrogen, iron phosphorous, sulfur, and other minerals. Many of these materials form salts, which are compounds that contain both a metal and a non-metal. Salts usually dissolve in water forming ions. Ions are particles that have a positive or negative charge. Water may also pick up metals such as lead or copper as they travel through pipes used to distribute water to consumers.

The principal application of TDS is in the study of water quality for streams, rivers and lakes, although TDS is not generally considered a primary pollutant (e.g. it is not deemed to be associated with health effects), but it is used as an indication of aesthetic characteristics of drinking water and as an aggregate indicator of the presence of a broad array of chemical contaminants.

**FINAL NOTE BEFORE STARTING REMINERALIZATION**: A civilized person always drinks purified and sterilized water, and always carries a pH meter or pH drops and a TDS meter with him/her, and manages the appropriate pH and TDS level in his/her drinking water. In general, this book recommends that purified water that is either neutralized (pH=7) or slightly alkalized (pH=7 to 7.25), and remineralized up to a TDS level of 200 ppm is the healthy drinking water.

# METHODS OF REMINERALIZATION [14, 15, 16, 17, 18, 19]
The following methods are being recommended to remineralize purified water at home:

(i) Adding **Himalayan pink salt** to purified water (RO water, distilled water, or zero water).
(ii) Adding **Celtic sea salt** to purified water (RO water, distilled water, or zero water).
(iii) Adding **ConcenTrace mineral drops** to purified water (RO water, distilled water, or zero water).

OTHER PRODUCTS FOR REMINERALIZATION OF DRINKING WATER
(iv) Pascalite Clay.
(v) Unflavored Green Blends.
(vi) Spa Water (Adding Veggies, Fruits, Herbs & Spices to Purified Water).

There are some other products, being used by some people, such as "Pascalite Clay, Unflavored Green Blends, and Spa Water (Adding Veggies, Fruits, Herbs & Spices to Purified Water)" to remineralize the drinking water. These product may be healthy if consumed with drinking water, but there are no confirmed reports or scientific data with regard to the mineral composition of these products if we want to add any of them to purified water in an attempt to remineralize it up to a TDS level of 200 ppm. Therefore these products will not be discussed in detail at this time in this book.

## ABOUT HIMALAYAN PINK SALT

### Introduction [20, 21, 22, 23]
Some people say that by adding half a teaspoon of unprocessed and unrefined Himalayan pink salt or Himalayan crystal salt or Celtic sea salt to a gallon of water, you can improve both TDS (total dissolved solids) level of purified water. [20] That is too much salt!

But in this book you will learn exactly how many milligrams of Himalayan pink salt should be added, like a civilized person, by measuring the weight of Himalayan pink salt and by monitoring the TDS level with a TDS meter.

**Why Himalayan pink salt?** The World Health Organization (WHO) warned the people based on scientific investigations that you should not drink demineralized water without minerals. It's because electrolytes are removed through the distillation or reverse osmosis processes. Electrolytes are foundational nutrients of the body, and they must be present to create water that's accessible for your body and cells. The solution is to add them back to your drinking purified water through the most popular Himalayan pink salt. [20]

Luckily, Himalayan pink salt contains all six electrolytes we require for health: sodium, potassium, chloride, magnesium, phosphorus and calcium. Therefore, you can replenish your body's natural supply of electrolytes by adding Himalayan rock salt to your drinking water or diet. This is especially helpful on hot days or after an intense workout when electrolytes are lost through sweat. You can make a natural "gatorade" with Himalayan rock salt by adding ¼ teaspoon (about 500 mg) of Himalayan rock salt to 1 quart (1 liter) of water, with the juice of half a lemon and some raw honey or green leaf stevia. [21] That 500 mg of Himalayan pink salt to 1 liter of purified water is the upper limit, you cannot do that every day. You should add a lot less than 500 mg.

The cost of adding minerals to distilled water or RO water by using Himalayan pink salt or Celtic sea salt is less than a penny per liter! Himalayan pink salt or Celtic sea salt contains 84 to 88 minerals, most of them are trace minerals with minute concentrations. [20]

Unprocessed and unrefined Himalayan pink salt comes from Khewra, Pakistan whereas Celtic sea salt comes from Brittany, France, and from where we import them directly. Himalayan salt, also known as Himalayan pink rock salt, is originally discovered in Pakistani salt mines, approximately 186 miles (300 kilometers) from the famous Himalayas Mountains. The rock has a pale pink color stemming from iron oxide deposits (rust) in the Himalayan mountains. Many people believe that it has many unbelievable health benefits and is the purest salt on Earth to be consumed. As with all varieties of salt, Himalayan rock salt is most commonly used for cooking. Research showed that in addition to boosting food flavor, Himalayan salt helps relieve migraines, increase energy and improve adrenal function. [21]

Himalayan pink salt is a very popular salt with 74,000 monthly searches on Google, followed by regular sea salt at 33,000 monthly searches, and Celtic sea salt at 5,400 monthly searches. Himalayan pink salt was first discovered around 326 BC. Centuries later, standardized salt mining practices were introduced in Khewra, Pakistan and were gradually improved to the "Room and Pillar" excavation method in 1827. Since then, Himalayan pink salt has been mined and sold for consumption and has evolved into one of the world's best-known food salts. Many people started using it to demineralize RO water and distilled water. [22]

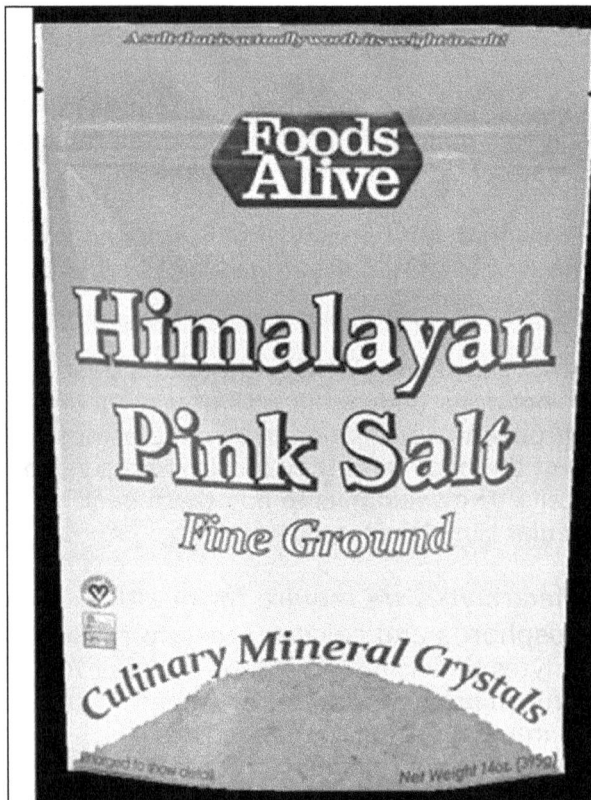

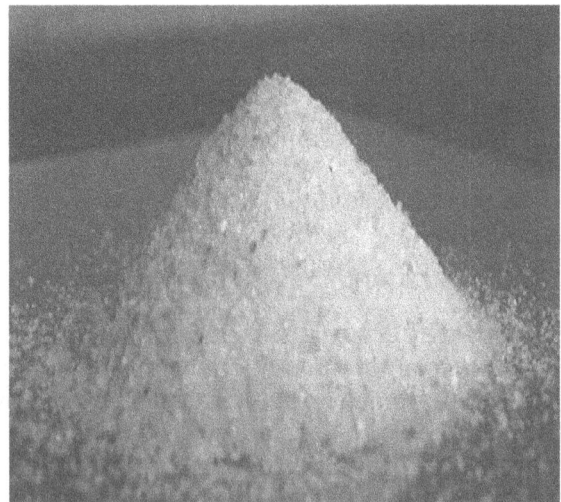

Unprocessed, unrefined and ground Himalayan crystal pink salt quickly dissolves and remineralizes the purified water.
Just add a tiny pinch to RO water or distilled water, and drink it!

Courtesy of Foods Alive

Figure 17.4 Himalayan pink salt (ground) quickly dissolves and remineralizes the purified water.

# HEALTH BENEFITS OF HIMALAYAN PINK SALT

## Health Benefits Posted by Brandi Black of PaleoHacks Blog [21]

Himalayan pink salt contains 84 to 88 trace minerals and electrolytes. Some of these minerals include calcium, iodine, potassium, magnesium and iron. In fact, Himalayan pink salt contains triple the amount of potassium per serving than Maldon or Celtic sea salt. This high mineral content in Himalayan rock salt attributes to many health benefits listed below:

● Electrolyste Balance: Himalayan salt contains all six electrolytes we require for health such as sodium, potassium, chloride, magnesium, phosphorus and calcium. Therefore, you can replenish your body's natural supply of electrolytes by adding Himalayan rock salt to your diet, your drinking water, and while cooking meals.

● Thyroid Function: Since Himalayan rock salt contains iodine, which is the element that your body needs to synthesize thyroid hormones, it is believed to promote and maintain healthy thyroid function. Doctors already linked iodine deficiency to hypothyroidism.

● Adrenal Glands Function: Your adrenals are two little glands sitting on top of your kidneys. They are responsible for regulating your body's stress response by producing the hormones cortisol and adrenaline. Your adrenal glands need minerals such as sodium and potassium for proper function. These minerals are abundantly found in Himalayan rock salt, which help proper function of adrenals. Ideal sodium and potassium balance is essential to adrenal health.

● Lamps Made With the Himalyan Pink Salt: Himalayan pink salt lamps are made with large Himalayan salt rocks by mounting lightbulbs inside them. Many people believe that these lamps have many health benefits. The soft pink glow of these lamps emits negative ions that cleanse the air in the room. These lamps are believed to help remove negative energy, improve blood flow, promote restful sleep, and boost serotonin levels in the brain.

## Health Benefits Posted by Empowered Sustenance [23]

● Himalayan salt is also mined from ancient sea beds, so it is pure from modern environmental toxins. It provides a whopping **84 trace minerals**, plus a unique ionic energy that is released when the salt is mixed with water.
● It is water-fully saturated with unrefined salt. When the ground Himalayan pink salt dissolves in water, it results in a concentrated, electrically charged matrix of the 84 trace minerals in the salt.
● The ionic salt and trace minerals nourish each cell in your body.
● It detoxifies the body by balancing systemic pH.
● It improves hydration by providing trace minerals.
● It improves mineral status of the body.
● It reduces muscle cramps by improving minerals and hydration.
● It helps balance blood sugar.
● It supports hormone balance for everyone, no matter what hormonal issues you face.
● It helps balance blood pressure because it provides unrefined, mineral-rich salt in an ionic solution.
● It improves sleep by supporting blood sugar and hormone balance.
● It acts as a powerful antihistamine.
● It supports weight loss by balancing hormones and improving energy.
● It supports thyroid and adrenal function (Source and read more benefits!).

## ⊙ Salt Therapy With Himalayan Pink Salt Inhaler
Spelotherapy, also called salt therapy, utilizes salt to address respiratory diseases and improve overall health. Although little known in the U.S., it is widespread in Europe. Since the 1800s, many people visit European salt mines to breathe in the salt-rich air. One modern form of salt therapy consists of sitting in a room pumped with salt-laden air. When the salty air is inhaled, the minute salt particles travel through the entire respiratory system. The antibacterial and antimicrobial properties purify and detox the lungs and sinuses. Studies show that salt therapy is widely effective for:

- Reducing asthma (many users report no longer needing their rescue inhaler)
- Reducing seasonal allergies by cleansing the sinuses
- Coughs and chest congestion
- Improving the respiratory systems of smokers
- Improving skin conditions like eczema and dermatitis
- Improving lung function in individuals with cystic fibrosis
- Also many people testify that salt therapy drastically improves snoring

## ⊙ Himalayan Pink Salt Is Also Widely Used in Neti Pot Application
By filling up the Neti Pot with Himalyan warm salt water, you can flush your sinuses away, as Neti Pot cleanses and purifies the sinuses. The salt also acts as an antimicrobial agent to ward off sinus infections. The health benefits of using a Neti Pot with Himalayan pink salt includes:
- Reducing or eliminating seasonal allergies
- Preventing or alleviating a sinus infection
- Clearing postnasal drip

## Health Benefits  Posted by Karen S. Garvin [24]
Himalayan pink salt is sold as a gourmet salt for use in cooking and adding at the dinner table. Because of its minerals content, Himalayan salt is considered healthier than regular table salt, which often has additives, such as the anti-caking agent sodium ferrocyanide. The need in human nutrition for many of the minerals found in Himalayan salt remains unknown, and many of the minerals are found only in minute quantities. Himalayan salt contains some minerals that are toxic in large quantities, including lead and plutonium, but which are safe in trace amounts.

**List of Elements (84 trace minerals):** The Meadow lists elements found in Himalayan salt in addition to sodium and chloride. In alphabetical order, they are: actinium, aluminum, antimony, arsenic, astatine, barium, beryllium, bismuth, boron, bromine, cadmium, calcium, carbon, cerium, cesium, chlorine, chromium, cobalt, copper, dysprosium, erbium, europium, fluorine, francium, gadolinium, gallium, germanium, gold, hafnium, holmium, hydrogen, indium, iodine, iridium, iron, lanthanum, lead, lithium, lutetium, magnesium, manganese, mercury, molybdenum, neodymium, neptunium, nickel, niobium, nitrogen, osmium, oxygen, palladium, phosphorus, platinum, plutonium, polonium, potassium, praseodymium, protactinium, radium, rhenium, rhodium, rubidium, ruthenium, samarium, scandium, selenium, silicon, silver, sodium, strontium, sulfur, tantalum, tellurium, terbium, thallium, thorium, thulium, tin, titanium, uranium, vanadium, wolfram, yttrium, ytterbium, zinc and zirconium.

All the above-mentioned 84 elements (trace minerals) can be found in our periodic tabe shown below:

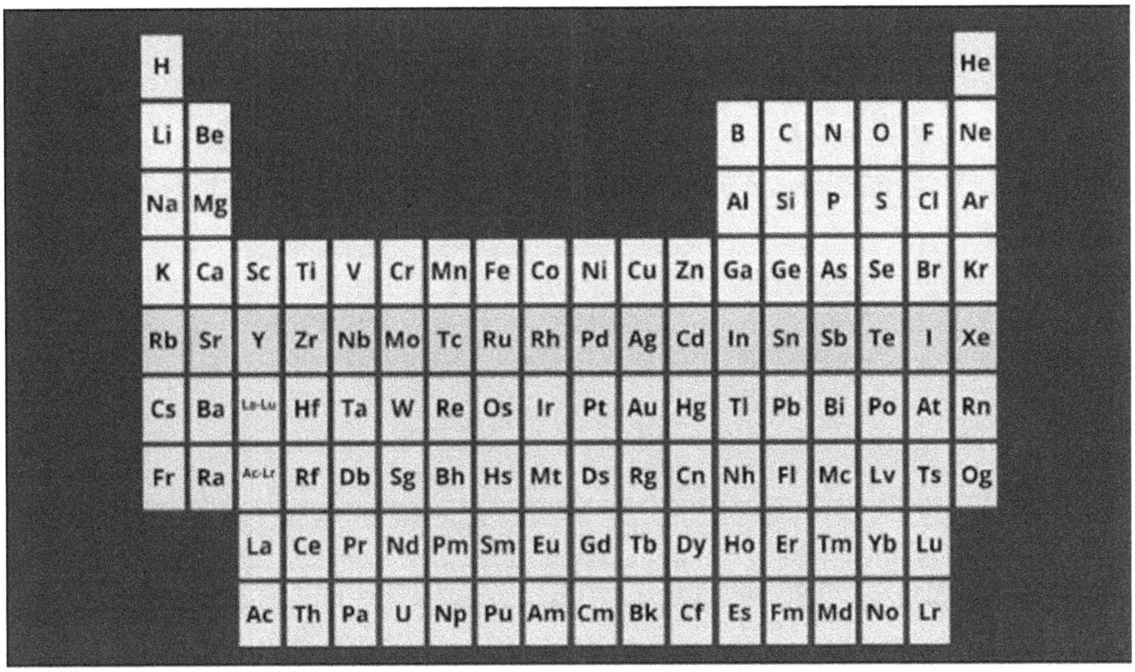

Figure 17.5  Periodic Table (there are about 118 elements discovered so far).

## IMPORTANT INFORMATION TO REMEMBER: All these minerals were originally manufactured in the burning cores of collapsing and exploding stars:

Please read through Stellar Nucleosynthesis, described in Chapter 1. Hydrogen was the primordial element, created in the Big Bang. Hydrogen was the primary element from which all other elements were created in the burning cores of earlier stars, dumped and scattered by supernovae explosions. A gigantic interstellar cloud known as "solar nebula" of space dust and primordial gas that was squeezed by a supernova explosion gave birth to our solar system. When our solar system began its formation 6 billion years ago, the space dust and interstellar gas were already enriched with all these elements that we found now on our Earth.

## CHEMICAL ANALYSIS OF HIMALAYAN PINK SALT [25, 26, 27]

The spectral analysis of Himalayan pink salt has been posted by several websites on the Internet. The list shows all the trace minerals, electrolytes, and elements contained in Himalayan salt. Himalayan pink rock salt is popular among health food advocates who seek it for the nutritional value of its fairly abundant trace minerals.

Spectral analyses done on Himalayan salt show that it contains both macrominerals, such as calcium and chloride, as well as trace minerals including iron and zinc. Mineral are naturally occurring inorganic elements with specific chemical compositions that have crystalline structure. Crystals have a very ordered arrangement of atoms, which gives them their unique shapes. Himalayan salt contains the minerals that are necessary for your health, including macrominerals and trace minerals. The macrominerals are needed in relative abundance and include calcium, chloride, iron, magnesium, phosphorus, potassium and sodium. The recommended daily amount of these macrominerals depends of your age, activity level and general health. Calcium is the most common mineral in your body and is found in your bones and teeth, as well as playing a vital role in nerve and muscle health. Trace minerals are needed in small amounts for health, and those found in Himalayan salt include boron, chromium, copper, fluoride, iodine, manganese, molybdenum, selenium and zinc. Other minerals in Himalayan salt include aluminum, carbon, platinum, selenium, sulfur and titanium. The complete list of minerals is shown below in a table.

100

Table 17.3  List of 88 macrominerals and trace minerals in Himalayan pink salt. [27]
Courtesy of The Medeau  https://themeadow.com
[ 1 ppm = 1 mg/L = 1 mg/Kg ]

| S No | Element | Symbol | Concentration |
|---|---|---|---|
| 1 | Hydrogen | H | 0.30 g/kg |
| 2 | Lithium | Li | 0.40 g/kg |
| 3 | Beryllium | Be | <0.01 ppm |
| 4 | Boron | B | <0.001 ppm |
| 5 | Carbon | C | <0.001 ppm |
| 6 | Nitrogen | N | 0.024 ppm |
| 7 | Oxygen | O | 1.20 g/kg |
| 8 | Flouride | F- | <0.1 g/kg |
| 9 | Sodium | Na+ | 382.61 g/kg |
| 10 | Magnesium | Mg | 0.16 g/kg |
| 11 | Aluminum | Al | 0.661 ppm |
| 12 | Silicon | Si | <0.1 g/kg |
| 13 | Phosphorus | P | <0.10 ppm |
| 14 | Sulfur | S | 12.4 g/kg |
| 15 | Chloride | Cl- | 590.93 g/kg |
| 16 | Potassium | K+ | 3.5 g/kg |
| 17 | Calcium | Ca | 4.05 g/kg |
| 18 | Scandium | Sc | <0.0001 ppm |
| 19 | Titanium | Ti | <0.001 ppm |
| 20 | Vanadium | V | 0.06 ppm |
| 21 | Chromium | Cr | 0.05 ppm |
| 22 | Manganese | Mn | 0.27 ppm |
| 23 | Iron | Fe | 38.9 ppm |
| 24 | Cobalt | Co | 0.60 ppm |
| 25 | Nickel | Ni | 0.13 ppm |
| 26 | Copper | Cu | 0.56 ppm |
| 27 | Zinc | Zn | 2.38 ppm |
| 28 | Gallium | Ga | <0.001 ppm |
| 29 | Germanium | Ge | <0.001 ppm |
| 30 | Arsenic | As | <0.01 ppm |
| 31 | Selenium | Se | 0.05 ppm |
| 32 | Bromine | Br | 2.1 ppm |
| 33 | Rubidium | Rb | <0.04 ppm |
| 34 | Strontium | Sr | <0.014 g/kg |
| 35 | Ytterbium | Y | <0.001 ppm |
| 36 | Zirconium | Zr | <0.001 ppm |
| 37 | Niobium | Nb | <0.001 ppm |
| 38 | Molybdenum | Mo | <0.01 ppm |

| S No | Element | Symbol | Concentration |
|------|---------|--------|---------------|
| 39 | Technetium | Tc | N/A unstable isotope |
| 40 | Ruthenium | Ru | <0.001 ppm |
| 41 | Rhodium | Rh | <0.001 ppm |
| 42 | Palladium | Pd | <0.001 ppm |
| 43 | Silver | Ag | 0.031 ppm |
| 44 | Cadmium | Cd | <0.01 ppm |
| 45 | Indium | In | <0.001 ppm |
| 46 | Tin | Sn | <0.01 ppm |
| 47 | Antimony | Sb | <0.01 ppm |
| 48 | Tellurium | Te | <0.001 ppm |
| 49 | Iodine | I | <0.1 g/kg |
| 50 | Cesium | Cs | <0.001 ppm |
| 51 | Barium | Ba | 1.96 ppm |
| 52 | Lanthanum | La | <0.001 ppm |
| 53 | Cerium | Ce | <0.001 ppm |
| 54 | Praseodymium | Pr | <0.001 ppm |
| 55 | Neodymium | Nd | <0.001 ppm |
| 56 | Promethium | Pm | N/A unstable isotope |
| 57 | Samarium | Sm | <0.001 ppm |
| 58 | Europium | Eu | <3.0 ppm |
| 59 | Gadolinium | Gd | <0.001 ppm |
| 60 | Terbium | Tb | <0.001 ppm |
| 61 | Dysprosium | Dy | <4.0 ppm |
| 62 | Holmium | Ho | <0.001 ppm |
| 63 | Erbium | Er | <0.001 ppm |
| 64 | Thulium | Tm | <0.001 ppm |
| 65 | Ytterbium | Yb | <0.001 ppm |
| 66 | Lutetium | Lu | <0.001 ppm |
| 67 | Hafnium | Hf | <0.001 ppm |
| 68 | Tantalum | Ta | 1.1 ppm |
| 69 | Wolfram | W | <0.001 ppm |
| 70 | Rhenium | Re | <2.5 ppm |
| 71 | Osmium | Os | <0.001 ppm |
| 72 | Iridium | Ir | <2.0 ppm |
| 73 | Platinum | Pt | <0.47 ppm |
| 74 | Gold | Au | <1.0 ppm |
| 75 | Mercury | Hg | <0.03 ppm |
| 76 | Thallium | Ti | <0.06 ppm |

| S No | Element | Symbol | Concentration |
|------|---------|--------|---------------|
| 77 | Lead | Pb | <0.10 ppm |
| 78 | Bismuth | Bi | <0.10 ppm |
| 79 | Polonium | Po | <0.001 ppm |
| 80 | Astatine | At | <0.001 ppm |
| 81 | Francium | Fr | <1.0 ppm |
| 82 | Radium | Ra | <0.001 ppm |
| 83 | Actinium | Ac | <0.001 ppm |
| 84 | Thorium | Th | <0.001 ppm |
| 85 | Protactinium | Pa | <0.001 ppm |
| 86 | Uranium | U | <0.001 ppm |
| 87 | Neptunium | Np | <0.001 ppm |
| 88 | Plutonium | Pu | <0.001 ppm |

# HOW TO REMINERALIZE THE PURIFIED WATER?
# EXPERIMENTS CONDUCTED AT HOME

## EXPERIMENT # 1

## Items needed:
(i) Purified Water
(RO water can be purchased in supermarkets at Refill Yourself Stations or from local vendors; And distilled water can be purchased in any pharmacy or from local vendors).
(ii) Himalayan pink salt
(This can be purchased at any local health food store, supermarket, or online).
(iii) TDS Meter
(Already discussed how to purchase it and how to use it at the beginning of this chapter).
(iv) Digital Kitchen Scale
(Discussed below on how to purchase an accurate digital scale to measure the weights of small or tiny amounts, or a pinch of Himalayan pink salt or Celtic sea salt).

### Digital Kitchen Scales Are Available on Amazon
Please do your own research, and purchase a reliable and accurate digital kitchen scale that has ultra fine accuracy in measuring the weights of salts with 0.01 g (or 0.001 oz) increments.

Make sure that you will be able to measure the the weights of Himalyan pink salt or Celtic sea salt as follows: 0.01 g (10 mg), 0.05 (50 mg), 0.1 g (100 mg), 0.2 g (200 mg), 0.5 g (500 mg), etc. with accuracy and without any difficulty.

You should also purchase calibration weights possibly covering 10 mg, 100 mg, 500 mg, 1 g, 2 g, 5 g, etc. so that you can test your digital kitchen scale while you are conducting these experiments, and make sure that the scale is reliable and trustworthy. If you don't find that kind of calibration weights in that range, you should at least find the calibration weights covering 0.5 g (500 mg) and 1 g so that you can test your scale every time you use it for these experiments.

The following digital scales are available on Amazon.com, and may be helpful, but the author never purchased them and tested them. It is your responsibility to purchase the appropriate digital kitchen scale to be used for your experiments being conducted on "Remineralization of Purified water with Himalayan pink salt and/or Celtic sea salt".

1. Smart Weigh Culinary Kitchen Scale 10 kilograms x 0.01 grams, Digital Food Scale with Dual Weight Platforms for Baking, Cooking, Food, and Ingredients, Smaller platform has a min readability of 0.01g and max capacity of 300g, ASIN # B01LXXBQWD, Available on Amazon.com.

2. Boldall Portable Digital Kitchen Food Scale with Black Cover, 500 Grams x .01g/.001oz, LCD Display, Tare Function, ASIN # B01HDONIOU, Available on Amazon.com.

3. Digital Kitchen Scale Multifunction Food Scale, 500g/0.01g Small Portable Electronic Precision Scale, Food Scale with Back-Lit LCD Display(Batteries Included), ASIN # B07BHGZN3L, Available on Amazon.com.

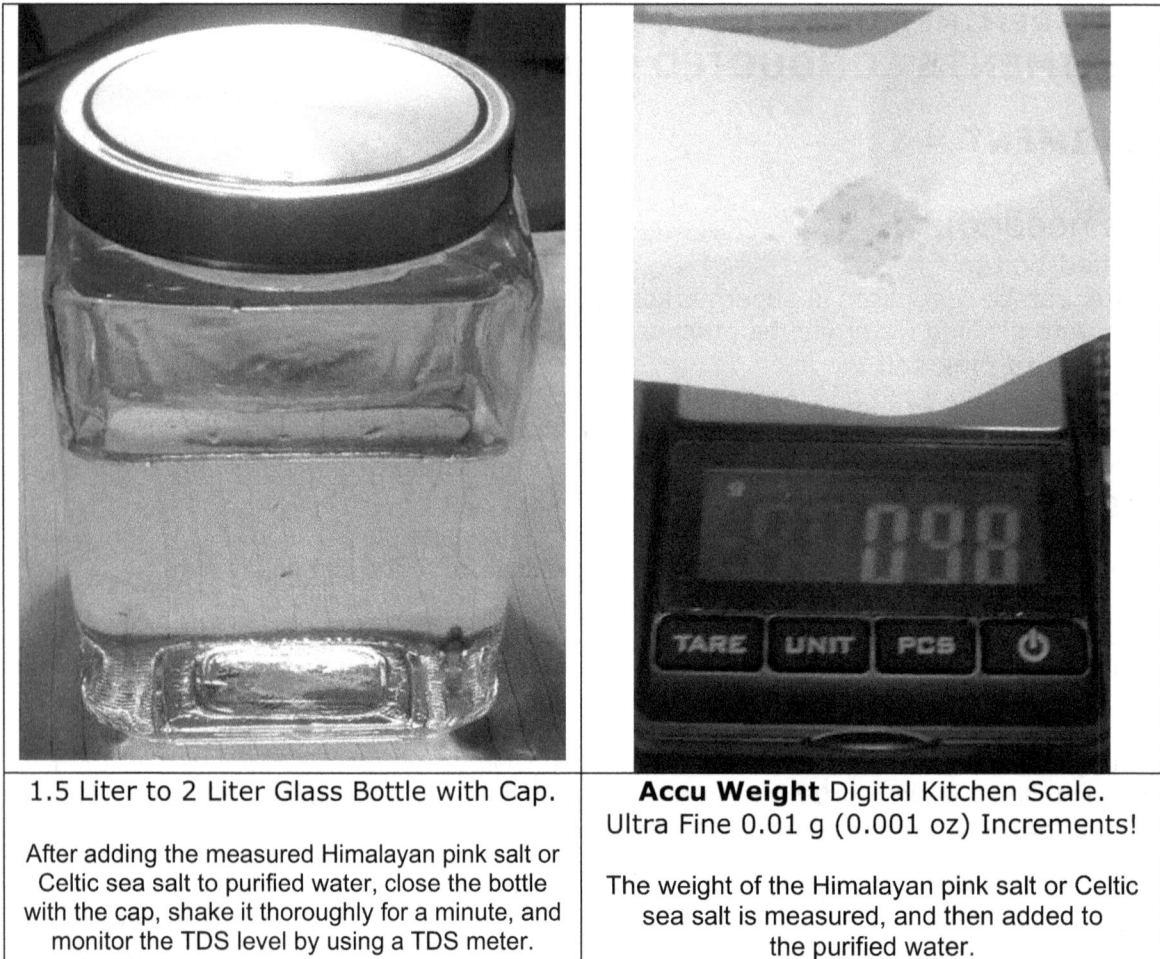

| 1.5 Liter to 2 Liter Glass Bottle with Cap. | **Accu Weight** Digital Kitchen Scale. Ultra Fine 0.01 g (0.001 oz) Increments! |
|---|---|
| After adding the measured Himalayan pink salt or Celtic sea salt to purified water, close the bottle with the cap, shake it thoroughly for a minute, and monitor the TDS level by using a TDS meter. | The weight of the Himalayan pink salt or Celtic sea salt is measured, and then added to the purified water. |

Figure 17.6  How to remineralize the purified water with Himalayan pink salt.

## HOW TO REMINERALIZE THE PURIFIED WATER?

(i) A clean and dry piece of paper (the computer paper purchased from Staples has been cut into small pieces and used) was placed on the digital kitchen scale, and the paper weight was measured (weight = 0.48 g). The Himalayan pink salt was added very slowly on to the paper until the digital reading hits exactly 0.98 g. That means the weight of the Himalayan pink salt to be added to the purified water was precisely 0.50 g (500 mg).

Weight of the Paper + Himalayan pink salt = 0.98 g (980 mg)          1 g = 1000 mg
Weight of the Paper                        = 0.48 g (480 mg)
Weight of the Himalayan pink salt          = 0.50 g (500 mg)

(ii) The bottle was filled with precisely 1 liter (4 cups) of purified water (distilled water or RO water).

(iii) The measured Himalayan pink salt (0.50 g or 500 mg) was added to the purified water (either distilled water or RO water), the bottle was closed tightly with the cap, and shaken thoroughly for a minute until the salt was perfectly dissolved. The purified water then became remineralized with the Himalayan pink salt. It is important to note that the Himalayan pink salt dissolved in the purified water very quickly and very easily.

(iv) The TDS level of the remineralized purified water was monitored by using a TDS meter. As expected, the TDS reading = 505 ppm or mg/L.

# HOW TO UNDERSTAND THE TDS METER READING?

● Try to understand the meaning of TDS conceptually from the units of TDS.
TDS is expressed in mg per liter (mg/L), which is the same as ppm (parts per million).

● Think about "how many milligrams of Himalayan pink salt is in 1 liter of purified water?".
That is TDS. If you can calculate how many milligrams of Himalayan pink salt is added to
1 liter of purified water, then you know the value of TDS.  Remember 1g = 1000 mg.

● 0.50 g (500 mg) of Himalayan pink salt was added to 1 liter (4 cups) of purified water
(distilled water or RO water). That means the concentration of the Himalayan pink salt in
the purified water should be 500 mg/L if there are no experimental errors.

● In scientific experiments, up to plus or minus 5% of error is reasonable and acceptable.
Sometimes even plus or minus 10% of experimental error is accepted depending on the
circumstances in which the experiment was conducted or performed.

● In this case, the true measured value of the concentration of the Himalayan pink salt in
purified water is 500 mg (if there is no error in the digital kitchen scale), which is added to
1 liter of purified water. The TDS meter reading is 505 mg/L. The error is (5/500)% or 1%.

## HOW TO EXPLAIN THAT "PPM IS THE SAME AS mg/L"?

We know that the density of water = 1 g/cm$^3$ = 1 g/mL = 1 kg/L.
Conversion Factors    1 L = 1000 mL  = 1000 cm$^3$
1 kg = 1000 g,        1 g = 1000 mg,        Therefore 1 kg = 1,000,000 mg

**SCIENTIFIC FACT:** If you measure 1 liter of water using a measuring flask, and weigh it
using an electronic balance or digital kitchen scale, you will find that 1 liter water weighs
exactly 1 kilogram. It is because the density of water is roughly 1 kg/L at room temperature.
Therefore for water, and for all dilute solutions, 1 liter is approximately the same as 1 kg.
We also know that 1 kg = 1,000,000 mg; Therefore 1 liter = 1 L = 1 kg for water.

## WHAT IS PPM?
PPM is a term used in chemistry to denote a very, very low concentration of a solution (It is
true in only dilute solutions). A dilute solution has the same physical properties as water.

PPM = Parts Per Million (One part per one million parts)
PPM = Parts Per Million (1 miligram per one million milligrams )
PPM = Parts Per Million (1 mg per 1,000,000 mg )

$$PPM = \frac{1\ part}{1\ million\ parts} = \frac{1\ part}{1,000,000\ parts} = \frac{1\ mg}{1,000,000\ mg} = \frac{1\ mg}{1\ kg} = \frac{1\ mg}{1\ L}$$

Since the density of water is 1, we can express both weight (in the numerator) and volume (in the
denominator) in milligrams. We also know that 1 cm$^3$ of water weights 1 gm, or 1 liter of water
weighs 1 kg (1 kg = 1 liter = 1 L).
Therefore 1 ppm = 1 mg/L
That is to say 1 ppm is the same as 1 mg/L in all dilute solutions.

# EXPERIMENT # 2  REMINERALIZATION OF DISTILLED WATER

In order to gain more experience on remineralization of purified water with Himalayan pink salt, more experiments were conducted as follows:

a. The water in the bottle of previous batch was discarded, the bottle was cleaned with distilled water, and filled precisely with 1 liter or 4 cups  (1 cup = 250 mL) of new distilled water.
b. The weight of Himalayan pink salt was measured, the amount is increased in the following pre-determined increments, and each time the TDS meter reading was recorded.

● 0.10 g (100 mg) of the Himalayan pink salt was measured, added to the water bottle, stirred well, and monitored the TDS level using a TDS meter.
● Another batch of 0.10 g (100 mg) of the Himalayan pink salt was measured, added to the same water bottle (previously used water was not discarded), (Total=200mg), stirred well, and monitored the TDS level using a TDS meter.
● Another batch of 0.10 g (100 mg) of the Himalayan pink salt was measured, added to the same water bottle (previously used water was not discarded), (Total=300mg), stirred well, and monitored the TDS level using a TDS meter.
● Another batch of 0.10 g (100 mg) of the Himalayan pink salt was measured, added to the same water bottle (previously used water was not discarded), (Total=400mg), stirred well, and monitored the TDS level using a TDS meter.
● Another batch of 0.10 g (100 mg) of the Himalayan pink salt was measured, added to the same water bottle (previously used water was not discarded), (Total=500mg), stirred well, and monitored the TDS level using a TDS meter. The results are tabulated as shown below:

Table 17.4  Remineralization of distilled water with Himalayan pink salt.

| Himalayan Pink Salt Added To 1 Liter of Distilled Water | TDS Level  Monitored With TDS Meter | Error (Plus or Minus) |
|---|---|---|
| 0.100 g (100 mg) | 96 ppm | 4.0% |
| 0.200 g (200 mg) | 190 ppm | 5.0% |
| 0.300 g (300 mg) | 310 ppm | 3.3% |
| 0.400 g (400 mg) | 393 ppm | 1.75% |
| 0.500 g (500 mg) | 492 ppm | 1.6% |

1 g = 1000 mg

## What If the TDS Meter Did Not Show the Reading As Expected?

a. That means the digital kitchen scale is not working perfectly. The digital kitchen scale should be calibrated with the calibration weights (100 mg, 200 mg, 500 mg, 1000 mg, 1 g,  2 g, etc).

b. The TDS meter is not working perfectly. The TDS meter should be calibrated and tested using the calibration solution. The calibration solution (NaCl solution) can be purchased at prescribed concentrations or several levels of ppm.

c. Himalayan pink salt was probably expired or it was not dissolving in the water properly. New Himalyan pink salt (ground) package has to be purchased from a different and reliable distributor, and the experiment should be repeated.

# EXPERIMENT # 3  REMINERALIZATION OF RO WATER

a. The water in the bottle of previous batch was discarded, the bottle was cleaned with distilled water, and filled precisely with 1 liter or 4 cups (1 cup = 250 mL) of RO water.
b. The weight of Himalayan pink salt was measured, the amount is increased in the following pre-determined increments, and each time the TDS meter reading was recorded.

◉ 0.10 g (100 mg) of the Himalayan pink salt was measured, added to the water bottle, stirred well, and monitored the TDS level using a TDS meter.
◉ Another batch of 0.10 g (100 mg) of the Himalayan pink salt was measured, added to the same water bottle (previously used water was not discarded), (Total=200mg), stirred well, and monitored the TDS level using a TDS meter.
◉ Another batch of 0.10 g (100 mg) of the Himalayan pink salt was measured, added to the same water bottle (previously used water was not discarded), (Total=300mg), stirred well, and monitored the TDS level using a TDS meter.
◉ Another batch of 0.10 g (100 mg) of the Himalayan pink salt was measured, added to the same water bottle (previously used water was not discarded), (Total=400mg), stirred well, and monitored the TDS level using a TDS meter.
◉ Another batch of 0.10 g (100 mg) of the Himalayan pink salt was measured, added to the same water bottle (previously used water was not discarded), (Total=500mg), stirred well, and monitored the TDS level using a TDS meter. The results are tabulated as shown below:

Table 17.5 Remineralization of RO water with Himalayan pink salt.

| Himalayan Pink Salt Added To 1 Liter of RO Water | TDS Level  Monitored With TDS Meter | Error (Plus or Minus) |
|---|---|---|
| 0.100 g (100 mg) | 95 ppm | 5.0% |
| 0.200 g (200 mg) | 205 ppm | 2.5% |
| 0.300 g (300 mg) | 316 ppm | 5.3% |
| 0.400 g (400 mg) | 390 ppm | 2.5% |
| 0.500 g (500 mg) | 506 ppm | 1.2% |

1 g = 1000 mg

The results turned out to be almost the same either for distilled water or RO water.

The TDS level of RO water is 2 ppm, 3 ppm or 4 ppm (in local supermarket).
The TDS level of distilled water is precisely zero (it is purchased in a pharmacy).
Both kinds of purified water are good enough to do the remineralization experiments.
It is up to the individual to choose either one or the other.

# ABOUT CELTIC SEA SALT [35]

The Celtic sea salt is naturally formulated in Guerande, Brittany, France. It was hand-collected according to an age-old ancestral Celtic method by highly experienced people. It has not undergone any physical or chemical modification of the original composition. It is completely unprocessed and unrefined very special sea salt. It comes in two different forms: (i) Unrefined coarse grey sea salt, and (ii) Unrefined fine grey sea salt.

Unrefined coarse or fine grey sea salt is obtained through the evaporation of seawater by the combined action of the wind and sun. It is hand-harvested from the clay-bottom pans of salt marshes, which gives it its natural grey colour as well as its richness in minerals and trace elements. Unrefined sea salt has a pleasing natural taste and contains none of the harsh overtones found in processed salt.

Per 10 g of Celtic sea salt, it contains 3860 mg of sodium (161%), 10% iron, 4% calcium, and all other ingredients being zero. The consumer should be extremely careful with the high sodium content, and should consume limited quantity only.

Light Grey Celtic® gets its light grey hue from the pure clay lining of the salt beds where it is harvested. It was harvested with three simple ingredients: Sun, wind and human skill, preserving the vast array of vital trace minerals.

Serve it in a bowl with a small spoon or season with pinches instead of shakes. If a shaker is to be used, it should have large holes and be nonmetallic. Use about one-third less than the recipe indicates or salt to taste. Unrefined fine sea salt or "so called Celtic sea salt" can be used for your everyday seasoning, as it possesses a variety of health benefits similar to Himalayan pink salt.

## Health Benefits Posted by Westpoint Naturals: [35]

- Celtic sea salt (unrefined fine grey salt) is an inexpensive and health-enhancing gift extracted from our planet Earth's ocean.
- Called "Living Salt of Life", Celtic sea salt is the only natural sea salt on the market which is healthy for the human body, certified organic, and graded according to quality.
- Celtic sea salt provides all minerals needed for the human body in the perfect ratio and composition.
- It is naturally iodized and therefore easily assimilated into the body.
- It maintains the proper electrolyte balance in body's fluids.
- It facilitates osmotic transfer of nutrients through the cell walls.
- It restores the optimum acid-alkaline balance in the body.
- It aids digestion by producing hydrochloric acid (HCL) in the stomach.
- It allows the body to extract as much as 7 times the nutrient value from food.
- It cleans arteries and veins.
- It stabilizes the blood pressure.
- It protects the body from radiation in the atmosphere.
- All the above-mentioned health benefits can be obtained for just pennies a day.

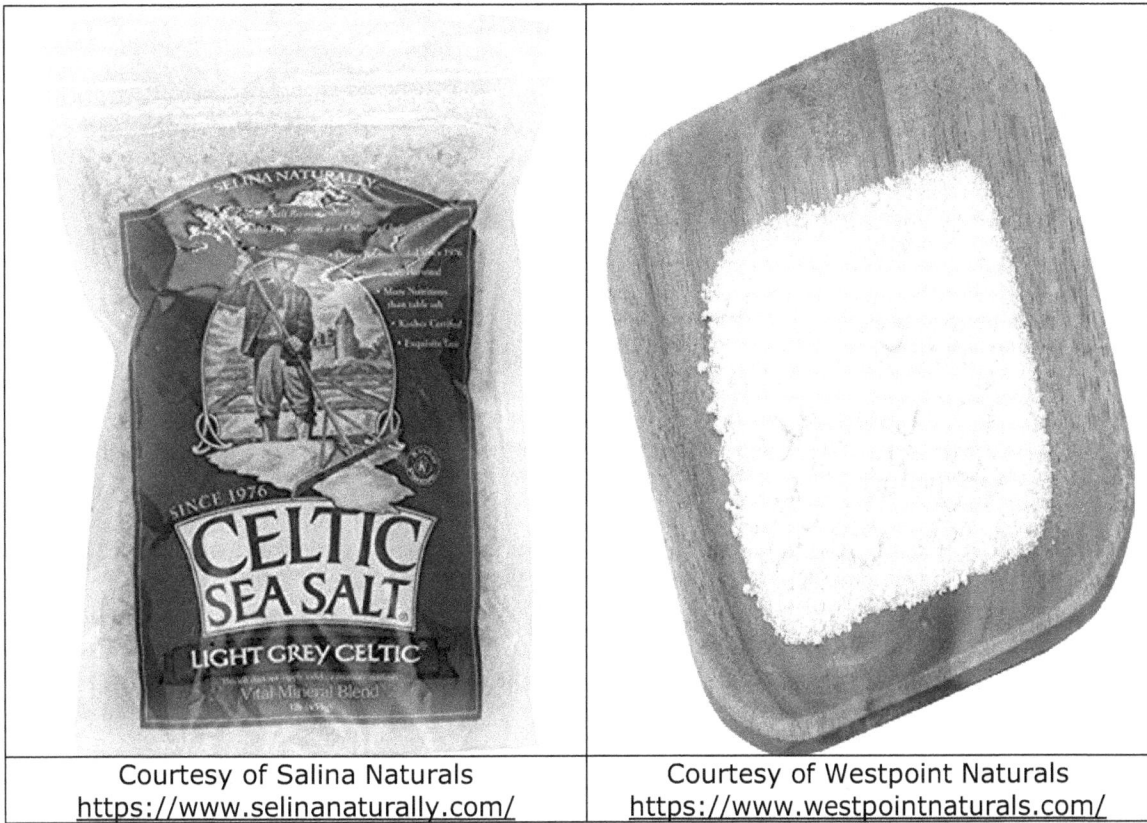

| Courtesy of Salina Naturals https://www.selinanaturally.com/ | Courtesy of Westpoint Naturals https://www.westpointnaturals.com/ |
|---|---|

Figure 17.7 Celtic Sea salt (fine grey) quickly dissolves and remineralizes purified water.

Table 17.6  Nutritional Information of Celtic sea salt (Unrefined fine grey sea salt)
Courtesy of Westpoint Naturals [35]

### Nutrition Facts (per 10 g)

| Amount | % Daily Value |
|---|---|
| Calories   0 | |
| Fat   0g | 0% |
| Saturated   0g | 0% |
| ⁏Trans   0g | |
| Cholesterol   0mg | |
| Sodium   3860mg | 161% |
| Carbohydrate   0g | 0% |
| Fibre   0g | 0% |
| Sugars   0g | |
| Protein   0g | |
| Vitamin A | 0% |
| Vitamin C | 0% |
| Calcium | 4% |
| Iron | 10% |

**Storage & Shelf Life**
When stored in a cool, dry location, unrefined sea salt should last indefinitely.

# Health Benefits Posted by Salina Naturally [36]

There are exciting reasons for their choice. All Celtic Sea Salt® Brand salts are authentic, unprocessed, whole salts, guaranteed to be optimally balanced in mineral content and to be free from pesticides, herbicides and harmful chemicals.

**Compare the trace mineral and moisture content of sea salts***
Celtic Sea Salt Brand Makai Pure ………….. 23.10%
Celtic Sea Salt® Brand Light Grey Celtic®... 17.50%
Himalayan and other leading salt brands…….4.12%, 3.96%, and 1.68%
*Results of third-party laboratory analysis, performed in 2014

• All of our gourmet salts are traditionally harvested to preserve their natural balance of minerals – a balance that fits ideally with the natural composition of the "natural salt water" that makes up as much as 60% of the human body.

• According to H.H. Mitchell, Journal of Biological Chemistry 158, the brain and heart are composed of 73% water, and the lungs are about 83% water (May 2, 2016). The composition of the minerals in the water of the body are, not only sodium, but a natural balance of potassium, calcium, magnesium, and a host of other essential minerals. In fact, it is the ionic charge across the cell wall between sodium and potassium, often referred to as the sodium pump, that creates the electric charge that accounts for life itself.

# Disadvantages of Celtic Sea Salt [37, 38]

**High Sodium Content:** As a natural salt, Celtic sea salt is high in sodium. It contains more of this essential mineral than any other nutrient. Sodium is needed by your body to function properly, as it helps your body control blood pressure and volume. It is also necessary for proper muscle and nerve function. However, the RDA (Recommended Daily Allowance) of sodium is to taken into serious consideration.

(i) The RDA (Recommended Daily Allowance) of sodium is 2,300 milligrams for healthy adults, and (ii) 1,500 milligrams for adults with a history of heart disease, who are over 51 years old or are African-American.

A diet that is high in sodium, if consumed in unlimited quantities beyond The RDA (Recommended Daily Allowance), can lead to atherosclerosis, heart disease, high blood pressure, high cholesterol levels and an increased risk of kidney disease. Keep in mind that many foods, especially prepared foods, contain too much added sodium. [37]

The bottom line is that Sel gris (Celtic sea salt), sea salt and common table salt all have undesirably high concentrations of sodium chloride (NaCl). Research showed that all these salts, if consumed in unlimited quantities beyond the suggested daily requirement, develop hypertension, osteoporosis, kidney stones, Menierre's Syndrome (ear ringing), insomnia, motion sickness, asthma, and a variety of cancers. [38]

# Himalan Pink Salt Vs Celtic Sea Salt [39]

◦ Himalayan pink salt comes from Khewra, Pakistan where there are several mines that supply the world. Celtic sea salt comes from Brittany, France from where the distributors import it.

◦ Celtic sea salt contains about 13% residual moisture compared to the 0.026% residual moisture found in Himalayan pink salt. In addition to its different mineral composition, the harvesting methods for Celtic sea salt differ from those used for Himalayan pink salt. It is typically gathered by evaporating seawater and collecting the salt in a salt pan.

◦ Like Himalayan Salt, Celtic sea salt can be used for a variety of different purposes. This salt has a fairly coarse grain but it can be used for both cooking and finishing. The density of Celtic sea salt is however much greater than that of the regular table salt so you do not need to use as much of it. Celtic sea salt also has a lot of residual moisture in it, so it will not suck the moisture out of food.

◦ Celtic sea salt contains relatively less number of minerals (more than 70 minerals were detected and analysed thus far, according to Salina Naturally) but with much higher concentrations compared to the Himalayan pink salt. Celtic sea salt contains about 84% sodium chloride in comparison to Himalayan salt's 98% concentration. This is due to the fact that Celtic sea salt contains a higher amount of natural brine (seawater).

◦ There are some unconfirmed reports such as: Himalayan salt is over 99% pure whereas Celtic sea salt typically contains some impurities that can easily be contaminated during harvesting. Himalayan sea salt is completely unrefined and requires no refinements or processing to be edible.

Table 17.7   List of over 70 macrominerals and trace minerals in Celtic sea salt. [40]
Courtesy of Salina Naturals
https://www.selinanaturally.com       https://www.celticseasalt.com/

| Analysis | Result mg/0.25 tsp 1.4g | Result mg/0.25 tsp 1.4g | Result mg/0.25 tsp 1.1g | Result mg/0.25 tsp 1.1g | Result mg/0.25 tsp 1.2g | Result mg/0.25 tsp 1.35g | Result mg/0.25 tsp 1.8g |
|---|---|---|---|---|---|---|---|
| Element | Celtic light grey coarse | Celtic light grey fine | Gourmet Kosher | Celtic Kosher coarse | Celtic Kosher fine | Makai pure | PINK |
| Aluminum | 0.18704 | 0.35756 | 0.008 | 0.015 | 0.019 | 0.02731 | 0.113 |
| Antimony | 0.00532 | 0.0035 | 0.007 | 0.013 | 0.006 | 0.00139 | <0.0006 |
| Arsenic | 0.0004746 | 0.0008442 | 0.000046 | 0.000069 | 0.000023 | 0.000139 | 0.000217 |
| Barium | 0.001162 | 0.000133 | 0.003 | 0.001 | 0.0008 | 0.00305 | 0.0017 |
| Beryllium | <0.0007 | <0.0007 | <0.0006 | <0.0006 | <0.0006 | 0.00225 | <0.0006 |
| Bismuth | <0.0007 | <0.0007 | <0.0006 | <0.0006 | <0.0006 | <0.00068 | <0.0006 |
| Boron | 0.01988 | 0.0238 | 0.049 | 0.024 | 0.01 | 0.05609 | 0.006984 |
| Cadmium | 0.0000014 | 0.0000028 | 0.000003 | 0.000004 | 0.0000012 | 0.000003 | <0.000002 |
| Calcium | 2.7986 | 3.7296 | 6.21 | 2.47 | 2.32 | 16.322 | 0.763 |
| Cerium | <0.000002 | <0.000002 | 0.000001 | 0.000002 | 0.000001 | 0.000003 | 0.000054 |
| Cesium | 0.0000882 | 0.001064 | 0.000001 | 0.000002 | 0.000001 | 0.000003 | 0.0000096 |
| Chloride | 581.4354 | 624.03 | 627.44 | 657.91 | 624.03 | 766.41525 | 707.372 |
| Chromium | 0.001134 | 0.00224 | 0.0009 | 0.0009 | <0.0006 | 0.00238 | <0.0006 |
| Cobalt | 0.00126 | 0.00154 | 0.00064 | <0.0006 | <0.0006 | 0.00296 | 0.000894 |
| copper | <0.0007 | <0.0007 | 0.0011 | 0.0011 | <0.0006 | 0.00252 | <0.0006 |
| Dysprosium | 0.0000224 | 0.0000266 | <0.000001 | <0.000001 | <0.000001 | 0.000003 | 0.00004 |
| Erbium | 0.0000098 | 0.0000126 | <0.000001 | <0.000001 | <0.000001 | <0.000001 | 0.00001 |
| Europium | 0.000007 | 0.0000084 | 0.000001 | <0.000001 | <0.000001 | <0.000001 | 0.00001 |
| Fluoride | 0.0006874 | 0.0013146 | 0.0088 | 0.0165 | 0.0275 | 0.00027675 | 0.00104 |
| Gadolinium | 0.0000364 | 0.0000392 | <0.000001 | <0.000001 | <0.000001 | <0.000001 | 0.000005 |
| Gallium | 0.0000462 | 0.0000518 | 0.000096 | 0.000057 | 0.000071 | 0.0000065 | 0.000142 |
| Germanium | <0.000002 | <0.000002 | <0.000001 | <0.000001 | <0.000001 | <0.000001 | <0.000002 |
| Gold | <0.0007 | <0.0007 | 0.0014 | 0.004 | 0.0024 | 0.00068 | <0.0006 |
| Hafnium | 0.000427 | 0.0001442 | 0.000102 | 0.000261 | 0.000164 | 0.000294 | 0.000049 |
| Holmium | 0.0000042 | 0.0000056 | 0.000002 | 0.000003 | 0.000001 | 0.000003 | 0.0000012 |
| Indium | <0.000002 | <0.000002 | <0.000001 | <0.000001 | <0.000001 | <0.000001 | <0.000002 |
| Iodine | 0.0002604 | 0.0003584 | 0.0154 | 0.0286 | 0.0209 | 0.0089113 | 0.001505 |
| Iridium | 0.000007 | 0.0000014 | 0.000001 | 0.000001 | 0.000001 | 0.000003 | <0.000002 |
| Iron | 0.26996 | 0.47054 | 0.008 | 0.0286 | 0.008 | 0.00528 | 0.0678 |
| Lanthanum | <0.0007 | <0.0007 | <0.0006 | <0.0006 | <0.0006 | 0.00273 | <0.0006 |
| 30 elements | | | | | | | |

| Analysis | Result mg/0.25 tsp | Result mg/0.25 tsp | Result mg/0.25 tsp 1.1g | Result mg/0.25 tsp | Result mg/0.25 tsp | Result mg/0.25 tsp | Result mg/0.25 tsp 1.8g |
|---|---|---|---|---|---|---|---|
| Element | Celtic light grey coarse | Celtic light grey fine | Gourmet Kosher | Celtic Kosher coarse | Celtic Kosher fine | Makai pure | PINK |
| Lead | 0.0006986 | 0.0010836 | 0.000028 | 0.0006986 | 0.000055 | <0.000001 | 0.00011 |
| Lithium | 0.00308 | 0.00378 | 0.005 | 0.0000028 | 0.002 | 0.00798 | <0.0006 |
| Lutetium | 0.0000028 | <0.000002 | <0.000001 | <0.000025 | <0.000001 | 0.00001 | <0.000002 |
| Magnesium | 6.986 | 8.4462 | 19 | 12.2 | 4.66 | 15.498 | 2.218 |
| Manganese | 0.00644 | 0.01176 | 0.002 | 0.0034 | 0.002 | 0.00229 | 0.00541 |
| Mercury | <0.000002 | <0.000002 | <0.000001 | <0.000001 | <0.000002 | <0.000001 | 0.000046 |
| Molybdenum | <0.0007 | <0.0007 | 0.00062 | 0.001 | 0.0009 | <0.00068 | <0.0006 |
| Neodymium | 0.000189 | 0.0001988 | <0.000001 | 0.000001 | 0.000001 | <0.000001 | 0.0000312 |
| Nickel | 0.0028 | 0.00518 | 0.002 | 0.0022 | <0.0006 | 0.0021 | 0.000816 |
| Niobium | 0.00266 | 0.00546 | 0.0044 | 0.0045 | 0.003 | 0.00255 | 0.00486 |
| Osmium | 0.0000042 | 0.0000028 | 0.000001 | 0.000002 | 0.000002 | 0.000001 | <0.000002 |
| Palladium | 0.0000168 | 0.000014 | 0.00006 | 0.00006 | 0.000006 | 0.000012 | 0.00092914 |
| Phosphorous | 0.01918 | 0.0224 | 0.007 | 0.014 | <0.0006 | 0.00218 | 0.000692 |
| Platinum | 0.0000014 | 0.0000014 | 0.00002 | 0.000002 | 0.000002 | 0.000003 | <0.000002 |
| Potassium | 2.73 | 2.52 | 7.02 | 4.73 | 2.14 | 11.204 | 2.12 |
| Praseodymium | 0.0000476 | 0.0000518 | <0.000001 | <0.000001 | <0.000001 | <0.000001 | 0.000006 |
| Rhenium | <0.000002 | 0.0000014 | <0.000001 | <0.000001 | <0.000001 | <0.000001 | <0.000002 |
| Rhodium | 0.000007 | 0.0000084 | 0.000048 | 0.000034 | 0.00005 | 0.000014 | 0.000004 |
| Rubidium | 0.0012488 | 0.0013944 | 0.000569 | 0.000283 | 0.000088 | 0.000998 | 0.00016908 |
| Ruthenium | 0.000035 | 0.000035 | 0.000089 | 0.000077 | 0.000079 | 0.000088 | 0.000126 |
| Samarium | 0.0000378 | 0.0000434 | <0.000001 | <0.000001 | <0.000001 | <0.000001 | 0.000006 |
| Scandium | 0.0003136 | 0.0002968 | 0.000182 | 0.000198 | 0.000215 | 0.000155 | 0.000191 |
| Selenium | <0.0007 | <0.00007 | <0.0006 | <0.0006 | <0.0006 | <0.00068 | <0.0006 |
| Silicon | 0.28056 | 0.45052 | 0.023 | 0.024 | 0.014 | 0.06506 | 0.14 |
| Silver | <0.0007 | <0.0007 | <0.0006 | <0.0006 | <0.0006 | 0.00185 | <0.0006 |
| Sodium | 459.2 | 435.12 | 257 | 207 | 234 | 341.685 | 449 |
| Strontium | 0.07546 | 0.091084 | 0.148 | 0.171 | 0.146 | 0.318 | 0.076 |
| Sulfur | 6.1166 | 7.343 | 13.1 | 8.21 | 3.96 | 22.005 | 1.85 |
| Tantalum | <0.000002 | <0.000002 | <0.000002 | 0.000003 | 0.000002 | 0.000003 | 0.000005 |
| Tellurium | <0.0007 | <0.0007 | 0.0073 | 0.0024 | 0.009 | 0.02491 | 0.00691 |
| Terbium | 0.0000042 | 0.0000056 | <0.000001 | <0.000001 | <0.000001 | <0.000001 | <0.000002 |
| Thallium | 0.00182 | 0.00504 | <0.0006 | 0.003 | 0.001 | 0.00908 | <0.0006 |
| Thorium | 0.00798 | 0.00952 | 0.026 | 0.016 | <0.0006 | 0.01994 | 0.000649 |
| Thulium | 0.0000014 | 0.0000014 | <0.000001 | <0.000001 | <0.000001 | <0.000001 | <0.000002 |
| 34 elements | | | | | | | |

| | | | | | | | |
|---|---|---|---|---|---|---|---|
| Tin | 0.000007 | <0.000002 | <0.000001 | <0.000001 | 0.000017 | <0.000001 | 0.000025 |
| Titanium | 0.01022 | 0.0133 | 0.0012 | 0.0022 | <0.0006 | 0.0026 | 0.0074 |
| Tungsten | <0.0007 | 0.001092 | 0.011 | 0.0013 | 0.021 | 0.00574 | 0.00176 |
| Vanadium | 0.00224 | 0.00434 | 0.012 | 0.014 | 0.018 | <0.00068 | <0.0006 |
| Ytterbium | 0.000007 | 0.0000098 | <0.000001 | <0.000001 | <0.000001 | <0.000001 | 0.0000012 |
| Yttrium | | | | | | | 0.00074 |
| | | | | | | | |
| Analysis | Result mg/0.25 tsp | Result mg/0.25 tsp | Result mg/0.25 tsp 1.1g | Result mg/0.25 tsp | Result mg/0.25 tsp | Result mg/0.25 tsp | Result mg/0.25 tsp 1.8g |
| Element | Celtic light grey coarse | Celtic light grey fine | Gourmet Kosher | Celtic Kosher coarse | Celtic Kosher fine | Makai pure | PINK |
| Zinc | 0.0035 | 0.00462 | 0.009 | 0.005 | 0.003 | 0.01263 | 0.00125 |
| Zirconium | <0.0007 | <0.0007 | <0.0006 | <0.0006 | 0.007 | 0.00146 | 0.00067 |
| Bromine 8 elements more | 0.0011424 | 0.0012754 | | | | 0.011804 | 0.00726 |
| pH | 8.53 | 9.94 | 9.2 | 8.75 | 8.43 | 9.93 | 9.54 |
| solubility | | | 35.66 | 35.28 | 35.79 | 34.95 | 40.58 |
| moisture | 8.4 | 1.6 | 9.71 | 6.52 | 4.28 | 5.06 | 4.187 |

Altogether there are 72 trace minerals identified and analysed thus far in Celtic sea salt. Courtesy of Courtesy of Salina Naturals.

**HOW TO REMINERALIZE DISTILLED WATER WITH CELTIC SEA SALT? EXPERIMENTS CONDUCTED AT HOME**

Just repeat Experiment # 1, Experiment # 2, Experiment # 3 by simply replacing the Himalayan pink salt with Celtic sea salt. All the remineralization procedure remains the same. Given below is an example of the same kind of experimentation.

# EXPERIMENT # 4

# **Items** needed:

(i) Purified Water

RO water can be purchased in supermarkets at Refill Yourself Stations or from local vendors; And distilled water can be purchased in any pharmacy or from local vendors.

(ii) Celtic salt

(This can be purchased at any local health food store, supermarket, or online).

(iii) TDS Meter

(Already discussed how to purchase it and how to use it at the beginning of this chapter).

(iv) Digital Kitchen Scale

(Already discussed how to purchase it and how to use it in the previous section).

a. The water bottle was filled with 1 liter or 4 cups (1 cup = 250 mL) of distilled water as precisely as possible.

b. The weight of the Celtic sea salt was measured, the amount is increased in the following pre-determined increments, and each time the TDS meter reading was recorded.

◉ 0.10 g (100 mg) of Celtic sea salt was measured, added to the water bottle, stirred well, and monitored the TDS level using a TDS meter.

◉ Another batch of 0.10 g (100 mg) of the Celtic sea salt was measured, added to the same water bottle (previously used water was not discarded), (Total=200mg), stirred well, and monitored the TDS level using a TDS meter.

◉ Another batch of 0.10 g (100 mg) of the Celtic sea salt was measured, added to the same water bottle (previously used water was not discarded), (Total=300mg), stirred well, and monitored the TDS level using a TDS meter.

◉ Another batch of 0.10 g (100 mg) of the Celtic sea salt was measured, added to the same water bottle (previously used water was not discarded), (Total=400mg), stirred well, and monitored the TDS level using a TDS meter.

◉ Another batch of 0.10 g (100 mg) of the Celtic sea salt was measured, added to the same water bottle (previously used water was not discarded), (Total=500mg), stirred well, and monitored the TDS level using a TDS meter. The results are tabulated as shown below:

Table 17.8  Remineralization of distilled water with Celtic sea salt.

| Celtic Salt Added To 1 Liter of Distilled Water | TDS Level Monitored With TDS Meter | Error (Plus or Minus) |
|---|---|---|
| 0.100 g (100 mg) | 95 ppm | 5.0% |
| 0.200 g (200 mg) | 188 ppm | 6.0% |
| 0.300 g (300 mg) | 289 ppm | 3.7% |
| 0.400 g (400 mg) | 390 ppm | 2.5% |
| 0.500 g (500 mg) | 495 ppm | 1.6% |

# HOW TO REMINERALIZE THE PURIFIED WATER WITH HIMALAYAN PINK SALT OR CELTIC SEA SALT USING TEASPOONS (WITHOUT SCALE OR TDS METER)

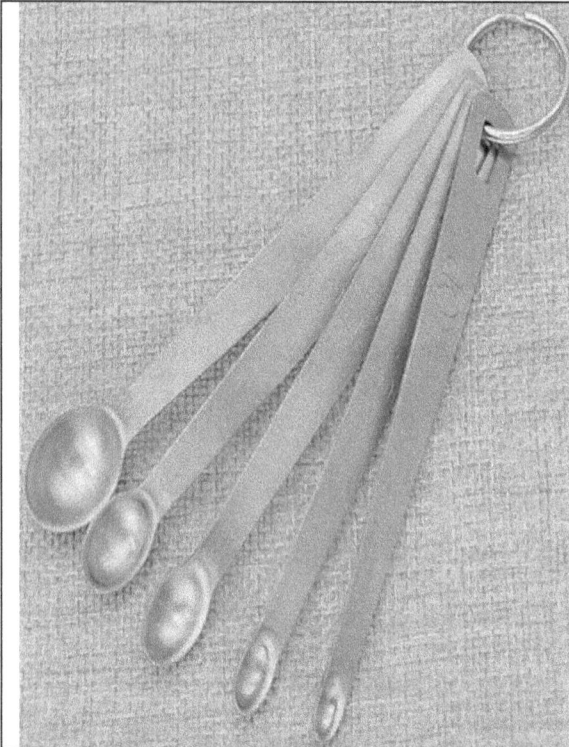

A set of Teaspoons in the descending order:
1 Teaspoon = 5.69 g
1/2 Teaspoon = 2.84 g
1/4 Teaspoon =1.42 g
1/8 Teaspoon = 0.71 g
1/16 Teaspoon = 0.36 g

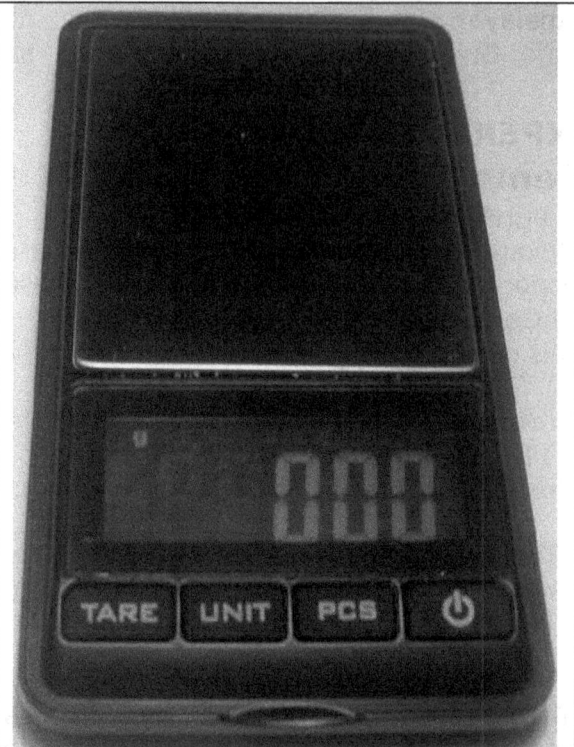

**Accu Weight** Digital Kitchen Scale. Ultra Fine 0.01 g (0.001 oz) Increments!

You should learn how to use these Teaspoons by practicing it with a digital kitchen scale until you become familiar.

The Scientific Definition for the Weight of One Teaspoon of Salt = 5.69 g
This definition is valid for all kinds of salts, including table salt, regular sea salt, Himalayan pink salt & Celtic sea salt.
**Be Careful When You Use Teaspoons:** For example, you want to use 1/4 Teaspoon in order to add 1.42 g of Himalayan pink salt to purified water. Scoop out the Himalayan pink salt with 1/4 Teaspoon, cut the salt flat on the top of the Teaspoon with a finger (cut it flat), place the salt on the digital scale, and measure the weight. It should be approximately 1.42 g. If it too high or too low, you have to do it again until you understand how Teaspoon is designed. Otherwise, you would be collecting erroneous amounts of Himalayan pink salt for the remineralization of purified water.

Figure 17.8 Remineralization of purified water can be done with the aid of teaspoons.

A set of these Teaspoons can be purchased in any local dollar store, on eBay.com or online. When you buy this pack, you can see the markings on each teaspoon as 1 Teaspoon, ½ Teaspoon, ¼ Teaspoon, 1/8 Teaspoon, 1/16 Teaspoon. They usually are chained together. Sometimes, they are sold along with tablespoon. A Tablespoon in this kind of experimentation is unnecessary, as it is too big to be used! The 1/4 Teaspoon, 1/8 Teaspoon, 1/16 Teaspoon, or even smaller Teaspoons are very useful in the remineralization of purified water.

**EXPERIMENT # 5 HOW TO REMINERALIZE THE PURIFIED WATER USING TEASPOONS?**

# Items needed:

(i) Purified Water (Distilled Water/RO Water)
(ii) Himalayan pink salt
(This can be purchased at any local health food store, supermarket, or online).
(iii) TDS Meter
(Already discussed how to purchase it and how to use it at the beginning of this chapter).
(iv) Digital Kitchen Scale
(Already discussed how to purchase it and how to use it in the previous section).
(v) A set of teaspoons (This can be purchased in any dollar store, supermarkets, or online).

a. The water bottle was filled with 1 liter or 4 cups (1 cup = 250 mL) of purified water (distilled water/RO water) as precisely as possible.
b. The 1/8 Teaspoonful of Himalayan pink salt (after cutting it flat on Teaspoon) was placed on the digital kitchen scale in order to make sure that the amount of salt in the Teaspoon weighs exactly or at least approximately 0.71 g (710 mg).
c. The measured 1/8 Teaspoonful of Himalayan pink salt was then dumped into the bottle of distilled water, closed with the cap and shaken thoroughly for a minute until all the Himalayan pink salt is perfectly dissolved in the purified water.
d. The TDS level of the remineralized purified water was monitored with the TDS meter.
e. The experiment was repeated by using 2 different Teaspoons 1/4 Teaspoon & 1/8 Teaspoon.

Table 17.9  Remineralization of the purified water using Teaspoons
(weight of the salt was measured and verified with a digital kitchen scale)

| Teaspoon Used | Himalayan Pink Salt Added | TDS Level Monitored | Error |
|---|---|---|---|
| | To 1 Liter of Distilled Water | With TDS Meter | (Plus or Minus) |
| 1/4 Teaspoon | 0.71 g (710 mg) | 694 ppm | 2.25% |
| 1/8 Teaspoon | 0.36 g (360 mg) | 346 ppm | 3.90% |

**EXPERIMENT # 6 HOW TO REMINERALIZE THE PURIFIED WATER USING TEASPOONS?**
EXPERIMENT # 5 was repeated without using digital kitchen scale and without verifying the weight of the Himalayan pink salt in the Teaspoon. The experiment was conducted like a lay person.

Table 17.10  Remineralization of the purified water using Teaspoons
(weight of the salt was not measured, and not verified with digital scale)

| Teaspoon Used | Himalayan Pink Salt Added | TDS Level Monitored | Error |
|---|---|---|---|
| | To 1 Liter of Distilled Water | With TDS Meter | (Plus or Minus) |
| 1/4 Teaspoon | Weight was not measured! | 755 ppm | 6.30% |
| 1/8 Teaspoon | Weight was not measured! | 384 ppm | 6.67% |

**CONCLUSION:** What we have learned from the above-mentioned 2 experiments is that if the Teaspoons were used without measuring the weight with a digital scale, the experimental error was relatively higher, but is still reasonable, and the Teaspoons can be used in the remineralization. However, a person should practice thoroughly on how to use a Teaspoon while scooping up the salt (Cut it flat!) when trying to remineralize the purified water.

**EXPERIMENT # 7** HOW TO REMINERALIZE THE PURIFIED WATER USING TEASPOONS?
# Items needed:
(i) Purified Water (Distilled Water/RO Water)
(ii) Celtic sea salt
(This can be purchased at any local health food store, supermarket, or online).
(iii) TDS Meter
(Already discussed how to purchase it and how to use it at the beginning of this chapter).
(iv) Digital Kitchen Scale
(Already discussed how to purchase it and how to use it in the previous section).
(v) A set of teaspoons (This can be purchased in any dollar store, supermarkets, or online).

a. The water bottle was filled with 1 liter or 4 cups (1 cup = 250 mL) of purified water (distilled water/RO water) as precisely as possible.
b. The 1/8 Teaspoonful of Celtic sea salt (after cutting it flat on Teaspoon with a finger) was placed on the digital kitchen scale in order to make sure that the amount of salt in the Teaspoon weighs exactly or at least approximately 0.71 g (710 mg).
c. The measured 1/8 Teaspoonful of Celtic sea salt was then dumped into the bottle of purified water (distilled water/RO water), closed with the cap and shaken thoroughly for a minute until all the Himalayan pink salt is perfectly dissolved in the distilled water.
d. The TDS level of the remineralized purified water was monitored with the TDS meter.
e. The experiment was repeated by using 2 different Teaspoons 1/4 Teaspoon & 1/8 Teaspoon.

Table 17.11  Remineralization of the purified water using Teaspoons
(weight of the salt was measured and verified with a digital kitchen scale)

| Teaspoon Used | Himalayan Pink Salt Added | TDS Level  Monitored | Error |
|---|---|---|---|
| | To 1 Liter of Distilled Water | With TDS Meter | (Plus or Minus) |
| 1/4 Teaspoon | 0.71 g (710 mg) | 687 ppm | 3.24% |
| 1/8 Teaspoon | 0.36 g (360 mg) | 343 ppm | 4.72% |

**EXPERIMENT # 8** HOW TO REMINERALIZE THE PURIFIED WATER USING TEASPOONS?
EXPERIMENT # 5 was repeated without using digital scale and without verifying the weight of the Himalayan pink salt in the Teaspoon. The experiment was conducted like a lay person.

Table 17.12  Remineralization of the purified water using Teaspoons
(weight of the salt was not measured, and not verified with digital kitchen scale)

| Teaspoon Used | Himalayan Pink Salt Added | TDS Level  Monitored | Error |
|---|---|---|---|
| | To 1 Liter of Distilled Water | With TDS Meter | (Plus or Minus) |
| 1/4 Teaspoon | Weight was not measured! | 759 ppm | 5.60% |
| 1/8 Teaspoon | Weight was not measured! | 388 ppm | 7.78% |

**CONCLUSION:** What we have learned from the above-mentioned 2 experiments is that if the Teaspoons were used without measuring the weight with a digital kitchen scale, the experimental error was relatively higher, but is still reasonable, and so the Teaspoons can be used in the remineralization. However, a person should practice thoroughly on how to use a Teaspoon while scooping up the salt (Cut it flat!) when trying to remineralize the purified water.

# HOW TO MAINTAIN A TDS LEVEL OF 200 PPM IN DRINKING WATER?

A TDS Level of 200 ppm = 200 mg/L
Which means 200 milligrams (0.20 g) of Himalayan pink salt or Celtic sea salt should be added to 1 liter of purified water (distilled water/RO water).

**METHOD 1 (By USING DIGITAL KITCHEN SCALE)**: You can use a digital kitchen scale to measure 200 mg of the Himalayan pink salt or Celtic sea salt precisely, and add it to 1 liter of purified water in order to maintain a TDS level of 200 ppm.

**METHOD 2 (By USING TEASPOONS)**: You can also use Teaspoons to measure 200 mg of the salt, and add it to 1 liter of purified water. For example 1/16 Teaspoon of Himalayan pink salt is equivalent to 0.36 g (360 mg). A little over 360 mg would be 400 mg. You can remineralize 2 liters of purified water by adding approximately 400 mg of Himalayan pink salt or Celtic sea salt by using a 1/16 Teaspoon. Or split that 400 mg into two equal portions (200 mg each), and add 200 mg of Himalayan pink salt or Celtic sea salt to 1 liter of purified water in order to maintain a TDS level of 200 ppm.

# HASSLE-FREE REMINERALIZATION OF THE PURIFIED WATER

## EXAMPLE 1  HASSLE-FREE REMINERALIZATION OF THE PURIFIED WATER

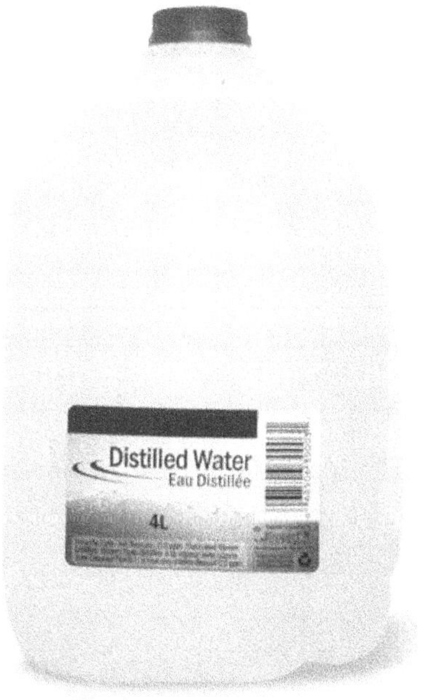

Distilled Water in a 4 Liter BPA-Free Plastic Bottle.

A person should drink at least 8 cups or 2 liters of purified water per day.

A TDS level of 200 ppm or 200 mg/L in drinking water is considered safe and healthy. So if you drink 8 cups or 2 liters of purified water per day, you should add 400 mg of Himalayan pink salt or Celtic sea salt per day, and 800 mg would be enough for 2 days.

1/8 Teaspoon = 0.71 g (710 mg)
A little over 710 mg would be equal to 800 mg.

AN EXAMPLE: When Peter gets up early in the morning, by using a 1/8 Teaspoon, he adds a little over 710 mg of Himalayan pink salt (which is close to 800 mg) to a 4 liters distilled water bottle. He also adds a few kernels of baking soda so that pH would be close to 7, and shakes it thoroughly until the salt dissolves perfectly. This 800 mg of Himalayan pink salt or Celtic sea salt is his dosage for 2 days.

He leaves that remineralized and slightly alkalized distilled water bottle (BPA-free) in the fridge. This remineralized distilled water would be enough for him for 2 days.

Figure 17.9  Hassle-free remineralization of the purified water.

# EXAMPLE 2  HASSLE-FREE REMINERALIZATION OF THE PURIFIED WATER

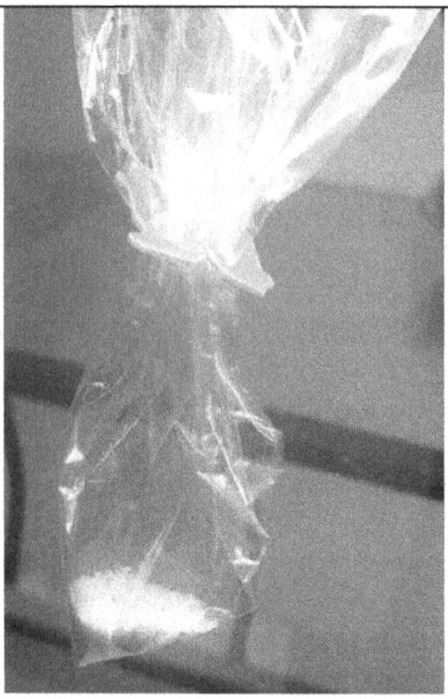

By using a 1/16 Teaspoon, about 0.40 g (400 mg) of Himalayan pink salt is placed in a sandwich bag, and safely kept in the kitchen drawer.

This pink salt would be enough for one person to remineralize 2 liters (8 cups) of the purified water for a day.

A person should drink at least 8 cups or 2 liters of purified water per day.

A TDS level of 200 ppm or 200 mg/L in drinking water is considered safe and healthy. So if you drink 8 cups or 2 liters of purified water per day, you should add 400 mg of Himalayan pink salt or Celtic sea salt to purified water.

1/16 Teaspoon = 0.36 g (360 mg)
A little over 360 mg would be equal to 400 mg.

AN EXAMPLE: When Maria gets up early in the morning, by using a 1/16 Teaspoon, she puts a little over 360 mg of Himalayan pink salt (which is close to 400 mg) in a sandwich bag, closes the bag firmly, and leaves it in her kitchen drawer.

Whenever she drinks the purified water, during the day (during 24-hour period), she adds a pinch of Himalayan pink salt from the sandwich bag to her cup of water. She does that several times a day until she finishes all that salt in that sandwich bag in a day. That is her daily dosage of Himalayan pink salt (400 mg of Himalayan pink salt per 8 cups of the purified water per day). She also adds a few kernels of baking soda so that pH would be close to 7. She drinks remineralized and slightly alkalized purified water every day that has a TDS level of approximately 200 ppm.

Figure 17.10  Hassle-free remineralization of the purified water.

# EXAMPLE 3  HASSLE-FREE REMINERALIZATION OF THE PURIFIED WATER

| RO Water in a 4 Liter BPA-Free Bottle. | RO Water in a 4 Liter BPA-Free Bottle. | RO Water in a 4 Liter BPA-Free Bottle. |
|---|---|---|

An adult should drink at least 8 cups or 2 liters of purified water per day. If there are 5 adults in a family, they would drink 10 liters.

A TDS level of 200 ppm or 200 mg/L in drinking water is considered safe and healthy.
If there are 5 adults living in a family, it would require 1000 mg (5 x 200 mg = 1000 mg = 1 g) of Himalayan pink salt or Celtic sea salt to remineralize the purified water.

AN EXAMPLE: Robert lives in a family of 5 adults, and they all drink only remineralized RO water every day. When Robert gets up in the morning, he weighs precisely 1 g (1000 mg) of Himalayan pink salt or Celtic sea salt using a digital kitchen scale, and adds it to 10 liters of RO water in a stainless steel container (stockpot), mixes thoroughly until the salt is dissolved perfectly. He also adds a few kernels of baking soda so that pH would be close to 7. He then transfers this remineralized and slightly alkalized RO water into two-and-half 4-Liter BPA-free water bottles, and leaves them in the fridge.

This remineralized and slightly alkalized RO water with a TDS level of 200 ppm would be enough for a family of 5 people for a day.

If Robert wants to reduce the TDS level to 100 ppm, he would add 500 mg of Himalayan pink salt to 10 liters of purified water. He can maintain any desired level of TDS in drinking water.

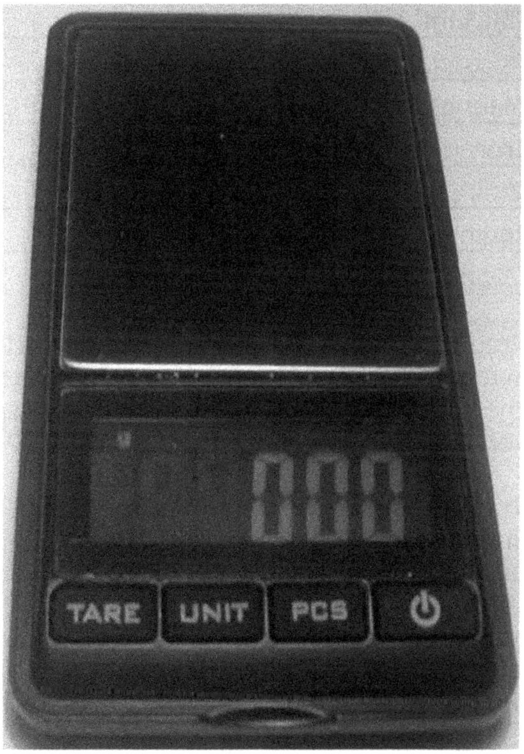

**Accu Weight** Digital Kitchen Scale. Ultra Fine 0.01 g (0.001 oz) Increments!

Figure 17.11  Hassle-free remineralization of the purified water.

# MOST COMMONLY ASKED QUESTION

The nagging question on everyone's mind could be "Are we getting all those essential minerals that our bodies need" through remineralizing the drinking water"? The straight answer has to be a resounding NO.

We are remineralizing the purified water to comply with the WHO's recommendation and requirement to convert purified water into mineral water. Our goal of remineralization like many think and believe mistakenly is not to consume essential minerals that our bodies require through drinking remineralized purified water. As a matter of fact, the mineral concentrations in Himalayan pink salt, Celtic sea salt are so minute that you would never be able to meet the RDA (Recommended Daily Allowance) standards. The RDA standards for minerals are as follows:

According to Dr. Willem Serfontein, an adult human body requires the following daily consumption of minerals through consuming foods: [41, 42]

Table 17.13 RDA (Recommended Daily Allowance) of typical minerals for a human body.

| Nutrient | Daily Requirement |
|---|---|
| Calcium | 800 mg |
| Phosphorous | 800 mg |
| Magnesium | 300 mg |
| Iron | 14 mg |
| Zinc | 15 mg |
| Iodine | 150 µg |
| Copper | 2 mg |

If you examine all the mineral water bottles being sold in supermarkets, all of those bottles have extremely low mineral content. And that bottled mineral water being sold in supermarkets does not contain 84 to 88 trace minerals like Himalayan pink salt has. Even the Celtic sea salt has more than 70 trace minerals.

For example Himalayan pink salt contains the following extremely low concentrations of minerals:
Calcium      4.05 g/Kg
Magnesium    0.16 g/Kg
Potassium    3.5 g/Kg
Iron         38.9 ppm (mg/Kg)
Sodium       382 g/Kg or 382 mg/g

Compared to the RDA (Recommended Daily Allowance) standards, these levels of mineral concentrations in Himalayan pink salt are negligibly low. There is no way that we can consume 800 mg of calcium, 800 mg of phosphorous, 300 mg of magnesium, etc. from consuming mineral water. If we try to do so, it would tremendously increase TDS level in drinking water, which could jeopardize the people's health. Extremely high TDS level in drinking water is harmful to health, as it negatively influences on kidneys. Howsoever, please bear in mind that the drinking water has no role on the RDA (Recommended Daily Allowance) standards on minerals. You should take multivitamins (supplements) so that your body would get sufficient vitamins and minerals.

## WHAT IS THE GOAL OF REMINERALIZATION OF PURIFIED WATER AFTER ALL?

Dr. Frantisek Kozisek, MD, PhD, whose research paper was endorsed by World Health Organization (WHO), published a paper scaring the consumers that demineralized water or low-TDS water leaches minerals from the body's cells and is potentially harmful to health. [43, 44, 45]

In order to combat this situation, if we can incorporate some trace amounts of minerals into the purified water or demineralized water we drink, the driving force to leach minerals from the body's cells can be avoided or at least minimized. If Dr. Frantisek Kozisek's research results were true, as there are no minerals at all in the demineralized water we drink, the minerals from the body's cells could have been forced to leach out due to the infinitely high driving force of mass transfer phenomenon that takes place between the body's cells and the demineralized water present in the body. Mass transfer takes place from higher concentration to lower concentration, and if the concentration gradient is infinite due to zero concentration in demineralized water, the driving force reaches an infinitely high value, thereby forcing the minerals to leach out from the body's cells. It is believed that this process of leaching minerals from body's cells to demineralized water present in the body can be either minimized or completely offset by incorporating some trace amounts of diversified minerals into the purified water that we wish to drink to protect our health from contaminants. This can be accomplished by remineralizing the purified water with the natural Himalayan pink salt or Celtic sea salt, which contain both macrominerals such as calcium and chloride, as well as very many diversified trace minerals (there are up to 88 trace minerals in Himalayan pink salt) including iron and zinc.

**How About Spring Water?** This aspect has been discussed earlier. As far as the spring water is concerned, Dr. RK shows in Chapter 8 through his experimental findings and scientific calculations that the mineral composition of spring water being sold in the supermarkets is not significant enough due to the depletion of the aquifer from which the spring water is being collected by distributors. But consumers never observed this scientific fact, and this tradition of selling and drinking spring water in supermarkets has been going on for decades. Many people like and drink spring water mostly based on the tradition and belief that the spring water has a wide spectrum of mineral composition and drink it because of its taste and natural occurrence, but there is no guarantee that spring water has no harmful chemicals and impurities in it. Our goal should be to drink the purified water that is one 100% free of contaminants.

**BOTTOM LINE:** By remineralizing the purified water (distilled water or RO water), we are simply mimicking and producing our own mineral water at home, similar to the bottled mineral water being sold in all supermarkets, but we are doing it without swallowing those dangerous contaminants. This book has repeatedly reminded that "bottled mineral water" being sold in supermarkets is made from tap water by adding artificial vitamins and minerals, and the investigative research teams proved time and time again that the bottled mineral water is highly contaminated and is extremely harmful to health, and so it is untrustworthy.

We are therefore making our own mineral water, which is one 100% pure and free of all contaminants, and one 100% safe to drink every day.

# RECOMMENDATIONS ON REMINERALIZATION (by Dr. RK)
[Remineralization of Purified Water Using Himalayan Pink Salt Or Celtic Sea Salt]

## 1. TRY TO UNDERSTAND THE MEANING OF PPM CONCEPTUALLY
The "PPM" is expressed in mg/L

$$PPM = \frac{1\ part}{1\ million\ parts} = \frac{1\ part}{1,000,000\ parts} = \frac{1\ mg}{1,000,000\ mg} = \frac{1\ mg}{1\ kg} = \frac{1\ mg\ (solids)}{1\ L\ (water)}$$

Table 17.14 How to remineralize the purified water (Just follow these hints).

| Desired TDS Level | How to Remineralize Purified Water |
|---|---|
| 10 ppm | If you want to drink purified water with TDS=10, then add 10 mg of Himalayan pink salt or Celtic sea salt to 1 liter of purified water. |
| 20 ppm | If you want to drink purified water with TDS=20, then add 20 mg of Himalayan pink salt or Celtic sea salt to 1 liter of purified water. |
| 30 ppm | If you want to drink purified water with TDS=30, then add 30 mg of Himalayan pink salt or Celtic sea salt to 1 liter of purified water. |
| 50 ppm | If you want to drink purified water with TDS=50, then add 50 mg of Himalayan pink salt or Celtic sea salt to 1 liter of purified water. |
| 100 ppm | If you want to drink purified water with TDS=100, then add 100 mg of Himalayan pink salt or Celtic sea salt to 1 liter of purified water, or add 200 mg to 2 liters of purified water. |
| 200 ppm | If you want to drink purified water with TDS=200, then add 200 mg of Himalayan pink salt or Celtic sea salt to 1 liter of purified water, or add 400 mg to 2 liters of purified water. |

 An adult should drink at least 8 cups or 2 liters of purified water per day. Therefore you double the amount of Himalayan pink salt or Celtic sea salt when you remineralize 2 liters of purified water. For example, if you want to maintain a TDS level of 200 ppm in 2 liters of purified water, then you add 400 mg of Himalayan pink salt or Celtic sea salt to 2 liters of purified water. You can do this by using a digital kitchen scale that allows 0.01 gm (10 mg) increments.

## 2. THE RECOMMENDED TDS LEVEL IN DRINKING WATER IS UP TO 200 PPM:
 A TDS level of greater than 500 ppm in daily drinking water (a lay person's recommendation as mentioned earlier) is dangerously high due to severe sodium content, and therefore it should be avoided.

 In the worst case scenario, a person could go to the maximum of 500 ppm. However, if you drink water with a TDS level of 500 ppm or higher daily, you are risking yourself, could face long-term health consequences, and you could be putting your health in jeopardy.

 A TDS level of "10 ppm to 200 ppm" suits most people. Each person is different as some people like more salts in drinking water than others. So each person should research on his/her body, and find out the suitable TDS level. A TDS level of approximately 10 ppm, 20 ppm, 30 ppm, 40 ppm, 50 ppm, 100 ppm, or 200 ppm is being recommended. Different people choose different levels. At least 10 ppm of salts should be there in drinking water in order to prevent any leaching effect.

🖎 For example, in Vancouver, British Columbia, Canada, the tap water has a TDS level of 11 ppm to 16 ppm. In USA, the tap water TDS varies from 50 ppm to 300 ppm or even more depending on the city. This book recommends that you should not drink tap water.

## 3. PRACTICE REMINERALIZATION EXPERIMENTS AT HOME
🖎 Please practice remineralization experiments for a few weeks until you master all the concepts discussed in this chapter. Please do not use teaspoons right from the first day to simplify your responsibility of remineralization. You should learn how to use the TDS meter, digital kitchen scale, and learn how to add the precise amount of measured Himalayan pink salt or Celtic sea salt to purified water. And learn how to calculate the concentration of the salt in ppm or mg/L in the remineralized purified water. You should be able to adjust and maintain any TDS level you wish in drinking water.

🖎 After learning everything, you can use Teaspoons to simplify the remineralization method. However every now and then, once every week or once every month, you should use your TDS meter and monitor TDS level of your drinking water, and make sure that everything is going well (make sure that the TDS level is below 200 ppm)!

🖎 You should make sure that you never remineralize the purified water by adding too much Himalayan pink salt. Every now and then, you should test your remineralized water using a TDS meter, and make sure it is under 200 ppm. Worls Health Organization recommended the maximum TDS is 500 ppm. Always make sure you never reach that 500 ppm limit.

## 4. CONCENTRACE MINERAL DROPS WOULD SIMULTANEOUSLY REMINERALIZE AND ALKALIZE THE PURIFIED WATER
🖎 "Remineralizatiion of the purified water using ConcenTrace mineral drops" is discussed with experiments in the next section of this chapter. If you decided to use the ConcenTrace mineral drops, you should not use Himalayan pink salt or Celtic sea salt because the ConcenTrace mineral drops increase both the TDS level (close to or more than 200 ppm) and pH in your drinking water. If you further add Himalayan pink salt or Celtic sea salt to your drinking water, the TDS level will be elevated to a dangerous level. So you should take a decision weather you want to use the Himalyan pink salt, Celtic sea salt, or the ConcenTrace mineral drops. It is important to note that ConcenTrace mineral drops would simultaneously remineralize and alkalize the purified water at home.

🖎 Please always bear in mind that Himalayan pink salt and Celtic sea salt increase the TDS level, but do not increase the pH (we cannot use them to alkalize purified water), whereas ConcenTrace mineral drops increase the TDS level as well as pH if dissolved in purified water.

## 5. HIGH SODIUM CONSUMPTION IS DANGEROUS
🖎 It is warned not to consume too much Himalayan pink salt and/or Celtic sea salt because of their high sodium content. The upper limit of sodium consumption is 2,300 milligrams for healthy adults and 1,500 milligrams for adults with a history of heart disease, who are over 51 years old or are belong to African-American race.

🖎 High sodium consumption beyond the RDA (Recommended Daily Allowance) can lead to atherosclerosis, heart disease, high blood pressure (hypertension), high cholesterol levels, kidney stones and kidney disease, osteoporosis, Menierre's Syndrome (ear ringing), insomnia, motion sickness, asthma, and also a variety of cancers. [37, 38]

Himalayan pink salt has 420 mg of sodium per gram.
Celtic sea salt has 386 mg of sodium per gram.

1 Teaspoon = 5.68 g
The sodium in 1 Teaspoon of Himalayan pink salt = 5.69 x 420 mg = 2389 mg.
The sodium in 1 Teaspoon of Celtic pink salt = 5.69 x 386 mg = 2196 mg.
Compare those values with the RDA (Recommended Daily Allowance) of 2,300 mg, and learn your lesson.

• If you maintain a TDS level at 200 ppm in drinking water in 2 liters (8 cups) of purified water you drink, you would be consuming 400 mg of Himalayan pink salt or Celtic sea salt per day.

The sodium content in 400 mg of Himalayan pink salt = (420/1000)(400) =168 mg
The sodium content in 400 mg of Celtic sea salt = (386/1000)(400) =154.4 mg
So the sodium intake would be very little if you maintain and stick to a TDS level of 200 ppm in the drinking water.

• Every person consumes sodium from all kinds of foods he/she consumes throughout the day. In addition, if a person consumes 1 Teaspoon of Himalayan pink salt or Celtic sea salt every day, he/she would be skyrocketing the sodium consumption, which could lead to serious health issues. Always keep an eye on sodium consumption whatever you consume.

## 6. DANGEROUSLY HIGH TDS LEVEL IS NOT RECOMMENDED
You can find several articles on the Internet on drinking water guidelines with regards to "How Much Himalayan Pink Salt or Celtic Sea Salt Should be Added to Drinking Water".

• The following lay person's suggestion (without any scientific calculations) is very commonly found: "Add half a teaspoon of unprocessed and unrefined Himalayan pink salt or or Celtic sea salt to a gallon of purified water or tap water to improve the TDS (Total Dissolved Solids).

If you follow this suggestion and drink remineralized water daily, you would be consuming Way Too Much Sodium! Please do not follow this lay person's suggestion. Here is more explanation:

1Teaspoon = 5.67 g = 5670 mg
1/2 Teaspoon = 2.84 g = 2840 mg          1 Gallon = 3.78 Liters = 15 Cups

If you add 2840 mg of Himalayan pink salt or Celtic sea salt to 1 gallon (3.78 liters) of purified water, the TDS level = (2840/3.87) = 751 mg/L = 751 ppm.

That 751 ppm of TDS level in drinking water is too much. It will have devastating long-term side effects. So please be careful!

# NEXT SECTION

# CONCENTRACE MINERAL DROPS

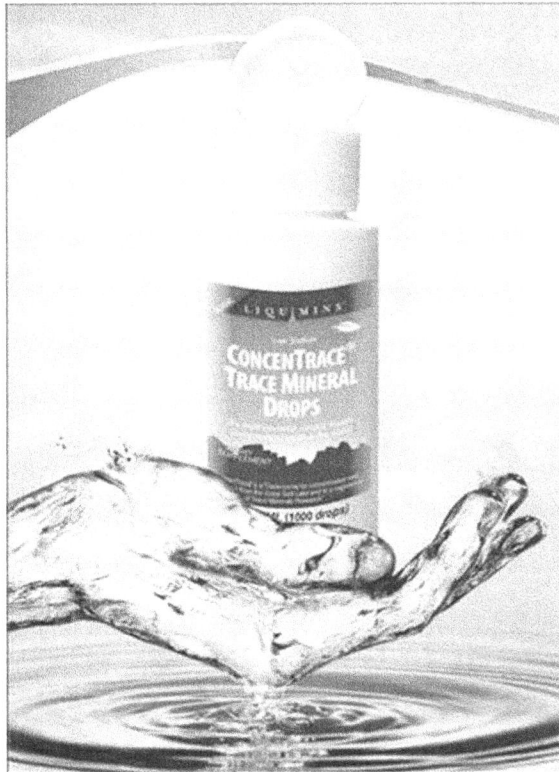

## ABOUT CONCENTRACE MINERAL DROPS [50, 51, 52, 53, 54, 55]

The most famous Utah's Great Salt Lake contains every known healthy element (mineral) known to mankind. The Great Salt Lake is located in the northern part of the state of Utah in the United States of America (USA). It is the largest salt water lake in the Western Hemisphere, and the eighth-largest terminal lake in the world. In an average year the lake covers an area of around 1,700 square miles (4,400 km$^2$), but the size of the lake fluctuates substantially due to its shallowness as the seasons change.

In today's continuously and rapidly changing fast-paced society, supplying our bodies with the minerals they require is not easy. Many of the plant-based foods we eat are grown in minerally deficient soil as the same soil is used repeatedly over and over again. In addition, modern food processing techniques further strip away important minerals like iron, calcium, magnesium, potassium and boron that play key roles in our health. It could be true that you may be eating a perfectly balanced diet and still could be deficient in minerals and trace minerals. Supplementing your diet with ConcenTrace drops can replenish your body with the important nutrients that your body might be lacking. Many people believe that the natural product ConcenTrace, available in the market today, is a liquid mineral supplement concentrated and balanced for greater energy, vitality and well-being.

These minerals are naturally occurring in almost the exact ratios as the major fluids of our own bodies and are the very same as were once found in our soils, but are now depleted. Just like the minerals found in the liquids of fresh fruits, vegetables and teas, the minerals in ConcenTrace are naturally ionic, which means that each independent element is either positively or negatively charged. This is extremely important for absorption since the body uses positive and negative charges to attract elements into the receptor cells present in the villi of the intestine. No other mineral supplement could possibly surpass the ionic mineral saturation of ConcenTrace and still remain in solution. At supersaturation ConcenTrace is in a class by itself. Elements in their ionic form are necessary each time for all of the trillions of cells in our body metabolize energy. Ionic elements are also vital for every electrical brain impulse or healthy nerve transmission. Only ionic minerals will combine to form energetic crystals. Trace minerals present in ConcenTrace drops provide the vitality and energy, vitamin assimilation, muscle, bone, joint and internal organ health, nerve transformation, enzyme function, emotional balance, and help maintain good memory and concentration.

The ConcenTrace is a naturally harvested supersaturated liquid mineral and trace mineral supplement from Utah's Great Salt Lake. It takes 2 years of concentration, through solar evaporation, to produce this product ConcenTrace drops. As the beneficial minerals are concentrated, the sodium chloride naturally forms crystals and precipitates out (99% sodium removed). ConcenTrace is 100% pure and nothing is added to it. The mineral drops of ConcenTrace is safe for the whole family, even for your pets and plants. So far up to 84 minerals (most of them are trace minerals) were identified, analysed and verified, but the certificate of analysis shows only 72 or 73 trace minerals.

## Advantages of ConcenTrace Mineral Drops [51, 52, 53]

● ConcenTrace mineral drops instantly dissolve and alkalize (pH goes up right away) purified water. Adding these trace minerals to drinking water energizes the body, improves the TDS (total dissolved solids) value and alkalinity (pH) of the water. Trace minerals are the catalysts for vitamins and other nutrients your body uses for promoting and maintaining healthy energy levels in your body by providing your body's entire electrical system with the minerals it needs to function properly.

● Your body needs minerals, especially if your daily calorie intake is not substantial enough. Mostly older people don't eat enough food every day, don't get enough vitamins and minerals necessary, and so they need to supplement their diet with high-quality multivitamins and minerals. If you are living in a hot climate, you sweat too much, your body loses minerals through sweat and urine, and you need to replace the lost minerals as often as possible throughout the day by drinking mineralized water. The primary minerals that your body needs to replenish on a daily basis are calcium, magnesium, potassium and salt (sodium), though there are many other trace minerals your body needs.

• Remineralized water quenches thirst better and is absorbed by your body faster. This is a point of contention but the argument for faster hydration states that adding minerals back into the water boosts the pH and brings it back to an alkaline state. The water becomes ionized, which makes the water molecules cluster into smaller groups, which makes it easier for your body to absorb.

• Remineralized water tastes better. Though this is subjective, it's true that the human palate is used to the flavor of water with minerals in it. It gives it a fuller flavor (that is to say, it gives favorable flavor) that many people find it preferable adding trace minerals to RO water or distilled water.

• Bones and Joints: Taken as directed, many people have stated they have experienced dramatic results in improving and strengthening bones and joints and teeth. ConcenTrace drops contain relatively higher amounts of magnesium, an essential mineral, which works closely with calcium in building and maintaining strong and healthy bones and joints.

• ConcenTace drops are available of premium quality, highly concentrated for 2 years, least expensive, all natural, nothing added to it, GRAS (generally recognized as safe), water soluble, low in sodium, easy to assimilate, exists in electrolyte form as liquid ionic supplement, no artificial colors, flavors, preservatives, contains no artificial ingredients whatsoever, and gives more energy, suitable for everyone, especially the young, sick , bed-reddened, and those on liquid diet, it is versatile, goes with everything and it is good for everyone, just add a few drops to drinking water, juices, coffee, tea, and you can also add to your cooking pot so that vegitables won't leach the minerals.

▶ However, World Health Organization (WHO) states that "drinking water provides less than 5% of total mineral intake necessary for the body". These elements include iron, zinc, copper, iodine, phosphorus and chloride among others. So if you think you have mineral deficiency, and if you are not getting sufficient calories from the food being consumed, you should supplement your diet with high-quality multivitamins and minerals such as calcium, magnesium, potassium, and others. ConcenTace drops contain only trace minerals (except magnesium). Drinking remineralized water alone would not take care of your body's mineral balance, but it protects you from leaching minerals from body's cells.

## TOP TWO CONCENTRACE BRANDS [54, 55, 56, 57, 58]
There are two famous brand names of ConcenTrace mineral drops, being manufactured and marketed today:
(i) Anderson's Health Solutions, Mineral Resources Int, Salt Lake City, Utah, USA
https://www.mineralresourcesint.com/
https://www.mineralresourcesint.com/international

(ii) Trace Minerals Research, Salt Lake City, Utah, USA
https://traceminerals.com/utah-sea-minerals/
https://traceminerals.com/ConcenTrace-trace-mineral-drops/

The Anderson's family of Anderson's Health Solutions has been harvesting this ConcenTrace mineral drops product since 1969. Originally both "Anderson's Health Solutions" and "Trace Minerals Research" used to be business partners and worked together, but later separated into two independent companied. These two companies went through long disputes and legal battles. Trace Minerals Research, Salt Lake City, Utah, USA moved forward, and started selling their own product of ConcenTrace drops, which became more famous than Anderson's. You can find 1000's of reviews on Amazon.com.

Trace Mineral Research - ConcenTrace Trace Mineral Drops, 8 Oz, There are more than 1240 Reviews on Amazon.com in August 2018.
https://www.amazon.com/Trace-Minerals-Research-ConcenTrace-Mineral/dp/B000AMUWLK/ref=sr_1_1_a_it?ie=UTF8&qid=1534103659&sr=8-1&keywords=ConcenTrace%C2%AE%2BTrace%2BMineral%2BDrops&th=1

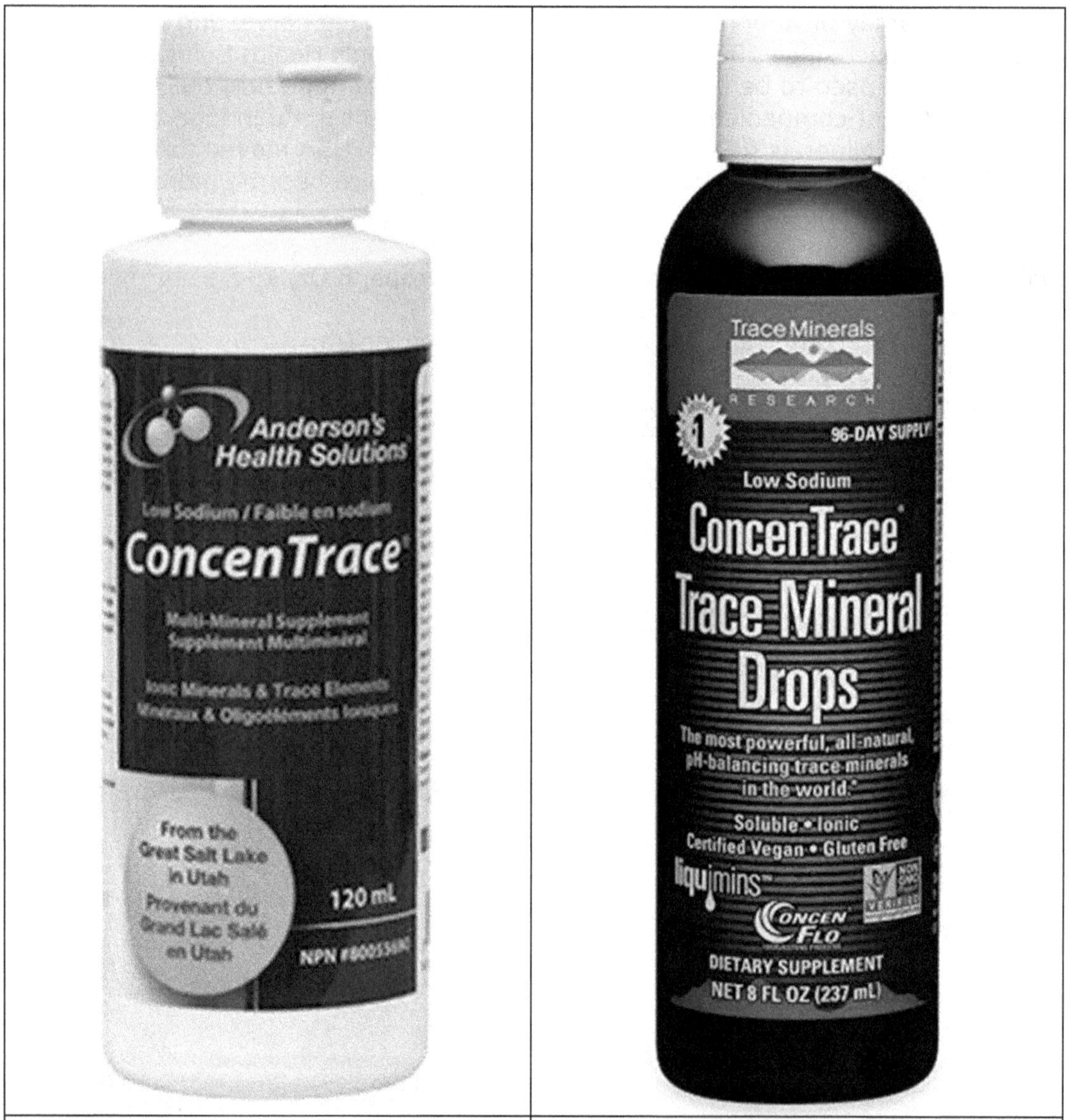

| Courtesy of Anderson's Health Solutions | Courtesy of Trace Minerals Research |

Figure 17.12 ConcenTrace mineral drops instantly dissolve in purified water, remineralize (TDS goes up), and alkalize (pH goes up right away) the purified water.

**List of 72 Minerals and Trace Minerals Present in Utah Sea Minerals™:** [56]
Aluminum, Antimony, **Arsenic (Inorganic)**, Barium, Beryllium, Bismuth, Boron, Bromide, Cadmium, Calcium, Carbonate, Cerium, Cesium, Chloride, Chromium, Cobalt, Copper, Dysprosium, Erbium, Europium, Fluoride, Gadolinium, Gallium, Gold, Hafnium, Holmium, Indium, Iodine, Iridium, Iron, Lanthanum, Lead, Lithium, Lutetium, Magnesium, Manganese, Mercury, Molybdenum, Neodymium, Nickel, Niobium, Osmium, Palladium, Phosphorus, Platinum, Potassium, Praseodymium, Rhenium, Rhodium, Rubidium, Ruthenium, Samarium, Scandium, Selenium, Silicon, Silver, Sodium, Strontium, Sulfate/Sulfur, Tantalum, Tellurium, Terbium ,Thallium, Thorium, Thulium, Tin, Titanium, Tungsten, Vanadium, Ytterbium, Yttrium, Zinc, Zirconium, plus other naturally-occurring trace minerals found in seawater.

# CHEMICAL ANALYSIS REPORT OF CONCENTRACE MINERAL DROPS

Anderson's Health Solutions, Salt Lake City, Utah, USA currently does not have chemical analysis report from a certified laboratory, and therefore their product is untrustworthy unless and until they provide chemical analysis report to consumers. The other company "Trace Minerals Research, Salt Lake City, Utah, USA" promptly provided the chemical analysis report from a certified laboratory, and there are 73 trace minerals in it as shown below:

Table 17.15 ConcenTrace Drops from Trace Minerals Research Certificate of Analysis.
Courtesy of Monnol (A Distribution Company in Canada)

| No | Element | Conc (mg/mL) | Conc (mg/L) | | No | Element | Conc (mg/mL) | Conc (mg/L) |
|---|---|---|---|---|---|---|---|---|
| 1 | Magnesium | 104.8 | 104800 | | 38 | Gold | 0.00004 | 0.04 |
| 2 | Chloride | 310.2 | 310200 | | 39 | Nickel | 0.00004 | 0.04 |
| 3 | Sulfate | 19.61 | 19610 | | 40 | Cobalt | 0.000018 | 0.018 |
| 4 | Sodium | 3.9 | 3900 | | 41 | Gallium | 0.000017 | 0.017 |
| 5 | Potassium | 1.3 | 1300 | | 42 | Lead | 0.000017 | 0.017 |
| 6 | Boron | 0.64 | 640 | | 43 | Tantalum | 0.000016 | 0.016 |
| 7 | Lithium | 0.638 | 638 | | 44 | Thallium | 0.000014 | 0.014 |
| 8 | Calcium | 0.0575 | 57.5 | | 45 | Rhenium | 0.000013 | 0.013 |
| 9 | Iodine | 0.014 | 14.0 | | 46 | Osmium | 0.000011 | 0.011 |
| 10 | Aluminum | 0.0077 | 7.7 | | 47 | Bismuth | 0.00001 | 0.01 |
| 11 | Phosphorus | 0.0075 | 7.5 | | 48 | Tin | 0.000008 | 0.008 |
| 12 | Fluoride | 0.004 | 4.0 | | 49 | Mercury | 0.000008 | 0.008 |
| 13 | Silicon | 0.0037 | 3.7 | | 50 | Platinum | 0.000007 | 0.007 |
| 14 | Zinc | 0.0031 | 3.1 | | 51 | Cerium | 0.000005 | 0.005 |
| 15 | Titanium | 0.0025 | 2.5 | | 52 | Ruthenium | 0.000005 | 0.005 |
| 16 | Vanadium | 0.0019 | 1.9 | | 53 | Lanthanum | 0.000004 | 0.004 |
| 17 | Zirconium | 0.0015 | 1.5 | | 54 | Palladium | 0.000004 | 0.004 |
| 18 | Rubidium | 0.001 | 1.0 | | 55 | Yttrium | 0.000004 | 0.004 |
| 19 | Copper | 0.0009 | 0.9 | | 56 | Neodymium | 0.000002 | 0.002 |
| 20 | Strontium | 0.0008 | 0.8 | | 57 | Cadmium | 0.000002 | 0.002 |
| 21 | **Arsenic** | 0.00055 | 0.55 | | 58 | Berylium | 0.000003 | 0.003 |
| 22 | Iron | 0.00058 | 0.58 | | 59 | Dysprosium | 0.000001 | 0.001 |
| 23 | Selenium | 0.00048 | 0.48 | | 60 | Erbium | 0.000001 | 0.001 |
| 24 | Thorium | 0.00048 | 0.48 | | 61 | Europium | 0.000001 | 0.001 |
| 25 | Molybdenum | 0.00045 | 0.45 | | 62 | Gadolinium | 0.000001 | 0.001 |
| 26 | Chromium | 0.00044 | 0.44 | | 63 | Germanium | 0.000001 | 0.001 |
| 27 | Antimony | 0.00042 | 0.42 | | 64 | Holmium | 0.000001 | 0.001 |
| 28 | Tungsten | 0.00034 | 0.34 | | 65 | Indium | 0.000001 | 0.001 |
| 29 | Scandium | 0.00033 | 0.33 | | 66 | Iridium | 0.000001 | 0.001 |
| 30 | Niobium | 0.00029 | 0.29 | | 67 | Lutetium | 0.000001 | 0.001 |
| 31 | Manganese | 0.00029 | 0.29 | | 68 | Praseodymium | 0.000001 | 0.001 |
| 32 | Silver | 0.00019 | 0.19 | | 69 | Rhodium | 0.000001 | 0.001 |
| 33 | Tellurium | 0.00016 | 0.16 | | 70 | Samarium | 0.000001 | 0.001 |
| 34 | Barium | 0.00013 | 0.13 | | 71 | Terbium | 0.000001 | 0.001 |
| 35 | Bromide | 0.00012 | 0.12 | | 72 | Thulium | 0.000001 | 0.001 |
| 36 | Cesium | 0.00012 | 0.12 | | 73 | Ytterbium | 0.000001 | 0.001 |
| 37 | Hafnium | 0.000053 | 0.053 | | | **Total (TDS)** | 0.000223 | 0.2230 |

# WARNING: BEWARE OF ARSENIC IN CONCENTRACE!
## THE PRODUCT "CONCENTRACE DROPS" HAS ARSENIC IN IT!

You should be very careful when you add mineral drops as this product contains arsenic in it, and do not exceed daily limit of mineral drops being added to your drinking water. You should exercise more caution when children and pregnant women are consuming these mineral drops. See below for more details.

## World Health Organization Posted the Following Information [59]

**IMPORTANT NOTE:** World Health Organization recommends intake of arsenic at levels no higher than 0.01 ppm.

Arsenic is a metalloid element, which forms a number of poisonous compounds. It is widely distributed throughout the Earth's crust, and is found in groundwater supplies in a number of countries. Soluble inorganic arsenic is acutely toxic. Intake of inorganic arsenic over a long period can lead to chronic arsenic poisoning (arsenicosis). Effects, which can take years to develop depending on the exposure level, include skin lesions, peripheral neuropathy, diabetes, cardiovascular diseases, and cancer.

Organic arsenic compounds, which are abundant in seafood, are less harmful to health, and are rapidly eliminated by the body. However human exposure to elevated levels of inorganic arsenic occurs mainly through the consumption of groundwater containing naturally high levels of inorganic arsenic, food prepared with this water, and food crops irrigated with high arsenic water sources. In one estimate, arsenic-contaminated drinking-water in Bangladesh alone was attributed 9,100 deaths.

Reduction in human exposure to arsenic can be achieved by screening of drinking-water supplies, clearly identifying those delivering water above the WHO guideline 10 micrograms arsenic per liter (0.01 mg/L or ppm) or national permissible limits, together with awareness-raising campaigns. Mitigation options include use of alternative groundwater sources, use of microbiologically safe surface water (e.g. rainwater harvesting), use of arsenic removal technologies, or dilution of high content arsenic source water with lower arsenic content source water that is microbially safe.

# HOW TO TEST THE DROPPER
## AND MAKE SURE IT IS CORRECTLY DESIGNED (by Dr. RK)?

If you use ConcenTrace mineral drops, you should learn how to test the dropper of the ConcenTrace bottle you purchased, and find out if it is properly working or not. If the dropper doesn't work correctly (not dropping the precise amount of ConcenTrace per each drop), everything will go wrong, and you may end up consuming inaccurate or dangerously excessive amount of arsenic through your water. See below to learn how to do this.

1 Fluid Ounce = 591.47 drops (this is the scientific definition)
I Fluid Ounce = 29.57 mL
1 mL = (1/29.57) Fluid Ounce = 0.0338 Fluid Ounce
1 Liter = 1000 mL = 33.81 Ounces

1 Cup = 8 Fluid Ounces = (8)(29.57) = 236.56 mL
1 Cup = (8)(591.47) = 4731.76 drops

I have just verified the definition "1 Fluid Ounce = 591.47 drops" by doing the following experiment: I purchased some measuring spoons in the pharmacy.
One small measuring Teaspoon is marked "¼ Teaspoon or 1.25 mL"
So for 1.25 mL of ConcenTrace, I calculated the number of drops.

1 mL = 0.0338 Fluid Ounce = (0.0338)(591.47) drops = 20 drops
1.25 mL = 25 drops          ( ¼ Teaspoon = 1.25 mL Teaspoon )

Then, I added 25 drops of ConcenTrace into the "¼ Teaspoon" or "1.25 mL Teaspoon", and that "¼ Teaspoon" was filled perfectly with 25 drops.

**That means the dropper was correctly designed.** If the dropper is not working, everything will go wrong, and I would be consuming inaccurate amount of ConcenTrace drops. From my calculations, I can confirm that I can use the dropper confidently whenever I add ConcenTrace drops to the distilled water or RO water whenever I make my own "mineral water". I should do this test every time I purchase a new bottle.

## HOW TO CALCULATE THE MAXIMUM NUMBER OF DROPS TO AVOID ARSENIC POISON (by Dr. RK)?

Because arsenic is present in concentrate drops, it is important to understand the upper limit of concentrate drops (maximum) that can be consumed. An 8-ounce bottle of trace mineral drops (see the picture below) is the natural mineral concentrate, ultra-concentrated, extracted from the waters of Utah's Inland Sea, the Great Salt Lake, Utah, USA. About 40 drops ConcenTrace equivalent to the mineral content of 1/2 cup sea water with 99% sodium removed and provides with a wide spectrum of health benefits to the consumers (contains only 5 mg of sodium per serving).

World Health Organization recommends intake of arsenic at levels no higher than 0.01 ppm or mg/L. So it is important that you should learn how to calculate the maximum number of ConcenTrace drops a person can consume per day so that you can protect yourself from exceeding the daily limit of arsenic (0.01 ppm). See below to learn how to calculate this.

Trace Minerals Research company emailed the mineral analysis results of their product ConcenTrace to Dr. RK. And Dr. RK made the following calculations to find out the maximum number of drops to be consumed to protect from arsenic poisoning.
Arsenic concentration in ConcenTrace product (from analysis) = 0.55 ppm or mg/L.

We know the following formula from the laws of physics and/or chemistry:
$(C1)(V1) = (C2)(V2)$
$C1$ = Concentration of Arsenic in the ConcenTrace = 0.55 ppm or mg/L (from analysis).
$V1$ = Volume of ConcenTrace liquid drops to be added to one cup of distilled water.
$C2$ = Maximum concentration of arsenic allowed in one cup of distilled water.
  = 0.01 ppm or mg/L (According to World Health Organization).
$V2$ = Volume of the one cup of distilled water (For example, 8 Ounces).
1 Cup = 8 Fluid Ounces = 250 mL
1 Fulid Ounce = 591.47 drops
$(C1)(V1) = (C2)(V2)$
$(0.55)(V1) = (0.01)(8 \text{ Fluid Ounces})$
$V1 = (0.01)(8)/(0.55) = 0.1455 \text{ Fluid Ounce} = (0.1455)(591.47) \text{ drops} = 86.03 \text{ drops}.$
That means, the maximum you can consume is 86 drops per one cup of distilled water.

Per 1 liter (4 cups) of distilled water, number of drops = 4 x 86 = 344 drops.
Per 2 liters (8 cups) of distilled water, number of drops = 8 x 86 = 688 drops.
An adult drinks 2 liters (8 cups) of water per day. Therefore 688 drops per day.

That is the maximum. When you reach maximum, you can have arsenic poison.
So stay away from maximum, and don't even reach halfway from maximum.
Trace Minerals Research company recommends a total consumption of 40 drops per day.

## IMPORTANT NOTES

(i) Please follow the dosage instructions on the label of the Mineral ConcenTrace bottle you purchased, and do not do the above-mentioned calculations unless you know what you are doing.

(ii) You might be getting arsenic from other liquids and foods you consume daily here and there, now and then, so you should take that into consideration, and stay as far away as possible from maximum limit of arsenic consumption (consume 10 times less than the maximum to be on the safe side).

(iii) **VERY IMPORTANT (HIGH IN MAGNESIUM):** There is significant amount of magnesium in Mineral ConcenTrace drops (105 mg/mL). You should take this amount of magnesium into consideration, and adjust the daily dosage if you have magnesium deficiency and if you are taking magnesium supplements. Or you may be overdosed by magnesium and may suffer from diarrhea and/or chronic gas in bowels.

## HOW TO REMINERALIZE AND ALKALIZE THE PURIFIED WATER WITH CONCENTRACE MINERAL DROPS?
## EXPERIMENTS CONDUCTED AT HOME

Dr. RK remineralized the purified water (both distilled water and RO water) by adding ConcenTrace mineral drops. Interestingly, Dr. RK noticed that after adding only 1 or 2 drops of ConcenTrace mineral drops to purified water, both the TDS level and pH level went up, revealing the fact that it is possible to remineralize and simultaneously alkalize the purified water by adding ConcenTrace mineral drops.

Dr. RK monitored and recorded both TDS level and pH level by increasing the number of drops. He added 2 drops of ConcenTrace mineral drops, monitored both the TDS level and pH. He then added 3 drops, and repeated the experiment. He then added 5 drops, and repeated the experiment. He then added 7 drops, and repeated the experiment until the TDS level reaches significantly higher than 200 ppm (which is the recommended TDS level).

Dr. RK conducted experiments by remineralizing and alkalizing both the distilled water and RO water. He did that by using the ConcenTrace mineral drops being distributed by two different companies "Adberson's Health Solutions" and "Trace Minerals Research". The results of his experimentation are shown below in two different tables.

Daily Maximum of ConcenTrace mineral drops recommended by both companies is 40 drops. If a person drinks 2 liters (8 cups) a day, he/she has to add 5 drops per cup. Dr. RK interpreted that it would be unnecessary to add 40 drops per day. If we add 40 drops to 2 liters (8 cups) of purified water, both TDS level and pH could be elevated. By adding approximately 20 drops to 2 liters (8 cups) of purified water, it is possible to neutralize or slightly alkalize and remineralize the purified water to a TDS level of 200 ppm (which is the recommended TDS level).

Table 17.16  Remineralization of purified water with Anderson's ConcenTrace mineral drops.

| Anderson's ConcenTrace | | |
|---|---|---|
| **Distilled Water** | | |
| ConcenTrace Drops Added | TDS (Total Dissolved Solids) | pH Measured |
| To 1 Cup (250 mL) of distilled Water | Monitored with TDS Meter | With Digital pH Meter |
| No Drops Added | 0 ppm | 6.3        (Acidic) |
| 2 Drops | 270 ppm | 7.2 (Light Green) |
| 3 Drops | 375 ppm | 7.3    (Pale Blue) |
| 5 Drops | 745 ppm | 7.6   (Light Blue) |
| 7 Drops | 838 ppm | 8.3        (Blue) |
| | | |
| **RO Water** | | |
| ConcenTrace Drops Added | TDS (Total Dissolved Solids) | pH Measured |
| To 1 Cup (250 mL) of RO  Water | Monitored with TDS Meter | With Enagic pH Drops |
| No Drops Added | 2 ppm | 6.4        (Acidic) |
| 2 Drops | 275 ppm | 7.1 (Light Green) |
| 3 Drops | 378 ppm | 7.3        (Green) |
| 5 Drops | 750 ppm | 7.5  (Light Blue) |
| 7 Drops | 842 ppm | 8.0        (Blue) |

Table 17.17 Remineralization of purified water with ConcenTrace mineral drops of Trace Minerals Research.

| Trace Mineral's ConcenTrace | | |
|---|---|---|
| **Distilled Water** | | |
| ConcenTrace Drops Added | TDS (Total Dissolved Solids) | pH Measured |
| To 1 Cup (250 mL) of distilled Water | Monitored with TDS Meter | With Digital pH Meter |
| No Drops Added | 0 ppm | 6.3        (Acidic) |
| 2 Drops | 163 ppm | 7.2 (Light Green) |
| 3 Drops | 252 ppm | 7.4    (Pale Blue) |
| 5 Drops | 425 ppm | 8.3   (Light Blue) |
| 7 Drops | 558 ppm | 8.8        (Blue) |
| | | |
| **RO Water** | | |
| ConcenTrace Drops Added | TDS (Total Dissolved Solids) | pH Measured |
| To 1 Cup (250 mL) of RO  Water | Monitored with TDS Meter | With Enagic pH Drops |
| No Drops Added | 2 ppm | 6.4        (Acidic) |
| 2 Drops | 166 ppm | 7.2 (Light Green) |
| 3 Drops | 256 ppm | 7.5        (Green) |
| 5 Drops | 422 ppm | 8.3  (Light Blue) |
| 7 Drops | 563 ppm | 8.7        (Blue) |

# THE RESULTS OF BOTH BRANDS COMPARED
# Dr. RK'S EXPERIMENTAL FINDINGS

ConcenTrace mineral drops are being manufactured and marketed by two different companies from Salt Lake City, Utah, USA.
(i) Anderson's Health Solutions, Mineral Resources Int, Salt Lake City, Utah, USA
(ii) Trace Minerals Research, Salt Lake City, Utah, USA

Both products represent the natural mineral concentrate, ultra-concentrated, extracted from the waters of Utah's Inland Sea, the Great Salt Lake, Utah, USA. Both companies recommend a daily dosage of 40 drops, which is equal to the mineral content of 1/2 cup sea water with 99% sodium removed and provides, only 5 mg of sodium per serving, with a wide spectrum of health benefits.

Dr. RK compared the TDS levels of both brands, and noticed that the Anderson's brand had much higher concentrations of minerals, and so the TDS levels were much higher. Based on these findings, the drops from Trace Minerals research are preferable because they don't raise TDS level too high (200 ppm is the recommended level), and at the same time they either neutralize or slightly alkalize the drinking water with minimal number of drops.

Table 17.18  Anderson's ConcenTrace and Trace Minerals ConcenTrace are Compared.

| ConcenTrace Drops Added to 1 Cup (250 mL) of Distilled Water | Anderson's ConcenTrace TDS (Total Dissolved Solids) Monitored with TDS Meter | Trace Minerals ConcenTrace TDS (Total Dissolved Solids) Monitored with TDS Meter |
|---|---|---|
| No Drops Added | 0 ppm | 0 ppm |
| 2 Drops | 270 ppm | 163 ppm |
| 3 Drops | 375 ppm | 252 ppm |
| 5 Drops | 745 ppm | 425 ppm |
| 7 Drops | 838 ppm | 558 ppm |

## ACCEPTABLE TDS LEVEL IN DRINKING WATER [6, 7, 8, 9, 10, 11, 12, 13]

KENT's Patented Mineral RO™ Technology has been manufacturing RO water systems that allow remineralization of purified water, to any desired TDS level, by the consumer. [60, 61]

Kent's Health Organization, a panel of tasters & health professionals proposed the following conclusions about the preferable level of TDS in drinking water:

Table 17.19  Acceptable TDS levels established by Kent's Health Organization. [10]

| TDS Level (ppm or mg/L) | Rating |
|---|---|
| 50 to 150 | Excellent! |
| 150 to 250 | Good! |
| 250 to 300 | Fair (Bad for kidneys)! |
| 300 to 500 | Poor (very bad for kidneys)! |
| Above 1200 | Unacceptable! |

# DISCUSSION AND RECOMMENDATIONS (by Dr. RK)
## [ConcenTrace Mineral Drops]

1. ConcenTrace mineral drops instantly remineralize and alkalize (pH goes up right away) the purified water (RO water, distilled water, or zero water), meaning that they increase both TDS level and pH level at the same time. Even by adding 2 drops of ConcenTrace mineral drops to a cup of purified water, we can either neutralize or slightly alkalize the purified water. We can call them "pH Booster Drops".
So go ahead and use them.

◉ Whereas the Himalayan pink salt and Celtic sea salt, though they quickly dissolve and remineralize and raise TDS level, do not alkalize the purified water (pH does not go up).

2. ConcenTrace mineral drops perfectly fit the message of this book. This book teaches that purified water that is either neutralized (pH=7) or slightly alkalized (pH=7 to 7.25), and remineralized up to a TDS (Total Dissolved Solids) level of 200 ppm is the healthy drinking water. We can obtain this kind of drinking water hassle-free by adding ConcenTrace mineral drops to purified water. ConcenTrace mineral drops from Trace Minerals Research brand suit more appropriately than Anaderson's ConcenTrace mineral drops because they don't raise the TDS level too high and interestingly they instantly raise the pH of drinking water. This is what our bodies exactly need!

3. From the experiments conducted by Dr. RK on ConcenTrace mineral drops, it can be understood that 2 drops per 1 cup of purified water (distilled water/RO water) would create a TDS level of approximately 200 ppm in drinking water.

## IMPORTANT POINTS TO KEEP IN MIND
◉ An adult must drink at least 8 cups (2 liters) of purified water, and so 16 drops of ConcenTrace mineral drops are required per day to remineralize the purified water.
◉ But the manufacturer of both brands recommend 40 drops per day. If we add 40 drops per day to 2 liters (8 cups) of drinking water, the TDS level with Anderson's ConcenTrace drops would be close to 500 ppm.
◉ If we add 40 drops per day to 2 liters (8 cups) of drinking water, the TDS level with Trace Minerals ConcenTrace drops would be close to 400 ppm.
◉ This book recommends that the safe TDS level for drinking water is 200 ppm, even though many people are accustomed to drink water up to a TDS level of 500 ppm.

However, it is up to the individual to choose how many drops are to be added to the drinking water, and how many drops would suit to feel healthy without any further complications. Every person has to research on his/her own body, and find out the correct dosage of concenTrace mineral drops.

4. When you do research and conduct experiments at home, with a TDS meter, on "number of drops versus the TDS level", you should not expect the same results every time you do it because each bottle you purchase from the health food store does not come from the same batch while manufacturing and packaging. So you may observe different TDS levels each time you research and find out the TDS levels by using a TDS meter.

5. **ANOTHER IMPORTANT POINT:** If you decided to use the ConcenTrace mineral drops, you should not use Himalayan pink salt or Celtic sea salt because the ConcenTrace mineral drops increase both the TDS level (close to or more than 200 ppm) and pH in your drinking water. If you further add Himalayan pink salt or Celtic sea salt to your drinking water, the TDS level will be elevated to a dangerous level, and also you would be consuming too much sodium. So you should take a decision weather you want to use the Himalyan pink salt, Celtic sea salt, or the ConcenTrace mineral drops.

• However you should bear in mind that the recommended TDS level in drinking water is close to 200 ppm. Please do not drink purified water with a TDS level beyond 500 ppm by adding too many ConcenTrace mineral drops or additional Himalayan pink salt or Celtic sea salt. That could have devastating effect on kidneys.

• A TDS level of 200 ppm in drinking water is recommended as the upper limit. It does not mean that every person should maintain 200 ppm in the drinking water. Each person should research, and find out by trial & error the ideal TDS level that suits the body. Each person is different. Any TDS level ranging from 10 ppm to 200 ppm can be used. Drinking water should be remineralized in order to prevent the leaching effect and to comply with the recommendation of the World Health Organization (WHO). For example in Vancouver area, British Columbia, Canada, the tap water has a TDS level between 10 ppm and 20 ppm. Even that low TDS level of 10 ppm to 20 ppm would help prevent leaching effect. Much higher TDS level could be beneficial as your body gets more trace minerals.

6. If you are planning to try these drops (ConcenTrace mineral drops, or pH Booster drops, or any other drops) for the first time, please get your drinking water tested after adding the drops by a certified laboratory in your area and make sure that these drops did not release any dangerous contaminants into your drinking water.

7. Please do not worry about the aforementioned scientific calculations of this section (howto test the dropper & how to calculate the maximum number of drops) unless you have a scientific background.

8. **pH Testing Drops (the Reagent used to observe color change while testing for Water pH):** You might be using the pH testing drops to test your drinking water pH. Please do not consume this reagent (testing drops) with drinking water, or do not get this chemical in your eyes or on your skin. This solution is combustible so keep it away from heat, flames, or fire. And keep it away from children [62]

9. It is highly recommended that you should use digital pH meter (instead of using pH testing drops) to measure the pH when you try to remineralize and alkalize the purified water at home.

# REFERENCES

1. Health Risks from Drinking Demineralized Water by Frantisek Kozisek, MD, PhD, National Institute of Public Health, Prague, Czech Republic, Endorsed by Word Health Organization (WHO). This paper can be found on the following hyperlinks:
a. http://www.who.int/water_sanitation_health/dwq/nutrientschap12.pdf      (PDF File)
b.https://www.researchgate.net/publication/252043662_Health_Risk_from_Drinking_Demineralized_Water

2. Health Risks from Drinking Demineralized Water by Frantisek Kozisek, MD, PhD.
http://citeseerx.ist.psu.edu/viewdoc/summary?doi=10.1.1.378.4667

3. Nutrients in Drinking Water: Water, Sanitation and Health Protection and the Human Environment, Refer to Chapter 12 for Kozisek's Paper (PDF File Contains 14 Chapters), World Health Organization, Geneva, Switzerland, 2005.
http://www.who.int/water_sanitation_health/dwq/nutrientsindw.pdf

4. Drinking Demineralized Water & The Health Risks by Nancy Hearn, Water Benefits Health, 2010-2018.
https://www.waterbenefitshealth.com/drinking-demineralized-water.html

5. HM Digital TDS-4TM Handheld Hydro Tester TDS and Temperature Tester.
ASIN # B001RK38LU, PART # HMDIGITALTDS4, Available at Amazon.ca, Price: $22.60 CAD.
https://www.amazon.ca/HM-Digital-TDS-4TM-Handheld-Temperature/dp/B001RK38LU/ref=sr_1_1?ie=UTF8&qid=1437459250&sr=8-1&keywords=TDS-4+Water+Tester+by+HM+Digital

## ACCEPTABLE TDS LEVELS

6. Drinking Water Standards.
http://www.tdsmeter.com/
http://www.tdsmeter.com/what-is-tds/

7. How to Check TDS Level of Water at Home? – 2 Easy Methods
https://www.bestrowaterpurifier.in/blog/how-to-check-tds-level-of-water/

8. Total Dissolved Solids in Drinking Water, World Health Organization (WHO) Report, 1996.
http://www.who.int/water_sanitation_health/dwq/chemicals/tds.pdf

9. The US Environmental Protection Agency (EPA) advises against consuming water containing more than 500mg/liter, US AOL MessageBoard Refugees>Social Gathering Place>General Discussion by Taptalk.com.
https://www.tapatalk.com/groups/usaolmessageboardrefugees/tds-total-dissolved-solids-t2544.html

10. What is the acceptable TDS level of drinking water? by Quora Discussion Board.
https://www.quora.com/What-is-the-acceptable-TDS-level-of-drinking-water

11. What should be the minimum TDS level for the drinking water and what should be the maximum in RO system? by Quora Discussion Board.
https://www.quora.com/What-should-be-the-minimum-TDS-level-for-the-drinking-water-and-what-should-be-the-maximum-in-RO-system

12. Minimum and Maximum Acceptable TDS Level in Drinking Water by Dr. Jagdev Singh, Posted On Sep 21, 2017.
https://www.ayurtimes.com/minimum-maximum-acceptable-tds-level-drinking-water/

13. What is the acceptable TDS level of drinking water?, Federation of Consumer Organizations of Punjab, India, Posted on Facebook on February 16, 2017.
https://www.facebook.com/fcopunjab/posts/what-is-the-acceptable-tds/1317633224964100/

## HOW TO REMINERALIZE PURIFIED WATER?
14. How to Remineralize Reverse Osmosis Water, by the Water Geeks, 2019.
https://thewatergeeks.com/how-to-remineralize-ro-water/

15. RO Water Remineralization 101: Full How to Guide by Best RO System by Derek, Posted on September 19, 2017
https://www.best-ro-system.com/add-minerals-back-into-water/

16. How To Re-Mineralize Water For Drinking by Theresa Crouse, Posted on April 14, 2015.
http://www.survivopedia.com/how-to-re-mineralize-water/

17. Adding Minerals to Distilled Water is very EASY by Distilled Water Association.
http://www.distilledwaterassociation.org/adding-minerals-to-distilled-water-is-very-easy/

18. 7 Easy Ways to Enliven Your Drinking Water with Minerals for Better Health by Karen Peltier.
http://wellgal.com/7-ways-add-essential-trace-minerals-drinking-water-health/

19. Our Reverse Osmosis Water with Liquid Minerals Liquid Eden Holistic Center, Posted on February 14, 2015.
http://liquid-eden.com/reverse-osmosis-water-with-liquid-minerals/

## HIMALAYAN PINK SALT
20. Water Secrets: The Truth About Water, Distilled Water, Reverse Osmosis, and More! by Superlife.com, Malibu, California, USA.
http://www.superlife.com/the-truth-about-water/

21. Pink Himalayan Salt VS Table Salt by Brandi Black, PaleoHacks Blog.
https://blog.paleohacks.com/himalayan-salt/#

22. Laboratory tests prove Healthy Salt far better than Himalayan pink salt by Eileen Durfee, Posted on Nov 23, 2017.
https://www.gohealthynext.com/blog/laboratory-tests-prove-healthy-salt-far-better-than-Himalayan-pink-salt/

23. How to use Himalayan Salt, Benefits of Himalayan Salt by Empowered Sustenance, Posted on Jan 13, 2014.
https://empoweredsustenance.com/himalayan-salt-benefits/

24. What Are 84 Minerals in Himalayan Salt? by Karen S. Garvin, October 03, 2017.
https://www.livestrong.com/article/534033-what-are-the-84-minerals-in-Himalayan-salt/

25. Minerals in Himalayan Pink Salt: Spectral Analysis by The Meadow.
https://themeadow.com/pages/minerals-in-Himalayan-pink-salt-spectral-analysis

26. Chemical Analysis of Natural Himalayan Pink Rock Salt by Salt News.
http://www.saltnews.com/chemical-analysis-natural-Himalayan-pink-salt/comment-page-1/

27. Certificate of the Analysis of the Original Himalayan Crystal Salt (PDF file), Institute of Biophysical Research, Las Vegas, Nevada, USA.
http://www.tervisekool.ee/tervisekool/failid/File/lugemist/tervislk%20toitumine/Certificate%20of%20the%20Analysis%20of%20the%20Original%20Himalayan%20Crystal%20Salt.pdf

There are no references between 28 and 34.

## CELTIC SEA SALT

35. The brochure that comes with the purchase of Celtic Sea Salt (Unrefined Fine Sea Salt), Westpoint Naturals (distributor), Vancouver, British Columbia, Canada.
https://www.westpointnaturals.com/

36. Why it's the choice of health experts, chefs, and all who truly know sea salt, posted by Salina Naturally.
https://www.selinanaturally.com/celtic-sea-salt

37. Health Benefits of Celtic Sea Salt by Lana Billings-Smith, Posted on Livingstrong.com.
https://www.livestrong.com/article/260852-health-benefits-of-celtic-sea-salt/

38. CELTIC SEA SALT (SEL GRIS): NOT EVEN A PINCH PALEO, Loren Cordain, PhD, Professor Emeritus, Posted on June 6, 2014
https://thepaleodiet.com/celtic-sea-salt/

39. Himalayan Salt vs Celtic Salts by Saltpur, Johannesburg, South Africa.
http://www.saltpur.co.za/index.php?route=information/information&information_id=14

40. Mineral Analysis of Celtic sea salt, provided by Salina Naturally.
https://www.selinanaturally.com
https://www.celticseasalt.com

## Demineralized Water & Lack of Minerals

41. Consumption of Low TDS and Low pH Water by Perfect Water, 19 Clinton Road, Alberton, Gauteng, South Africa, Posted on November 1, 2014.
http://www.perfectwater.co.za/consumption-low-tds-ph-water/

42. Publications on Consumption of Low TDS and Low pH Water, The Russian Report on Minerals Intake Discussed, RO Water Units Described, and Other Stuff.
http://www.mondeorpw.co.za/

## Frantisek Kozisek's Papers on Dangers of Demineralized Water

43. Health Risks from Drinking Demineralized Water by Frantisek Kozisek, MD, PhD, National Institute of Public Health, Prague, Czech Republic, Endorsed by Word Health Organization (WHO). This paper can be found on the following hyperlinks:
 a. http://www.who.int/water_sanitation_health/dwq/nutrientschap12.pdf (PDF File)
 b. https://www.researchgate.net/publication/252043662_Health_Risk_from_Drinking_Demineralized_Water

44. Health Risks from Drinking Demineralized Water by Frantisek Kozisek, MD, PhD.
http://citeseerx.ist.psu.edu/viewdoc/summary?doi=10.1.1.378.4667

45. Nutrients in Drinking Water: Water, Sanitation and Health Protection and the Human Environment, Refer to Chapter 12 for Kozisek's Paper (PDF File Contains 14 Chapters), World Health Organization, Geneva, Switzerland, 2005.
http://www.who.int/water_sanitation_health/dwq/nutrientsindw.pdf

There are no references between 46 and 49.

## CONCENTRACE MINERAL DROPS
50. Great Salt Lake, from Wikipedia.
https://en.wikipedia.org/wiki/Great_Salt_Lake

51. Anderson's Health Solutions ConcenTrace Ionic Mineral Drops, Being Advertised by Abaco Health, Kelowna, British Columbia, Canada.
https://www.abacohealth.com/anderson-s-health-solutions-concen-trace-ionic-mineral-drops-60ml.html

52. Anderson's Health Solutions ConcenTrace Ionic Mineral Drops, 120 mL, Being Advertised by Nature's Fare Markets.
https://shop.naturesfare.com/health-wellness-vitamins-supplements-minerals/7000-anderson-s-ConcenTrace-ionic-mineral-120-ml-.html

53. Anderson's Concentrated Mineral Drops With the Picture of the Great Salt Lake, Utah, USA.
http://www.omega3global.com/cmd-full-spectrum-supplement.html

## CONCENTRACE DROPS FROM ANDERSON'S HEALTH SOLUTIONS
54. Anderson's Family Home Page, MRI (Mineral Resources International, Inc.).
https://www.mineralresourcesint.com/about-us/
https://www.mineralresourcesint.com/international

55. Anderson's Sea M.D. Concentrated Mineral Drops, 4 Ounces Bottle, Available at Amazon.com.
https://www.amazon.com/Andersons-Concentrated-Mineral-Drops-ounce/dp/B0028BW0IO/ref=cm_cr_arp_d_product_top?ie=UTF8

## CONCENTRACE DROPS FROM TRACE MINERALS RESEARCH
56. ConcenTrace Trace Mineral Drops, Utah Sea Minerals, Manufactured by Trace Minerals Research.
https://traceminerals.com/utah-sea-minerals/

57. Trace Mineral Research - ConcenTrace Trace Mineral Drops, 8 Oz, There are more than 1240 Reviews on Amazon.com in August 2018.
https://www.amazon.com/Trace-Minerals-Research-ConcenTrace-Mineral/dp/B000AMUWLK/ref=sr_1_1_a_it?ie=UTF8&qid=1534103659&sr=8-1&keywords=ConcenTrace%C2%AE%2BTrace%2BMineral%2BDrops&th=1

58. ConcenTrace Trace Mineral Drops, Trace Minerals Research, Available in Canada from Monnol.
http://www.monnol.com/en/products/ConcenTrace

59. Arsenic, International Programme on Chemical Society, World Health Organization.
http://www.who.int/ipcs/assessment/public_health/arsenic/en/

60. Kent Reverse Osmosis (RO) Systems to Produce Remineralized Water.
http://www.kentrosystems.com/ro-water-purifier.php

61. KENT's Patented Mineral RO ™ Water Purifiers
https://www.kent.co.in/water-purifiers/ro/

62. Testing the Accuracy of pH Reagent Drops by Alkaline Water Plus, Posted on August 13, 2011.
https://www.alkalinewaterplus.com/blog/testing-the-accuracy-of-ph-reagent-drops/

# CHAPTER 18: ALKALINE WATER
## [A Very Important Chapter]

YOU WILL LEARN: HOW TO MAKE YOUR OWN HASSLE-FREE ALKALINE WATER AT HOME, HOW TO PURCHASE AND USE CONCENTRACE MINERAL DROPS, pH BOOSTER DROPS, ALKALINE WATER PITCHERS, WATER IONIZERS, KANGEN WATER MACHINES, HYDROGEN WATER MACHINES, REVERSE OSMOSIS ALKALINE WATER SYSTEMS, ETC.

# TABLE OF CONTENTS

149

# How to Know If The Water Is Acidic or Alkaline?

By monitoring the pH water pH, a person can determine if the water is acidic or alkaline. pH is a value that rates how acidic or how alkaline the water is on a scale from 0 to 14. In the same manner, a person can measure the pH of urine, saliva or any other solution, and can conclude if it is acidic or alkaline, and what exactly is the pH value.

If the water pH is less than 7 (pH < 7), the water is considered to be acidic.
If the water pH is equal to 7 (pH = 7), the water is considered to be neutral.
If the water pH is greater than 7 (pH > 7), the water is considered to be alkaline or basic.
Pure water at 25 °C is neutral, meaning that the pH is exactly 7.

## Scientific Definition of pH

pH is the negative logarithm of hydrogen ion concentration.

$$pH = - \log [H^+]$$

On the pH scale, the difference between adjacent numbers represents a tenfold difference in acidity or alkalinity. For instance, the water with a pH of 5 is 10 times more acidic than the water with a pH of 6 and 100 times more acidic than the water with a pH of 7. For instance, also, the water with a pH of 7 is 10 times more alkaline than the water with a pH of 6, and the water with a pH of 8 is 100 times more alkaline than the water with a pH of 6, and so on. When the water pH is exactly 7.0, the water is said to be neutral (neither acidic nor alkaline).

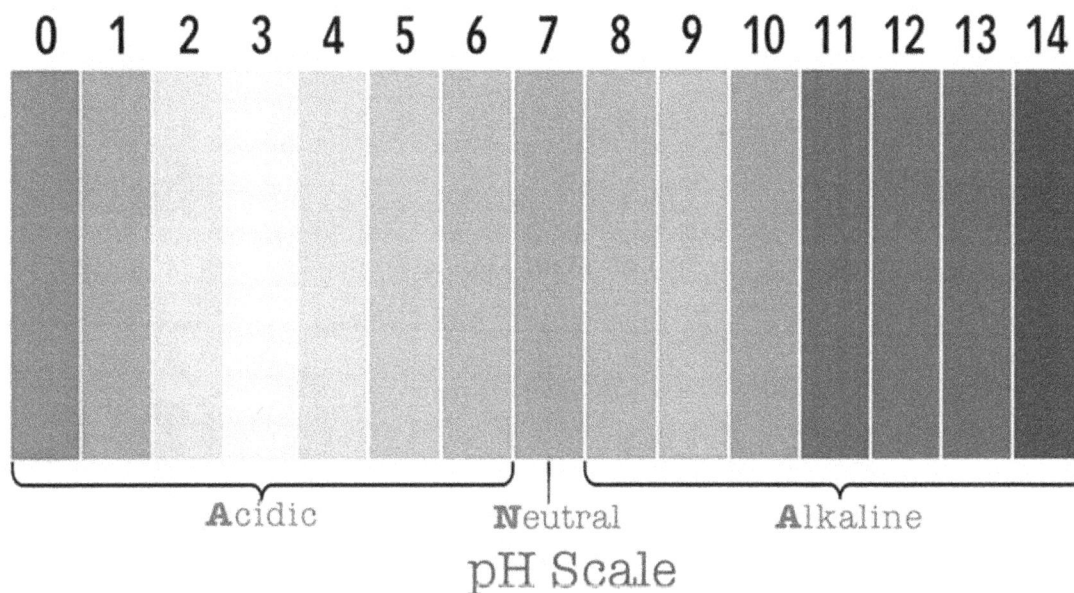

Figure 18.1 The colors of pH scale varies from 0 to 14 (Courtesy of Mokshamantra.com).

## pH indicators [1]

pH indicators are substances that change color when they are added to acidic or alkaline solutions or water. There are two types of pH indicators: (i) Universal indicator, and (ii) Litmus paper commonly used in the laboratory or at home. Universal indicator is a mixture of several different indicators, and can show us exactly how strongly acidic or alkaline a solution is. This is measured using the pH scale. The pH scale runs from pH 0 to pH 14. Universal indicator has many different colour changes, from red for strong acids to dark purple for strong bases. In the middle, neutral pH 7 is indicated by green color. Again each color varies from light-color to dark-color. Whereas litmus indicator strip turns red in acidic solutions and blue in alkaline solutions, and purple in neutral solutions.

## How to Measure the Water pH Using pH Testing Drops? [1]

All you need do is purchase a bottle of "pH testing drops for water". It comes with a bottle of reagent (drops) along with a pH color chart, as shown in the picture below. It is usually sold in a pet store or aquarium store. If you can find **Enagic office** (Kangen water company) in your area, you can purchase their pH testing drops and color chart. These drops indicate whole numbers of pH only. If you want decimal point accuracy, you need to use digital pH meter. Fill up a small cup with water, and pour 3 or 4 drops of colored solution into the water, and stir or shake the cup of water. The water color in the cup changes immediately. By looking at the color chart, and by comparing the water color in the cup, you can recognize the approximate pH value of the water being tested. The digital pH meters indicate more accurate pH values with decimal point.

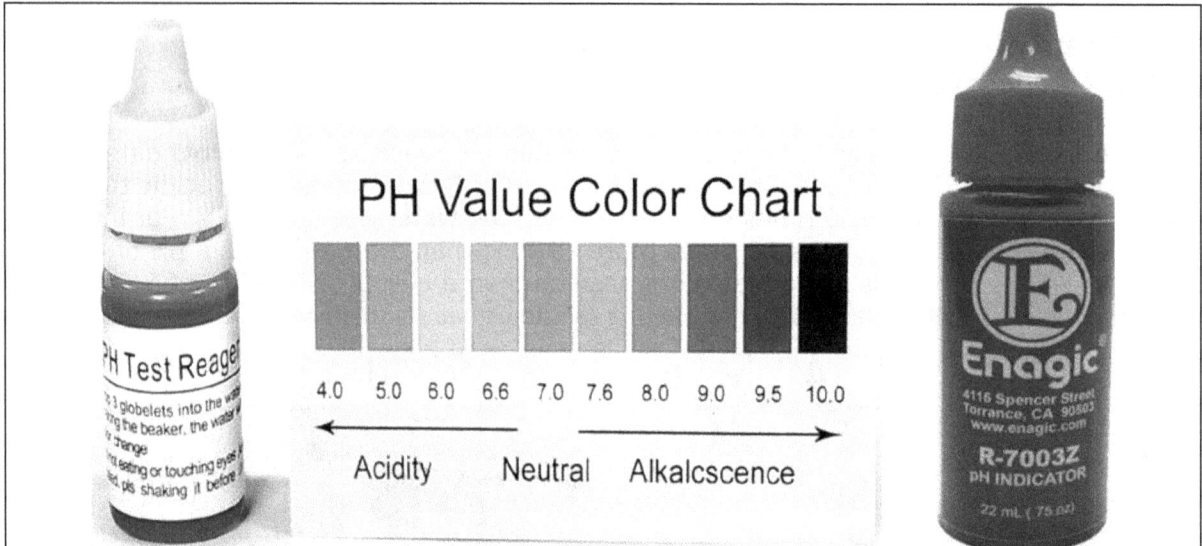

Figure 18. 2  On the Left is pH Testing Reagent Drops with color chart to measure the water pH.
Figure 18. 3  On the right is the Enagic pH Testing Drops; Courtesy of Enagic Co.

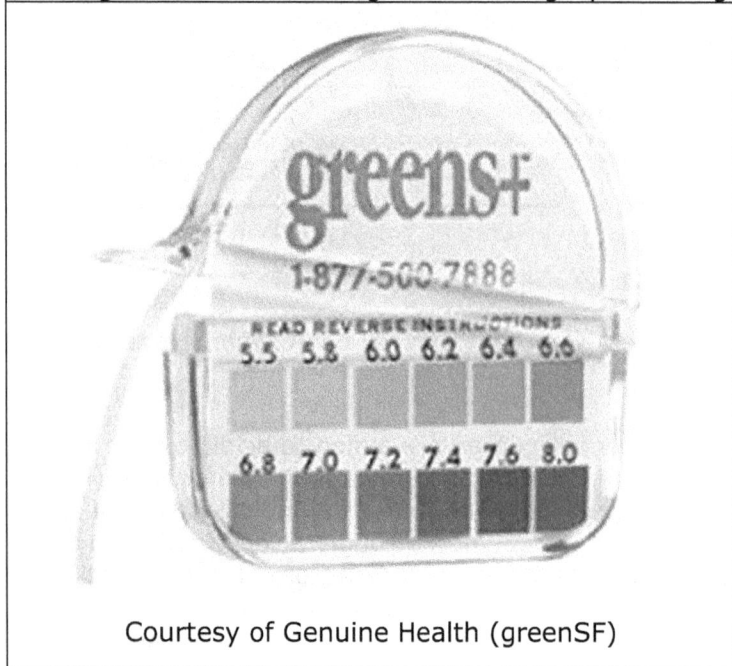

Courtesy of Genuine Health (greenSF)

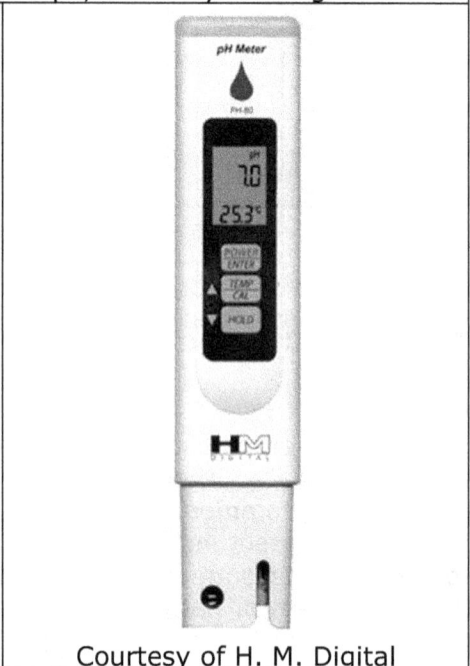

Courtesy of H. M. Digital

| Figure 18.4 A roll of pH paper to test urine/saliva. | Figure 18.5 Digital pH meter. |

## How to Measure the Water pH Using Digital pH Meter (H. M. Digital) [3]

You can purchase this digital pH meter on Amazon (ASIN # B0096N8OWI). Also purchase several calibration solutions (pH=4, 7 & 9). To use this meter, press the power button and it turns on. Dip the pH meter probe in a small cup filled with calibration solution-I, and press CAL button, it will show precisely the pH of that calibration solution-I. Repeat the same with other calibration solutions, and then test your real water samples, and record the pH. The pH value slowly progresses and becomes steady. This digital pH meter is more accurate than using pH testing drops.

## How to Measure the Urine pH?

Please note that the pH paper used to monitor the "urine pH" is very different from that used to monitor the water pH. So be extremely careful when you use pH paper! Genuine Health pH paper role is good to monitor urine pH. Tear a piece of pH paper from the roll, and pass the paper through your running urine stream. Read and compare against the provided color chart. By comparing and recognizing the color on the pH scale, you would know the approximate pH value of your urine.

## How to Measure the Saliva pH?

You can use the same Genuine Health pH paper to test the saliva. Just collect saliva under your tongue, and apply saliva on the strip. The color of the strip changes. By comparing and recognizing the color on the pH scale, you would know the approximate pH value of your saliva.

## SAFE pH LEVEL FOR DRINKING WATER [4, 4b, 5, 6, 7, 8]

The U.S. Environmental Protection Agency (EPA) does not regulate the pH level in drinking water. It is classified as a secondary drinking water contaminant whose impact is considered aesthetic. However, both the EPA and World Health Organization (WHO) recommend that the safe pH level for drinking water is between 6.5 and 8.5, including for the well water. [4, 4b, 5]

All the municipality water processing plants must meet the government regulations, and therefore they voluntarily test the pH of their water to monitor for pollutants, which may be indicated by a changing pH. When pollutants are present, the municipal water companies treat their water to make it safe to drink again by filtering and by taking adequate steps to adjust the pH level between 6.5 and 8.5. The tap water in most cities has a pH close to 6.5.

Pure water has a pH of 7 and is considered "neutral" because it has neither acidic nor basic qualities. But the artificially purified water such as RO water, distilled water, or zero water, because of their high purity, reacts with the carbon dioxide if exposed to the atmospheric air, and form carbonic acid, thereby lowering the pH level to below 7 (sometimes it may drop to a pH of 6). By boiling the purified water (RO water, distilled water, or zero water), and by storing it in a sealed glass container, it may be is possible to restore the pH between 6.5 and 7.

Table 18.1 Typical pH levels of drinking water. [7]

| Water Type | pH Level |
|---|---|
| 1. Tap water | 7 to 7.5 |
| 2. Distilled Water / RO Water | 5 to 7 |
| 3. Bottled Water | 6.5 to 7.5 |
| 4. Alkaline Water (bottled) | 8 to 9 |
| 5. Ocean Water | 8 |
| 6. Acid Rain | 5 to 5.5 |

If your drinking water pH level falls outside the aforementioned safe range, it's time to act. You should call your local drinking water supply company and alert them about your test findings, or you should adjust your drinking water pH with your own efforts by slightly alkalizing it.

Dr. RK tested the TDS level and pH level of several types of water at home and recorded:
Table 18.2 TDS level and pH level of several types of water at home.

| Water Type | TDS (ppm) | pH Level |
|---|---|---|
| 1. Tap water in Burnaby, BC, Canada | 16 | 6.5 to 6.9 |
| 2. RO Water (as purchased) | 0 to 2 | 5.8 to 6.3 |
| 3. RO Water (after boiled & cooled) | 0 to 2 | 6.6 to 6.7 |
| 4. Distilled Water (as purchased) | 0 | 5.9 to 6.4 |
| 5. Distilled Water (after boiled & cooled) | 0 | 6.7 to 6.9 |

Please notice that the pH of RO water and distilled water when purchased from supermarkets is not in the safe pH range. It is rather acidic. The safe pH level for drinking water is between 6.5 and 8, as recommended by EPA and WHO. You therefore should take action, and improve the pH of purified water you purchased before drinking. Boiling the purified water would improve the pH a little. **As shown in the table, boiling improved the pH significantly.** Adding a tiny bit of baking soda or minerals could further increase the pH. It could become a healthy water-drinking habit if you could patiently neutralize the purified water by raising the pH to 7 or close to 7. It is up to the individual habit if he/she wants to further alkalize the purified water by raising the pH beyond 7.

Alkalinity is a measure of the capacity of water to neutralize acids. It measures the presence of carbon dioxide, carbonate, bicarbonate, and hydroxide ions that are naturally present in water. At normal drinking water pH levels, bicarbonate, and carbonate are the main contributors to alkalinity. The pH and alkalinity of well water can be affected by natural geologic conditions at the site, acid rain, coal or other mining operations, landfill, factory, gas station, dry-cleaning operations, and water treatment processes. [4, 5]

Water with a low pH can be acidic, naturally soft and corrosive. Acidic water with pH level less than 6.5 can leach metals from pipes and fixtures, such as copper, lead and zinc. It can also damage metal pipes and cause aesthetic problems, such as a metallic or sour taste, laundry staining or blue-green stains in sinks and drains. Water with a low pH may contain metals in addition to the before-mentioned copper, lead and zinc. [4, 5]

Drinking water with a pH level above 8.5 indicates the presence of high levels of alkaline minerals. High alkalinity does not pose a health risk, but can cause aesthetic problems, such as an alkali taste to the water that makes coffee taste bitter, scale build-up in plumbing, and lowered efficiency of electric water heaters. [4, 5]

Therefore, maintaining water pH level between 6.5 and 8.5 is of utmost importance. The pH of any tap water, supplied by local municipalities, most commonly ranges between 6.5 and 7. Any water with a pH greater than 7 is considered alkaline water. Alkaline bottled water being sold in supermarkets typically has a pH of 8 or 9 (but you cannot simply rely on labels, it has to be tested and verified as most labels of bottled water are misleading or falsifying).

According to a Wilkes University study, the association of pH with atmospheric gases and temperature is the primary reason why water samples should be tested on a regular basis. The study says that the pH value of the water is not a measure of the strength of the acidic or basic solution, and alone cannot provide a full picture of the characteristics or limitations with the water supply. [8]

While the ideal pH level of drinking water should be between 6.5-8.5 (According to the standards set by EPA), the human body maintains pH equilibrium for several parts of the body on a constant basis and will not be affected by water consumption. No matter what kind of water you drink, the human body has an amazing ability to maintain a steady pH in the blood between 7.35 and 7.45. Also our stomachs have a naturally low pH level of 2, which is a beneficial acidity that helps us with food digestion, and also that acidity of low pH kills bacteria and viruses.

# HOW TO OBTAIN ALKALINE WATER?

## Introduction [9, 10]

Any water that has a pH greater than 7 is considered alkaline water. Alkaline water is somewhat controversial. Not everybody agrees with drinking alkaline water for a long time. The alkalinity of water is a measure of its ability to neutralize acids. Many health experts believe that water alkalinity can have a profound effect on the health. Regardless of pH level (the water pH is not that important), the Mayo Clinic recommends that regular water is the best for most people, and that any water you drink must first be free from toxins. Some proponents have suggested that drinking alkaline water can help boost energy and metabolism, lose weight, neutralize acid in the bloodstream, cure cancer and resist disease. There is no scientific evidence to fully verify these claims of sellers and business people. According to Mayo Clinic nutritionist Katherine Zeratsky, some research indicates that alkaline water may slow bone loss, but more studies are needed before further benefits can be established. You can obtain or have access to alkaline water as described below in 10 possible ways:

Table 18.3 Methods of obtaining alkaline water.

| METHOD OF ALKALINE WATER | COMMENTS |
|---|---|
| **1. Add Lemon Juice** to purified water. Or, consume one lemon a day. Lemon does not alkalize the water. The urine pH does not rise above 7 (pH < 7). | The best natural method to live healthy. Upon drinking, urine pH rises up to 7 only. Lemon slightly neutralizes your body and does not alkalize. Lemon has wonderful health benefits other than alkalization. |
| **2. Add a Pinch of Baking Soda** to purified water. It is perfectly alkaline water. Even 10 mg of baking soda raises a liter of purified water pH to 7. Purified water can be easily neutralized by adding only a tiny amount of baking soda (that is 10 mg). pH can be raised or adjusted up to 8.5 by adding more. | Upon drinking, urine pH rises up to 8.5. You can make your own alkaline water at home. This method has side effects (gastrointestinal distress) so make sure it suits your body. By adding only the optimal amount, you can avoid side effects. Only 10 mg per liter would do the job (you can have your purified water neutralized). |
| **3. Add ConcenTrace mineral drops** to the purified water (RO water, distilled water, or zero water). You can purchase a bottle of drops in any health food store or online. There are two brands (Anderson's & Trace Mineral Research). | Easy to make alkaline water hassle-free at home. These drops raise both TDS level and pH level instantly. Highly recommended. Please refer to Chapter 17, read and learn. Get your alkaline water tested for contaminants by a certified lab. |
| **4. Purchase Alkaline water from local vendors.** They make alkaline water by passing purified water (RO water) through industrial size calcite pitchers, or through pitcher loaded with minerals such as calcium, magnesium, potassium, etc. | Some local vendors make both RO water and alkaline water and sell. Please research and find out their addresses in your area. They test the unit every day and make sure that the unit is working, and so this alkaline water is reliable & trustworthy. |
| **5. Purchase pH Booster Drops**, and add the drops to purified water. It is perfectly alkaline water. pH can be adjusted up to 9, 10, or even more. | pH drops are unreliable unless the company provides the report of analysis. Drops may contain contaminants or toxins. Get your alkaline water tested for contaminants by a certified lab. |

| | |
|---|---|
| **6. Purchase an Alkaline Water Pitcher** that adds minerals to tap water or purified water and raises water pH, making it alkaline. | Do not believe their labels and verbal promises. Test it and make sure it works, using a TDS meter and pH testing drops or digital pH meter before using it. It is not reliable until you test it. Get your alkaline water tested for contaminants by a certified lab. |
| **7. Purchase a Water Ionizer** that turns your tap water to alkaline water (pH adjustable) at the touch of a button by electrolysis or electrodialysis. pH can be adjusted up to 9, 10, or more. | Maintaining this kind of unit at home is tedious. You need to test drinking water every day and make sure it is working. You never know if the machine is working or broke down. Get your alkaline water tested for contaminants by a certified lab. |
| **8. Purchase a Kangen Water Machine** that turns your tap water to alkaline water and acidic water (pH adjustable). | Maintaining this kind of unit at home is tedious. You need to test drinking water every day and make sure it is working. You never know if it is working or broke down. Please get your final product (Kangen water) tested, and make sure it is one hundred percent free of contaminants. |
| **9. Purchase a Hydrogen Water Generator.** (Not necessarily alkaline water, neutral pH). | It produces either alkaline water or non-alkaline water depending on the brand name. Needs to check for H2 concentration frequently. Please get your final product (H2 water) tested, and make sure it is one hundred percent free of contaminants. |
| **10. Purchase a Reverse Osmosis System** that remineralizes and pours alkaline water (pH adjustable) into your jug at the touch of a button. | Maintaining this kind of unit at home is tedious and a hussle. You need to test drinking water every day and make sure it is working. You never know if the machine is working or broke down. Please get your final product (remineralized alkaline water) tested, and make sure it is one hundred percent free of contaminants at least once or twice a year. |

# METHOD 1: ADD LEMON JUICE TO PURIFIED WATER

**IMPORTANT NOTE:** Lemon has a very low pH of 2.2, and so we cannot simply make alkaline water with lemon juice. In order to make alkaline water, you need a basic substance such as baking soda (sodium bicarbonate $NaHCO_3$) or other. Lemon or lime juice is not a base, and so is definitely not an alkalizing agent, it does not neutralize acids, and more importantly does not produce alkaline water if added. However both lemon and lime are healthy citrus fruits, and when consumed by a person, and after digested and metabolized in the stomach, they help slightly improve the urine pH level, as the citrus fruit contains minerals that can create alkaline byproducts within the body once digested and metabolized. Adding a squeeze of lemon or lime to a glass of water is a healthy water-drinking habit as it can give power to neutralize your body once the lemon water is digested. Please read the following demonstration.

## HOW TO NEUTRALIZE YOUR BODY'S URINE BY CONSUMING LEMON
Just by eating one large lemon a day directly after peeling off the skin and seeds removed, or by squeezing and drinking the juice obtained from a large lemon directly, or by drinking the purified water with added lemon juice, you can enjoy countless benefits from the citrus fruit lemon, and you can also neutralize your body. However, achieving alkaline state is not possible with lemon.

Lemon juice does not raise the pH level of your urine significantly, it may raise urine pH from 6.5 to 7.0, and doesn't rise beyond 7. This fact has been experimentally verified by Dr. RK from his own urine tests done at home.
++++++++++++++++++++++++++++++++++++++++++++++++++++++++++++++++++
Dr. RK monitored his urine pH several times a day, several days, and recorded as follows:
22-Aug-2018  7:00 am   pH (before consuming lemon) = 6.7.
22-Aug-2018  7:05 am   Dr. RK consumed one large lemon (lemon juice made from purified water).
22-Aug-2018  9:00 am   Dr. RK monitored his urine pH several times during the day and next morning.
                       His urine pH, during the day, rose from 6.7 to 7.0 (did not go up more than 7).
23-Aug-2018  7:00 am   Dr. RK consumed one large lemon (lemon juice made from purified water) again.
23-Aug-2018  9:00 am   Dr. RK monitored his urine pH several times during the day and next morning.
                       His urine pH, during the day, rose from 6.7 to 7.0. (did not go up more than 7).
24-Aug-2018  7:00 am   Dr. RK consumed one large lemon (lemon juice made from purified water) again.
24-Aug-2018  9:00 am   Dr. RK monitored his urine pH several times during the day and next morning.
                       His urine pH, during the day, rose from 6.6 to 6.9 (did not go up more than 7).

Dr. RK interpreted that the lemon or lemon juice with purified water did not influence his urine pH. But the foods (vegetables, fruits, nuts & egg whites) he has been eating kept his urine pH level close to 7 all the day. pH=7 means your body is in neutral state. The lemon juice does not have much impact on urine pH. Lemon juice neutralizes your body. However, lemon has many reported health benefits.
++++++++++++++++++++++++++++++++++++++++++++++++++++++++++++++++++
## Journal Publication: Influence of Lemon Juice on Urine pH [11, 12]
In vitro and in vivo study of effect of lemon juice on urinary lithogenesis,
Authors: Oussama A1, Touhami M, Mbarki M., Arch Esp Urol. 2005 Dec;58(10):1087-92.
https://www.ncbi.nlm.nih.gov/pubmed/16482864
CONCLUSION: After the ingestion of lemon juice, the urine pH increased from 6.7 to 6.9.
++++++++++++++++++++++++++++++++++++++++++++++++++++++++++++++++++
Maintaining the urine pH close it 7 may not be possible to everybody because it greatly depend on what kind of foods a person consumes throughout the day. If a person consumes too much animal meat, the urine remains in acidic state. For those who consume a lot of vegetables, fruits, nuts and egg whites (not whole eggs) for the protein requirement, it would be very easy to keep the urine pH close to 7 all the day.

Many authors have been suggesting with many articles on the Internet that alkaline water can be prepared by adding lemon juice to purified water or tap water (which is not correct). From his own experiment, Dr.RK found that drinking lemon juice directly or drinking purified water with lemon juice does not raise the pH level of the urine more than a few decimal points (not even one point). Dr. RK monitored his urine pH repeatedly, after ingestion of lemon juice, and found that the urine pH level did not go up more than 7. Dr. RK's experimental findings match well with the results of the aforementioned scientific journal publication.

If you suffer from kidney stones, lemon juice might be helpful. It certainly won't do you any harm (well, except possibly to your tooth enamel). A generally healthy diet is always beneficial. Lemon juice might have a very tiny effect on urine pH. However if it does, the result is only to raise the pH a tiny bit closer to pH 7 (i.e. neutral). It does not make your urine alkaline. [12]

## NORMAL RANGE FOR URINE pH [13, 14, 15, 16]
The normal range for human urine pH is between 4.5 to 8, although it can change depending on your diet, certain disease processes and the medications you take. Normally in the morning the urine ph is around 6.0, meaning it is acidic. Later during the day, the pH rises depending on what you eat, either acidic foods or alkaline foods. By eating one lemon, you can raise your urine pH close to 7, which is neutral.

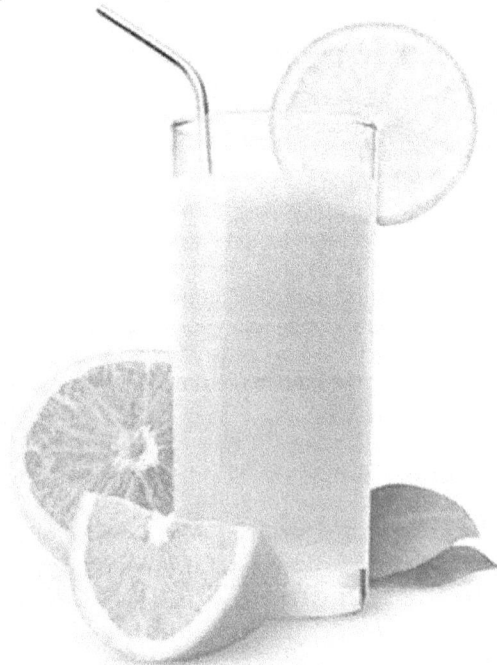

Figure 18.6  Eating one lemon a day, or drinking purified water with lemon juice is healthy.

## PRECAUTIONS WHILE CONSUMING LEMON JUICE
a. Use fresh whole lemons or limes (preferably organic) when eating directly or when making the juice and when mixing with purified water. Do not use store-bought lemon juice when making the drinking water with lemon juice. Use a lemon squeezer made from glass (not metal).

b. When making the drinking water with lemon juice, use purified water (RO water, distilled water, or zero water). Make sure you store the drinking water with lemon juice in a glass jar with an airtight lid if you are planning to prepare the drink for the entire day.

c. Do not expose the lemon pieces to air, after cutting, for more than a few minutes (maximum 30 minutes). Lemon juice will oxidize from air, light, and heat, and you may not get all the benefits possessed by raw lemons if you leave the cut lemon for a long time. If left exposed to air, lemons lose their antioxidizing properties and vitamin C. It would be the best practice consuming the lemon or lemon juice immediately after cutting.

d. Always use a straw when drinking lemon juice. The acids in lemons can damage your teeth because they cause the enamel on the surface to wear away, leaving you more susceptible to cavities and teeth decay.

## WONDERFUL BENEFITS OF CONSUMING WHOLE LEMON OR LEMON JUICE

● Lemons before consumption are acidic (pH = 2.2 approximately) and play a great role in digestion process, and produce many beneficial byproducts after consumption for your body.

● Lemons contain both citric acid and ascorbic acid (otherwise known as Vitamin-C), and as these weak acids easily metabolize after consumption, the mineral content of lemons help increase the urine pH as well as blood pH.

● Lemon is a powerful disinfectant and antibacterial agent that can treat numerous diseases and conditions and even cancer! So start drinking water with lemon juice regularly, to boost your health. [17]

● Lemons are high in heart-healthy vitamin-C, and several beneficial plant compounds that have been shown to lower cholesterol. The high vitamin-C and citric acid content helps you absorb non-heme iron from plants, ultimately preventing anemia. Studies show that lemon extract and plant compounds promote weight loss. Lemon juice also helps prevent kidney stones from re-forming. More importantly, some plant chemicals from lemons, such as limonene and naringenin, have been shown to prevent cancer. Research reveals the fruit lemon has a whopping 22 anti-cancer properties! Studies have shown that the compounds prevented malignant tumors from developing in tongues, lungs, and colons. It is also powerful disinfectant and anti-bacterial compound, which helps in the treatment of numerous conditions from bad breath to cholera. The soluble fiber in lemons also helps improve digestive health. [18]

● One lemon provides about 31 mg of vitamin C, which is 51% of your recommended daily intake (RDI). Animal studies show that lemon extract and plant compounds may promote weight loss, but the effects in humans are unknown. Lemon juice may help prevent kidney stones from re-forming. However, more quality research is needed. Lemons contain vitamin C and citric acid, which help you absorb non-heme iron from plants. This may help prevent anemia. Some plant chemicals from lemons have been shown to prevent cancer in animal studies. However, human studies are needed. The soluble fiber in lemons could help improve digestive health. However, you need to eat the pulp of the lemon, not just the juice. Not only are lemons a very healthy fruit, but they also have a distinct, pleasurable taste and aroma that make them a great addition to all kinds of foods and drinks. [19]

● "Citrus" refers to a large genus of flowering plants that are cultivated globally for their fruit. Oranges, lemons, grapefruits, limes and tangerines have all been featured in diets and medicinal practices of various cultures since far back in history. Citrus fruits are often juiced, either mechanically or by hand, the result is a fibrous and nutritious byproduct called pulp that has numerous health benefits. Citrus pulp is rich in vitamin C, which is a potent antioxidant that may help support numerous bodily systems. A study published in the journal "Epidemiology" found that vitamin C had an inverse effect on mortality for cancers and cardiovascular diseases. Citrus pulp also contains beta-carotene, which is converted by the body into vitamin A, as well as small amounts of vitamins B-1, B-2, B-3, B-5, B-6 and E. Citrus pulp also contains flavonoids, limonoids and coumarins, chemicals produced by plants to protect themselves from viral, bacterial and fungal invasions. [20]

● Citrus pulp contains high levels of calcium, magnesium, phosphorus and potassium, which may improve brain function, heart health and bone strength. Potassium also contributes to kidney function. Citrus fruit additionally provides small amounts of copper, iron, manganese and zinc. Lemons uniquely offer sodium, chlorine and sulphur. The thick, fibrous attribute of pulp is derived from high concentrations of a dietary fiber called pectin. Pectin helps lower cholesterol, ease digestion and improve the removal of fat and harmful chemicals from the body. [20]

● The entire fruit lemon, from peel to pulp is good for you, boost your metabolism, which is why the editors at "Eat This, Not That!" researched exactly what happens when you eat one lemon a day, and outlined many stomach-slimming tips with lemon. If you eat one lemon a day: you look younger, your blood pressure goes down, your cholestrol levels improve, you won't feel hungry (lemon is hunger suppressant), you lose weight, you fight off inflammation and cold quickly, you won't get kidney stones, and you will have fresh breath and feel good about yourself! [21]

● A 2014 study published in BioMed Research International found that essential oils in citrus fruit, such as lemons, can help protect against certain types of cancer. Limonoids are organic substances in citrus fruits that help determine their bitterness or sweetness. The compounds work by protecting your cells from damage that can lead to the formation of cancer. A 2013 article published in the academic journal Food & Function notes that limonoids have anti-proliferative and anti-aromatase properties in human breast cancer cells. [22]

● Lemons boost your immune system, and contribute to balancing your urine pH. Warm lemon water aids digestion. Lemons are diuretic, and therefore increase the rate of urination in the body, which helps purify it, and toxins are easily flushed out at a faster rate which helps keep your urinary tract healthy. Warm lemon water helps get rid of chest infections and halt those pesky coughs. It's thought to be helpful to people with asthma and allergies too. Vitamin-C is one of the first things depleted when you subject your mind and body to stress, and at this difficult time of distress, lemons keep you zen (provides you instant intuition and meditative state), as lemons are chock full of Vitamin-C. [23]

● Lemon juice in warm tea helps kick the coffee habit. Drinking warm water is more beneficial than cold water according to Chinese medicine so enjoy lemon juice in warm purified water (RO water, distilled water, or zero water)! [23]

# METHOD 2: ADD BAKING SODA TO PURIFIED WATER

**PREPARATION:** Alkaline water can be easily prepared at home by mixing purified water (RO water, distilled water, zero water) with baking soda. Even a tiny bit of banking soda (sodium bicarbonate) improves the pH of purified water. The pH of the purified water can be gradually increased by adding a tiny bit of baking soda. We know that the pH of baking soda is 9. So we can increase the alkalinity (pH) of distilled water up to 9.

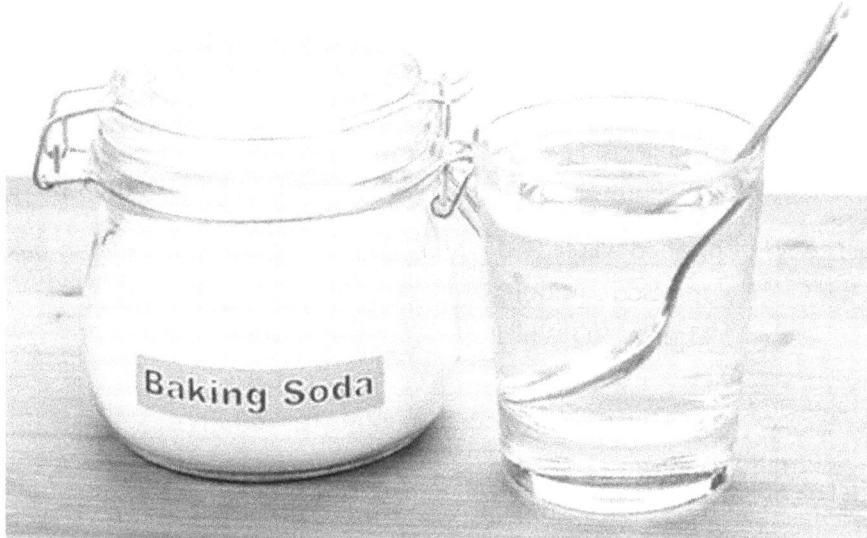

Figure 18.7   Baking soda instantly alkalizes (pH goes up) purified water, but does not fully dissolve.

## EXPERIMENTS CONDUCTED AT HOME OF Dr.RK

Dr. RK conducted an experiment at the comfort of his home. By using the digital kitchen scale, he added 0.125 g (125 mg) of baking soda to RO water, and measured the pH by using Enagic pH testing drops. He gradually added baking soda in the increments of 0.125 g (125 mg) of baking soda to RO water, stirred well and shook it in a closed container for 30 to 60 seconds, and measured both pH level and TDS level. He recorded the results as shown in the table below:

Table 18.4 The pH of purified water (RO water) can be increased by adding baking soda.

| Baking Soda Added To 1 Liter of RO Water | pH of RO Water Measured (pH) | TDS Level of RO Water ppm |
|---|---|---|
| 0 g | 6.0 to 6.5 | 2 |
| 0.125 g (125 mg) | 8.0 | 55 |
| 0.250 g (250 mg) | 8.5 | 102 |
| 0.375 g (375 mg) | 8.5 | 162 |
| 0.50 g (500 mg) | 8.5 | 260 |
| 1.0 g | 8.5 | 530 |
| 1.5 g | 8.5 | 786 |
| 2.0 g | 8.5 | 960 |
| 2.5 g | 8.5 | > 1000 |
| 3.0 g | 8.5 | > 1000 |

**IMPORTANT NOTE:** It is important to note from the above-mentioned table that the TDS levels did not match with the amount added. For example, when 125 mg of baking soda was added, TDS=55 ppm, indicating the fact that the baking soda does not fully dissolve in water at room temperature. In Chapter 17, when Dr. RK conducted his experiment with Himalayan pink salt, the weight of the salt added (125 mg) perfectly matched with TDS level monitored as 125 ppm. But with baking soda, different TDS levels recorded.

Dr. RK conducted more experiments to see what would be the minimal amount of baking soda required to neutralize or slightly alkalize the purified water. It was astounding to note that even 10 mg of baking soda increased the purified water pH to 7. Even a tiny bit (10 mg) would be enough to neutralize or slightly alkalize the purified water. He even repeated the same experiment with 2 liters of purified water, and observed the same results. He also measured the pH, using pH testing drops and digital pH meter, and observed the same results.

Table 18.5 The pH of purified water (RO water) can be increased by adding baking soda.

| Baking Soda Added To 1 Liter of RO Water | pH of RO Water Measured (pH) |
|---|---|
| 0 g | 6.5 |
| 0.010 g (10 mg) | 7.0 (turned green) |
| 0.020 g (20 mg) | 7.5 (turned pale blue) |
| 0.040 g (40 mg) | 8.0 (turned light blue) |

## Urine Test Results of Dr. RK After Consuming Purified Water With Baking Soda

a. Dr. RK prepared alkaline water by adding only a tiny bit of baking soda (up to 50 mg) to 1 liter of distilled water, stirred well, and monitored the pH as approximately 8.5.
b. He monitored his urine pH before consuming this alkaline water, and it was 6.7.
c. He then consumed 1 liter (4 cups) of this alkaline water (pH=8.5), and started monitoring his urine pH after an hour.
d. He found that his urine pH level increases by 1 point (pH rose to 7.7) after 2 hours and remained close to 8 for more than 12 hours. After 12 hours, his urine pH dropped back to 6.7. This reveals the fact that he accomplished alkaline state by drinking alkaline water even with a tiny bit of baking soda , and lived for 12 hours in the alkaline state. By consuming this alkaline water twice a day, he maintained his alkaline state of urine for 24 hours.

**Research shows** that raising the pH of your urine by just 1 point (for example by raising the pH from 6 to 7 or from 7 to 8) can prevent or eliminate the symptoms of metabolic syndrome: obesity, high blood pressure, high blood cholesterol, high blood sugar and kidney stones. [27]

## The Meaning of the pH of Baking Soda [24]

pH is a measure of the concentration of hydrogen ions. The more hydrogen ions present, the higher the acidity. The mathematical relationship between pH and hydrogen ions is: $pH = - \log [H^+]$
In this this equation, $H^+$ represents the molar concentration of hydrogen ions. Since pH is all about hydrogen ions in an aqueous (water-based) solution, and baking soda is a dry powder, it doesn't really have a pH as such by itself. To get a pH reading, you need to mix baking soda with purified water. The chemical formula for baking soda is $NaHCO_3$. After dissolved in water, each molecule of baking soda ($NaHCO_3$) splits into the positive sodium ion ($Na^+$) and the negative bicarbonate ion ($HCO3_-$), which float freely in the water-based solution. In water, baking soda being mildly alkaline neutralizes the acid, reduces the hydrogen ion concentration, thereby increasing pH. If you dip pH paper into the solution or add pH testing drops, it will indicate the pH. The more baking soda you add, the higher the pH would be.

## HOW TO ALKALIZE YOUR BODY AND YOUR URINE!
## (BEING RECOMMENDED bY Dr. RK)

**1.** Add 50 to 100 mg of baking soda to 1 liter (4 cups) of purified water (RO water, distilled water, or zero water) in a glass jar that comes with airtight lid.

**2.** Also add lemon juice, extracted from 1 fresh organic whole lemon using a glass squeezer, to the same purified water, which is about to become alkaline water. You can also add finely cut organic cucumber chunks, organic ginger pieces and other greens if you wish.

**3.** Stir or shake well the glass jar until the baking soda in completely dissolved in the purified water.

**4.** Monitor the pH of the alkaline water you just prepared. It should be close to 8.5. If the pH of alkaline water is less than 8.5, add more baking soda (a tiny pinch), and monitor pH again. Repeat this procedure until the pH of the alkaline water reaches approximately 8.5. By trial and error, you should be able to achieve the pH of alkaline water to be roughly 8.5.

**5.** Monitor your urine pH just before you consume the alkaline water, and record it.

**6.** Consume this alkaline water you just prepared, all 4 cups at a time or in several batches. This alkaline water should raise your urine pH by 1 point. Monitor and record your urine pH every few hours throughout the day until you become familiar with what is happening with the alkaline water you just drank and your urine pH. Your goal is to raise your urine pH by 1 point, and keep it raised for a day. If the urine pH is not raised by 1 point, prepare a new batch of alkaline water by adding a little bit more baking soda this time, and repeat the experiment next day. The amount of baking soda to be consumed depends greatly on the size of the body (mostly body weight). As each person is different, you need to find out your own optimal dosage of baking soda required by trial and error. It is important to consume only the optimal amount of baking soda (as little as possible) or you may experience negative side effects. You can also divide the daily dosage of baking soda into several parts, and consume alkaline water several times a day to avoid side effects.

**7.** By using trial and error procedure, by preparing alkaline water with baking soda and lemon juice, by adding a little bit more baking soda next day, by monitoring the pH of alkaline water, by consuming the alkaline water, by monitoring the urine pH every few hours, and  by repeating the experiment, you should be able to raise your urine pH by 1 point, and keep it steady for the entire day.

**8.** The daily requirement of water consumption for an adult is 8 cups per day, though some people drink 16 cups a day. You drink 4 cups of alkaline water as the medication for the first 12 hours, and another 4 cups of alkaline water water for the reminder of the day to achieve your urine pH raised by one point and keep it steady for the entire day. In addition, you can drink the regular water (purified water or any water of your choice) as much as you want whenever you are thirsty or while consuming lunch and meals.

**9.** Once you mastered the concept of preparing alkaline water in order to increase the urine pH by 1 point, you can maintain your own schedule for drinking alkaline water. You can drink it every day, every other day, every other week or you can drink occasionally as needed. You can discontinue alkaline water and start consuming it again after a few months. It all depends on what you want, and what kind of health conditions, disorders or diseases you are trying to resolve.

**10.** If you experience continuing and persistent side effects of baking soda (listed below), you should discontinue alkaline water, start drinking regular water, and evaluate your medical situation. Always drink purified water, not tap water!

**11.** No matter what kind of water you drink, the human body has an amazing ability to maintain a steady pH in the blood between 7.35 and 7.45 unless you have a disorder or disease.

## SIDE EFFECTS OF BAKING SODA [25]
- Excess gas release, stomach upset, chronic indigestion, constipation
- Frequent urge to urinate, trouble starting urination, nausea or vomiting
- Unpleasant taste, increased thirst, stomach cramps
- Loss of appetite (continuing), headache (continuing)
- Unusual tiredness or weakness
- Muscle pain or twitching
- Mood or mental changes
- Nervousness, restlessness, slow breathing
- Swelling of feet or lower legs

## BAKING SODA ENHANCES ATHLETIC PERFORMANCE [26]
- Baking soda, also known as sodium bicarbonate ($NaHCO_3$), has been actually a popular workout supplement. According to the *American College of Sports Medicine*, sodium bicarbonate is among the leading ergogenic (performance enhancement) aids. Athletes and individuals participating in vigorous exercise are using baking soda to help delay muscle fatigue and improve performance. Baking soda has been widely researched and appears to also help stiff muscles during intense workouts.

- Sodium bicarbonate ($NaHCO_3$) supplementation is especially popular during short bouts of high-intensity exercise. Sprinters, swimmers, and rowers have realized improved performance taking baking soda prior to their competitive sport.

- During high-intensity workouts, our body releases chemicals into the muscle tissue. Metabolic byproducts lactate and hydrogen form in the muscle cells. While most of the byproducts are buffered, some do remain in the muscle cells and create an acidic environment. Increased acidity lowers pH levels, causing our muscles to burn and feel fatigued. According to research, taking sodium bicarbonate ($NaHCO_3$) before exercise helps neutralize acids and flushes metabolic byproducts from the muscle tissue. Published in the *International Journal of Sports Nutrition and Exercise Metabolism,* "NaHCO3 ingestion has been proposed to enhance performance by increasing extracellular buffering capacity." This means taking baking soda works on a cellular level in our body creating a better chemical environment for our muscles.

- Baking soda ingestion is believed to have the ability to reduce the acidic environment caused by high-intensity exercise. When the environment in our body becomes too acidic we can experience adverse health effects. The heart, liver, and kidneys can be overworked which can lead to chronic health conditions. Too much acidity can also contribute to muscle impairment and atrophy (wasting). Baking soda has become well-known for balancing acidity in our body, healing, and good preventative medicine. Athletes and fitness enthusiasts are appreciating the health benefits and use it often to power their workouts.

- Recommended Dosage for Athletes: 0.3 grams per kilogram of bodyweight is the recommended dosage for athletes. This appears to be the optimal amount to balance acidity (pH) in the blood and muscle tissue. According to the study, it's also recommended that baking soda (sodium bicarbonate) be taken 120 to 150 minutes before exercise and combined with a small high carbohydrate meal. This reduces the chance of unwanted gastrointestinal (GI) symptoms. Not everyone is able to use sodium bicarbonate to enhance athletic performance. Approximately 10% of users will experience gastrointestinal (GI) distress. Some athletes have tried to divide the recommended dosage 0.3 grams per kilogram of bodyweight into several parts, and consumed throughout the day to eliminate this problem. Other athletes have reduced the amount of sodium bicarbonate and were successful using a dosage of 0.2 grams per kilogram of bodyweight prior to exercise.

## METHOD 3: ADD CONCENTRACE MINERAL DROPS TO PURIFIED WATER
### [Simultaneously Remineralize and Alkalize the Purified Water]

Please refer to "**Chapter 17 Remineralization of the Purified Water,**" read and learn all the contents. Chapter 17 teaches how to remineralize purified water by adding Himalayan pink salt or Celtic sea salt, and how to make alkaline water by adding ConcenTrace mineral drops. Please read through the experiments conducted at home by Dr. RK, and learn what to do exactly to make your own alkaline water at home from RO water or distilled water. Just follow the same experiments to make your own alkaline water by adding a few ConcenTrace mineral drops to purified water, and conduct your own experiments until you gain full concept.

**ConcenTrace mineral drops, if added to purified water, increases both TDS and pH at the same time.** After making the alkaline water, please test it by using pH testing drops or digital pH meter, and make sure that the pH is a little over 7. If you want to make alkaline water at a much higher pH (8.5 or 9), you can do so but the TDS level would be elevated. It is recommended to keep TDS level close to 200 ppm. If the TDS level is below 200 ppm, try to add Himalayan pink salt or Celtic sea salt to adjust the TDS level close to 200 ppm. You can do that by using TDS meter and pH meter at the same time.

● You are being recommended not to drink alkaline water at a high pH (pH=8.5) every day, but drink it periodically or for the therapeutic purposes only.

● If you are trying the ConcenTrace mineral drops for the first time, please get your final product (after adding drops to purified water) tested by a certified laboratory in your area, and make sure that the water you drink is one hundred percent free of contaminants. You should do that at least once or twice a year.

## METHOD 4: PURCHASE ALKALINE WATER FROM LOCAL VENDORS
### IN REUSABLE WATER BOTLES

Please research in your area, and find out the addresses and phone numbers of local vendor who sell both RO water and alkaline water. These vendors make fresh RO water and alkaline water every day, test the water, and make sure that the unit is working perfectly. Therefore the RO water and/or alkaline water you purchase from these local vendors is reliable and trustworthy.

(i) Some vendors use industrial size calcite pitchers to produce alkaline water from RO water.

(ii) Some other vendors use industrial size pitchers loaded with minerals such as calcium, magnesium, potassium and others, and produce alkaline water from RO water.

● Whenever you purchase alkaline water, please test it by using pH testing drops or digital pH meter, and make sure that the pH is at least 8.5. Also monitor TDS level by using a TDS meter. If TDS level is below 200 ppm, add some Himalayan pink salt or Celtic sea salt so that the final TDS level is approximately 200 ppm.

● Please do not purchase alkaline water in bottles being sold in supermarkets, health food stores and pharmacies. This kind of bottled water is untrustworthy and there is a good chance that the alkaline water being sold could have been made from contaminated tap water or spring water by adding some minerals.

● You are being recommended not to drink alkaline water at a high pH (pH=8.5) every day, but drink it periodically or for the therapeutic purposes only.

● Please get your alkaline water tested by a certified laboratory in your area, and make sure that the water you drink is one hundred percent free of contaminants. You should do that at least once or twice a year.

# METHOD 5: ADD pH BOOSTER DROPS TO PURIFIED WATER

## pH BOOSTER DROPS EXPLAINED [27]

Alkaline drops, also called pH booster drops, are an easy way to raise the pH of your drinking water one cup at a time whenever you drink water. The pH booster drops bottle is easy to carry with you wherever you go. You can conveniently add these drops to tap water, purified water, coffee, tea, juice or any other liquid to raise the pH level. You just need to follow the dosage instruction on the label, and do not exceed the daily dosage or upper limit. By using a pH paper or pH strip, or litmus paper, you can monitor the pH of alkaline water, and make sure you that the pH of your drinking water is at the desired level.

The pH booster drops are formulated by adding highly concentrated and potent alkaline minerals to deionized water, demineralized water or distilled water. The booster drops contain either one or some of the minerals such as calcium, magnesium, zinc, selenium, phosphate, potassium citrate, sodium citrate, potassium bicarbonate, bicarbonate, potassium lactate, tripotassium citrate, potassium hydroxide, or others.

These drops turn the ordinary tap water into antioxidant-rich mineral water that helps combat free radicals. When regular water is contaminated by pollutants, medications, chloride, fluoride and a host of other water pollutants, it becomes more acidic lowering the pH level to a very low value. If you add pH booster drops to that acidic water, the alkalinity of the water is improved significantly by neutralizing the free radicals and potent healthy cells. When the acids are neutralized, regular water becomes alkaline water with pH above 7. The more drops you add, the more the pH level would be and more the alkalinity of the drinking water would be. By trial and error, it is possible to adjust and achieve the desired pH of alkaline water.

There are many companies selling pH booster drops, and you can find them by searching on the Amazon.com website. The most popular distribution companies are discussed below.

1. ALKALIFE pH BOOSTER DROPS
2. ALKAZONE pH BOOSTER DROPS
3. ALKAVISION PLASMA pH DROPS
4. PIPINGROCK BOOSTER pH PROTECTOR DROPS
5. ALKALINE WATER DROPS from HealthyWiser

# 1. ALKALIFE pH BOOSTER DROPS [28]

ALKALIFE
8888 SW 129 Terrace , Miami, FL 33176, USA.
http://www.alkalife.com/
https://alkalifestore.myshopify.com/

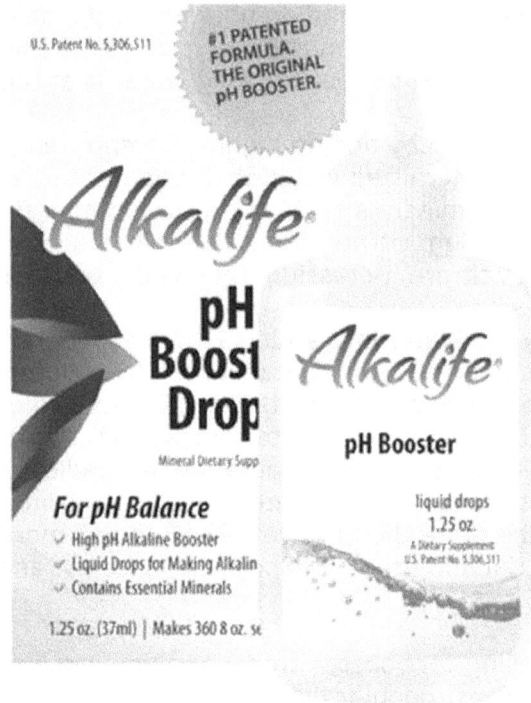

Figure 18.8  Alkalife pH Booster Drops (Courtesy of Alkalife).

## The website of Alkalife claims that:

◉ Two decades ago, scientist, inventor and Reverse Aging author Sang Whang developed Alkalife, the first pH water booster for the human body after researching health issues related to high levels of acid in the body. Today, Alkalife continues to be the leading brand of alkaline enhancers and remains the top choice of wellness experts and health enthusiasts around the world.

◉ Alkalife® provides you with a daily dose of alkaline mineral supplementation that promotes peak bodily performance and ultimate well-being.

◉ Alkalife is a natural, dietary supplement that plays an important part in neutralizing acid. Alkalife pH boosters are the foundation of an alkaline diet lifestyle and enable your body to eliminate harmful toxins. Left unchecked, these waste products become cholesterol, fatty acid, uric acid, kidney stones, urates, phosphates, and sulfates.

◉ Just a few drops of Alkalife turns ordinary drinking water into high pH alkaline water! One bottle of Alkalife creates 360 8 oz. servings of fresh alkaline water with a pH value of 10. Taken 5 times daily, that works out to more than 2 months of Alkalife per bottle!

# 2. ALKAZONE pH BOOSTER DROPS [29]

ALKLAZOE
200 South Newman Street,
Hackensack, NJ 07601, USA
https://alkazone.com/alkaline-drops/

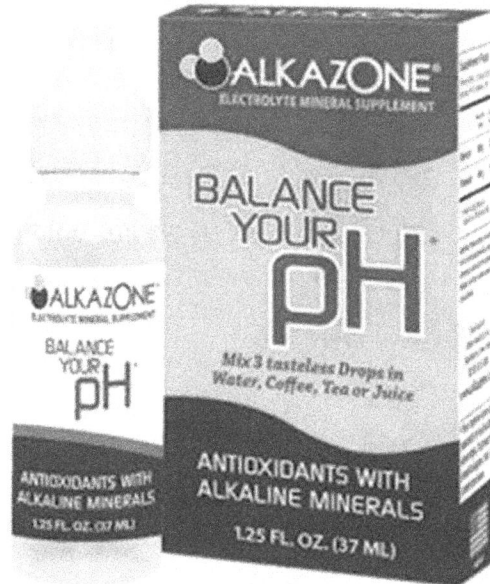

Figure 18.9  Alkazone pH Booster Drops (Courtesy of Alkazone).

## The website of Alkazone claims that:

⊕ Since 1994, we have been the pioneer in promoting good health and a healthy lifestyle with our Flagship Product "Balance Your pH" Booster Drops. Our mission is to fulfill the needs of people wanting to improve their health and to promote a healthy lifestyle.

We are proud to bring you our healthy lifestyle products from our flagship "Balance Your pH" Drops to our Award Winning Water Ionizers and now our new line of Mineral Drops!

⊕ ALKAZONE Antioxidant Alkaline Mineral Drops are designed to raise the pH of your water to improve alkalinity and reduce acidic waste. Formulated with key minerals like magnesium, zinc, phosphate and calcium, these drops turn ordinary water into antioxidant-rich mineral water that help fight free radicals.

⊕ **The Secret is in the water:** The pH balance is key to healthy living. The human body maintains a very delicate pH balance. This is increasingly a challenge! Stress, the environment and everyday foods that you eat here and there bring acids into our systems.

⊕ ALKAZONE  Booster Drops help balance your body's pH level. Just a few drop (3 drops in a glass of water) is enough to make your own alkaline water for healthy living. The essential alkaline minerals will enhance immune system of your body and elevate the pH of your drinking water to 9.5 or more. The essential alkaline minerals will enhance immune system of your body and 9.5+ pH level of your water will help to balance your pH level.

# 3. ALKAVISION PLASMA pH DROPS [30]

AlkaVision, Inc,
2910 Business One Dr,
Kalamazoo, MI 49048, USA
https://alkavision.com/
https://alkavision.com/plasma-ph-drops/

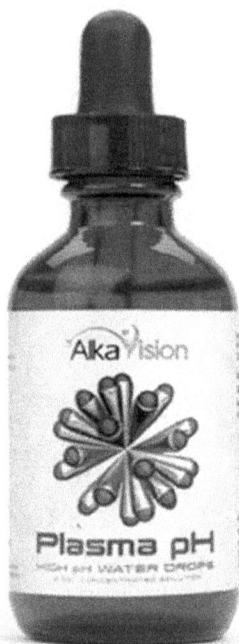

Figure 18.10  Alkavision Plasma pH Drops (Courtesy of Alkavision, Inc.).

## The website of Alkavision claims that:

● AlkaVision Plasma pH Drops contain a unique combination of the most alkaline minerals and compounds. You may have heard of pH drops before and maybe you've tried some. Some users of "other" pH products have reported testing the products for pH, only to find that the products were not at all what they claimed. We've confirmed this unfortunate fact with our own tests. Luckily, for you there's a better way.

● The Plasma pH drops are the best product of this kind on the market. This product delivers the most honest, effective, affordable and reliable method of increasing the pH of fluids in one's body. You can try a one-month supply of Plasma pH drops for free. If you want to experience the benefits of alkalizing your body through diet and supplementation, then you owe it to yourself to try Plasma pH drops today. See for yourself what a difference you can make in your own life.

● We always use glass bottle because concentrated alkaline formulas can leach plastic chemicals out of the plastic bottles. Our drops have no bitter taste, smell or color so you will enjoy them without any discomfort. Ours is by far the best product on the market. But don't just take our word for it. Listen to what your blood says.

## 4. PIPING ROCK BOOSTER pH PROTECTOR DROPS [31]

Piping Rock Health Products, LLC.
2120 Smithtown Avenue,
Ronkonkoma, NY 11779 USA
https://ca.pipingrock.com/alkaline/alkaline-booster-ph-protector-drops-2-fl-oz-59-ml-dropper-bottle-40646

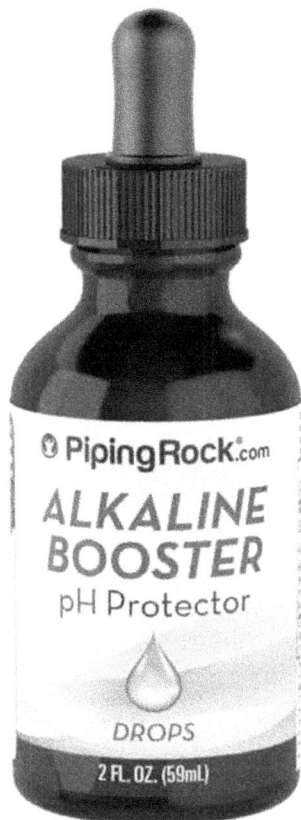

Figure 18.11  Piping Rock Booster pH Protector Drops (Courtesy of Piping Rock Health Products, LLC.).

### The website of Piping Rock Health Products claims that:

● The product contains demineralized water and potassium hydroxide. Serving size: 3 drops. Directions: For adults, take 3 drops in 8-12 oz. of water or beverage as needed. Shake before using.

● Add a boost to your water or drink today with Piping Rock's Alkaline Booster pH protector drops! In each serving, you can make your own alkaline water – convenient enough to take with you anywhere you go. Just throw 3 drops in, and you are set.

● WARNING: Do not use undiluted pH Protector drops. If you are pregnant, nursing or taking any medications, consult your doctor before use. If any adverse reactions occur, immediately stop using this product and consult your doctor. If outer seal is damaged or missing, do not use. Keep out of reach of children. Store it in a cool, dry place.

# 5. ALKALINE WATER DROPS from HealthyWiser [32]

Alkaline Water Drops With Natural Antioxidant 2oz (from HeatthyWiser), ASIN:
B01M337KL3, Available on Amazon.com.

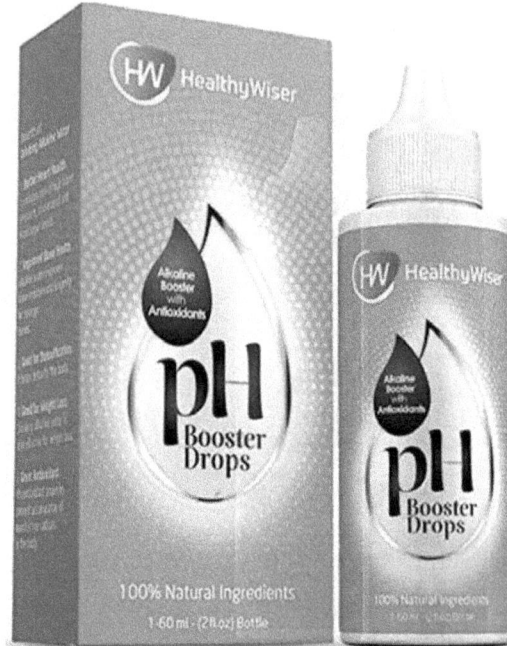

Figure 18.12  Alkaline Water Drops from HealthyWiser (Courtesy of HealthyWiser).

## The Product Owner HealthyWiser claims that:

● CONVENIENT, AFFORDABLE, AND EASY TO USE. Just add pH booster drops to alkalize your normal drinking water and to safely boost your pH levels. No need to buy expensive bottled alkaline water when you can get the same effect using alkaline drops.

● RAISES YOUR WATER'S PH TO OPTIMAL LEVELS. Just add 6 drops to 8oz of water four times per day and feel the difference. Offset acidity by adding drops to your coffee or tea or your favorite beverage. Shake the bottle before adding drops.

● GREAT FOR PHYSICALLY ACTIVE PEOPLE. pH water helps replace electrolytes and trace minerals lost during exercise or heavy physical activity. The bottle of water purifier is portable and easy to tuck into your pocket, backpack, or gym bag so you'll always have access to great tasting alkaline water wherever you go.

● HELPS NEUTRALIZE ACIDITY. Coffee, tea, soda and diet can increase the acidity in your system and can cause acidosis. Adding alkalized water drops immediately boosts your pH level and helps reduce acidity in your system.

● PERFECT FOR ALKALINE AND DETOX DIETS. These pH booster drops are infused with 100% natural antioxidants and alkalizing fruit extracts that go perfectly with your alkaline or detox diet. Flavorless formula doesn't interfere with the taste of your beverage or food so they can be virtually used in everything.

## Advantages of Alkaline Drops

● The pH booster drops, when ingested, act as buffering substances and induce alkalosis and so counteract and limit reduction in pH during the consumption of acidic foods and physical activity.

● Alkaline booster drops also provide your body with the essential minerals that are needed for healthy bones.

● If you feel sluggish and suffer from brain fog, these highly concentrated mineral drops provide you with the energy boost and help you focus on the daily activities.

● You don't need to buy mineral water in plastic bottles which contribute to waste development in landfills. All you need do is add a few drops of pH booster drops to your re-usable glass of water, and you would be saving our planet from waste accumulation.

● Preparing alkaline water by adding pH drops are very cheap compared to purchasing alkaline water in bottles or alkaline water systems.

## Disadvantages of Alkaline Drops

● Keep in mind that while pH drops increase the alkalinity of your water, they do not filter out any of the things like chlorine or fluoride that can be found in your tap water. You need to install an adequate filter to your tap water faucet or use purified water instead.

● These drops change the taste of your water so you may not like the bitterness. You need to be patient until you get used to the taste of highly concentrated minerals and salts.

● Overtime, the pH drops may become depleted and become ineffective. You cannot simply rely on these pH drops by simply believing that you are drinking alkaline water. You need to monitor the pH of your alkaline water, after adding drops, every now and then and make sure the that the the drops are not depleted and that the water you drink is at the desired pH level (which is a hassle!).

● There is no documented peer-reviewed evidence which has been internationally accepted and endorsed by the World Health Organization (WHO) and/or any accredited Medical Community Association, indicating that pH booster drops would contribute to good health better than drinking regular water.

● The statements and claims, posted by the pH booster drops distribution companies or printed on the labels of pH booster drops bottles, have not been evaluated by the FDA or WHO. This product is not intended to diagnose, treat, cure or prevent any disease. If you have a condition, disorder or disease, please consult a licensed medical practitioner.

## RECOMMENDATION ON pH BOOSTER DROPS (by Dr. RK)

Please have your final product (alkaline water obtained by adding these pH booster drops to your tap water or purified water) tested by sending a sample to a certified water testing laboratory in your area, and make sure from the water analysis report that the pH booster drops did not add any impurities or contaminants to your drinking water, and that the water you drink is one hundred percent safe and free of contaminants. Simply relying on these pH booster drops by trusting that they are good for your health would be naïve. Protect your health before it's too late.

# METHOD 6: PURCHASE AN ALKALINE WATER PITCHER

## WHAT IS ALKALINE WATER PITCHER & HOW DOES IT WORK?
Alkaline water pitchers are designed with a high-quality filter that filters the tap water from all kinds of contaminants (such as heavy metals, chemicals, pesticides and and all other toxins) and adds healthy minerals to the filtered water so that the final product would be the purified and alkalized drinking water. The pitcher comes with a drip filter system that allows you to pour tap water directly from the faucet to the top compartment of the pitcher. The pitcher filters the tap water and delivers the mineral-rich alkaline water with a pH level higher than 7, and the added minerals improve the TDS (Total Dissolved Solids) value to 100 ppm, 200 ppm or more. The taste of the resulting water is supposed to be similar to the natural spring water, but with much higher pH level and much higher TDS value. Some pitchers deliver mineralized water that is bitter than you expect, and it may take some time to get used to the alkaline water. The filter embedded in the pitcher has a lifespan (40 – 90 gallons of filtered water), and the consumer needs to replace the filter once every 3 months or 6 months depending on how frequently the pitcher is being used, and how many people are drinking the water from the pitcher.

## BENEFITS OF ALKALINE WATER PITCHER
◉ Alkaline water pitcher does two jobs at a time: (i) it filters and removes all contaminants, toxins from tap water, and (ii) it adds minerals to the filtered water improving both pH level and TDS level. The final product from the pitcher is the alkalized mineral-rich water.

◉ By using a properly designed and highly reputable real alkaline water pitcher (please do not buy a junk pitcher) , you would receive and enjoy all the benefits of alkaline water.

◉ Studies indicated that the alkalized water feeds your body with more oxygenated water, making you feel energized. If the pitcher is equipped with a good water filter, the filter should lower the ORP (Oxidation-Reduction Potential), increasing the water's ability to break down contaminants, thereby promoting higher cell growth.

◉ Keeping your body pH balanced prevents the growth of maligns cells, making it hard or impossible for diseases like cancer to fester in your body. It also prevents the development of diabetes because the pancreas is highly dependent on correct alkaline diet. In Japan, they are using alkaline water to bring down sugar levels. Research showed that alkaline water neutralizes the skin and reduces the symptoms of psoriasis.

◉ Our bodies work hard to maintain pH balance, and often pulls the alkalizing minerals from our tissues and bones to restore the required pH balance in the blood. If you drink slightly alkalized water, your body doesn't need to work that hard and you will not be stressed out from the lack of minerals. Mineral-rich water without toxins can be hard to find on the planet, and if the pitcher is working perfectly as it is designed (Beware! Most pitchers don't work perfectly, there are many junk pitchers in the market), it is a great gift to your body.

◉ It is convenient, reasonably inexpensive, and easy to manufacture your own alkaline water at the comfort of your home. The convenience of having filtered water at your home when you need it is worth the small investment in time and especially in your health. Filtering out those unseen bacteria and toxic contaminants is worth the peace of mind in filtering your own tap water. You just need to replace the filter once every few months.

◉ You don't need to buy mineral water in plastic bottles which contribute to waste development in landfills. All you need do is add a few drops of "pH booster drops" to your re-usable glass of water, and you would be saving our planet from waste accumulation.

# HOW TO SELECT AN ALKALINE WATER PITCHER? [43]

A good customer always does his/her home work before buying an alkaline water pitcher in today's competitive market. It is not hard to research and identify a great alkaline water filter pitcher in the market. More help is available now than ever before. You need to look for and analyze the following 8 criteria while buying an alkaline pitcher:

● **pH Level of Alkaline Water:** As the filter runs longer, the pH level will deteriorate. Be sure to get a pitcher which can maintain constant pH level (between 7 and 9) throughout the lifespan. Be prepared to test the pH of the alkaline water every now and then. You can get this information by talking to the manufacturer.

● **High Quality Filter to Purify the Tap Water:** Make sure the filter is of high quality and is capable to filter the toxic contaminants. The systems should not just add in alkaline remineralization. It should be removing unseen bacteria and toxic contaminants such as chlorine, chloramines, heavy metals, toxic chemicals, etc. Get the water analysis report from the manufacturer that would indicate that there are not contaminants and harmful chemicals in the filtered water.

● **High Quality Raw Material:** Beware of the poor quality pitcher which will leak and breaks. A great pitcher should be built with high-quality BPA-free material and consists of ISO quality certification.

● **Replacement Cost & Frequency:** Some products have low investment cost but unaffordable maintenance cost due to the low quality of the cartridge. Calculate the replacement cost before you buy the system.

● **Size and Capacity:** Depending on the size of your household, select the appropriate jug to serve your family. Some pitchers are great but the capacity is low which only suitable for single occupants.

● **Well Established Brand:** It is important to look for a well-established brand to make sure that you won't have trouble to search for filter replacement after 1 year of usage. Google the company and search for their website. Make sure that it has been in business for la long time.

● **Customer Reviews:** Customer ratings are often the strongest signals whether a pitcher is great or a junk. Spend some time reading the reviews of the water filter jug to determine the quality. The reviews are available on Amazon.com, Amazon.ca, Amazon.co.uk, and many other marketplaces. Read the reviews and pick the one that best suits your needs.

● **Warranty and Customer Service:** Make sure that the pitcher comes with 30-day money-back guaranty from a local store. Test it immediately after you receive it using pH paper and TDS meter, and return it immediately if it fails the tests. If you buy it online, and if you want to return the product, you may end up paying too much for shipping. Don't get into that kind of dilemma. Make sure the company has a toll free number so that you can talk to customer service whenever you encounter technical problems in using the pitcher.

# SOME SELECTED ALKALINE WATER PITCHERS

There are many companies selling pH booster drops, and you can find them by searching on the Amazon.com website. The following pitchers have good reviews so you can trust them:

## 1. pH Restore Pitcher by Invigorated Water

pH Range: 9.0-10.0, Filter Capacity/Lifespan: 96 Gallons (1500 Cups)
Price: $49.97 + Shipping Cost

1. pH RESTORE Alkaline Water Pitcher Ionizer With 2 Long-Life Filters, Water Filter Purifier, Water Filtration System, High pH Alkalizer Machine, Enhanced 4th Gen. Model, 118oz, 3.5L (White), ASIN: B011M7AQPS, 1932 Customer Reviews, Available on Amazon.com. Click Here to Visit.

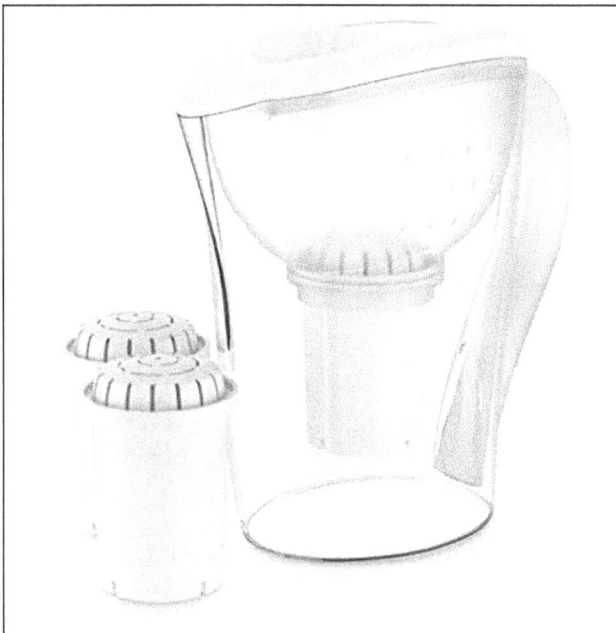

| Figure 18.13  pH RESTORE Alkaline Water Pitcher (Courtesy of Invigorated Water). | Figure 18.14 BIOCERA Pitcher (Courtesy of Biocera). |
| --- | --- |

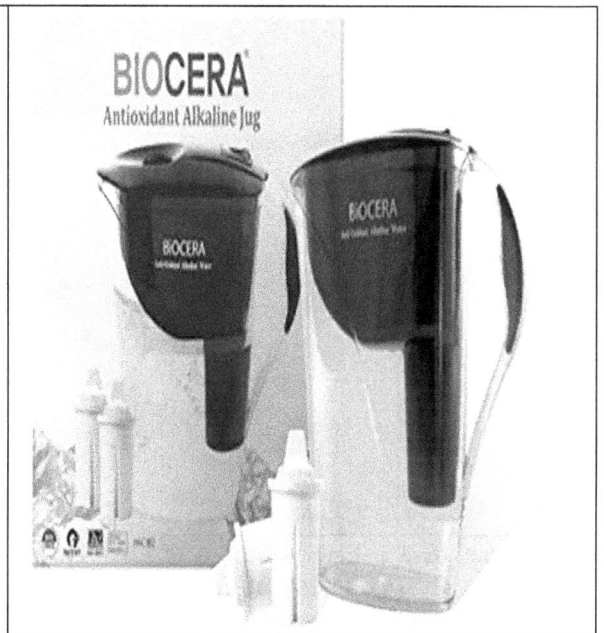

## 2. BIOCERA Alkaline Anti-Oxidant Jug Filter

pH Range: 8.5-9.5, Filter Capacity/Lifespan: Lasts 4 months
Price: $107.80 + Shipping Cost

BIOCERA Alkaline Anti-Oxidant Jug Filter (Includes 2 FREE Cartridges - Lasts 4 Months) by BIOCERA, ASIN: B008TSBFCW, 23 Customer Reviews, Available on Amazon.com. Click Here to Visit.

## 3. EHM ULTRA Premium Alkaline Water Pitcher

pH Range: 8.5-9.5, Filter Capacity/Lifespan: 6 to 8 Weeks.
Price: $39.95 + Shipping Cost

3. EHM ULTRA Premium Alkaline Water Pitcher by EHM, 3.5L Pure Healthy Water Ionizer With Activated Carbon Filter, Healthy, Clean & Toxin-Free Mineralized Alkaline Water In Minutes, ASIN: B00HYEIJLW, 666 Customer Reviews, Available on Amazon.com. Click Here to Visit.

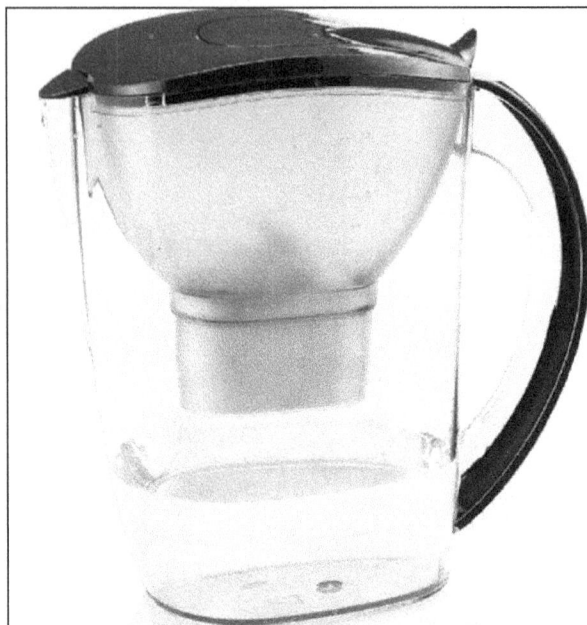

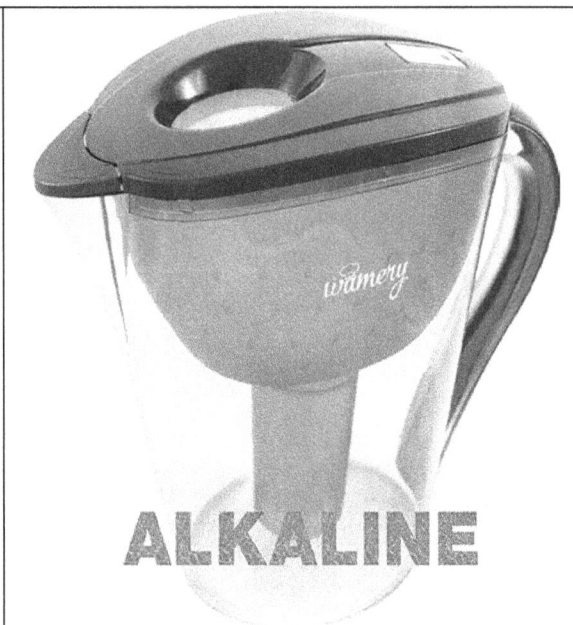

| Figure 18.15  EHM Alkaline Water Pitcher (Courtesy of EHM). | Figure 18.16 Wamery Pitcher (Courtesy of Wamery). |

## 4. Wamery Alkaline Water Pitcher

pH Range: Maintains 8.5 Optimal pH, Filter Capacity/Lifespan: 42 gallons, equivalent to 1 month of use if you fill it 3 times a day or 2 months if you fill it twice a day.
Price: $39.95 + Shipping Cost

Alkaline Water Pitcher. 2 liters or 8 cups, Portable Filter System for Tap Water, Ionize, Filter, Clear, Increase PH and Improve Kitchen Faucet Water Taste. Avoid bottles and machines. Free cartridge by Wamery, ASIN: B01N9CYVM0, 164 Customer Reviews, Available on Amazon.com. Click Here to Visit.

## 5. Lake Industries The Alkaline Water Pitcher

pH Range: 8.5-9.5, Filter Capacity/Lifespan: 6o Days.
Price: $39.95 + Shipping Cost

Lake Industries The Alkaline Water Pitcher - 3.5 liters, Free Filter Included, 7 Stage Filteration System to Purify and Increase PH Levels, ASIN: B0719JX1QG, 122 Customer Reviews, Available on Amazon.com. Click Here to Visit.

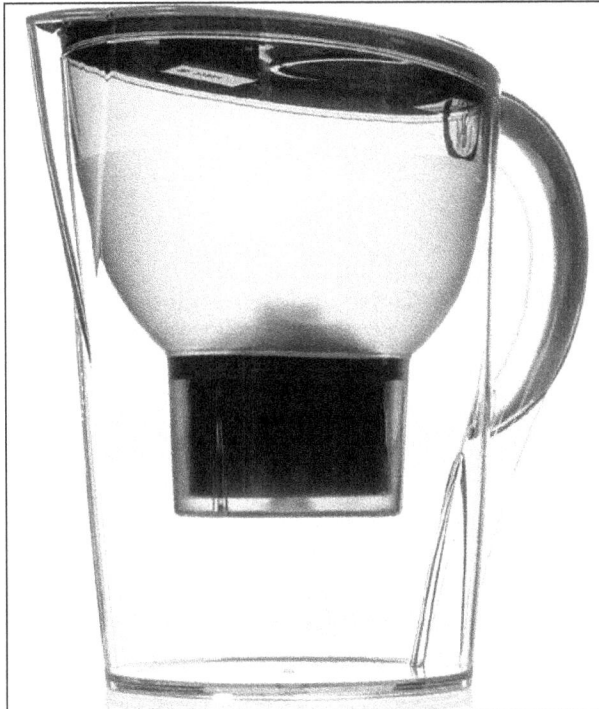

| Figure 18.17 Lake Industries Alkaline Water Pitcher (Courtesy of Lake Industries). | Figure 18.18 Reshape Pitcher (Courtesy of Reshape). |

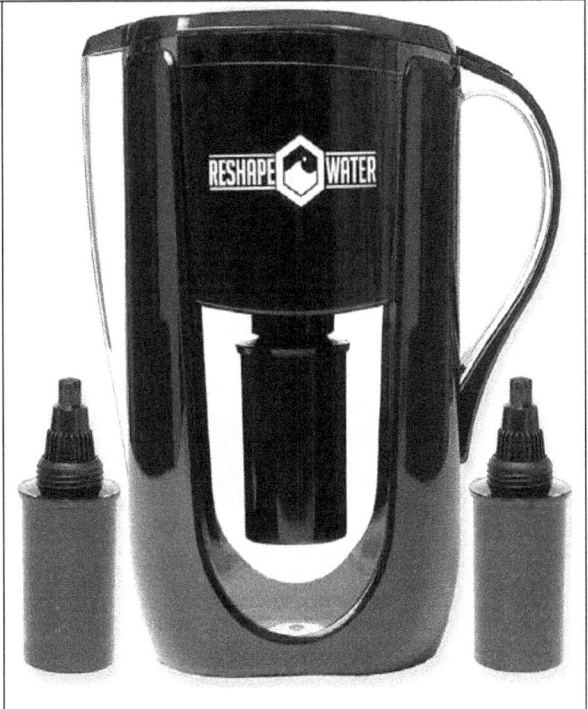

## 6. Reshape Alkaline Water Pitcher

pH Range: Up to 9.5, Filter Capacity/Lifespan: 79 Gallons or 300 Liters, 75 Days.
Price: $125.92 + Shipping Cost

Alkaline Water Pitcher With Fluoride Filter - 3.5 liter Negative ORP 6 Stage Filtration With 2 Replacement Filters, Removes Chlorine and Heavy Metals While Raising pH For Great Tasting Filtered Water, ASIN: B01N5ERFRI, 198 Customer Reviews, Available on Amazon.com. Click Here to Visit.

# RECOMMENDATIONS ON ALKALINE WATER PITCHERS (by Dr. RK)

• Some junk alkaline water pitchers are out there in the market readily available to be purchased and used. Please do not rely on verbal promises and labels, and please test the pitcher before drinking filtered alkaline water. Many of them are not at all what they were claimed to be. Please do not drink water from an alkaline water pitcher without testing it properly. Most of them don't work. Many people purchase and use them without knowing how to test them, and they remain satisfied from the taste of the water. If the water tastes bitter compared to tap water, many people believe that that the pitcher is good. That is the naive way of testing the water.

• For example, when Dr. RK purchased and tested Santevia water pitcher available in Health Food Stores in Burnaby, British Columbia, Canada, the alkaline water pitcher failed miserably. The pitcher was supposed to add minerals and raise the water pH. It did not raise the tap water pH at all. The pH and TDS value of filtered water were found to be unchanged from tap water. The company manager, when questioned, was found suspicious, and refused to provide any further information, but issued a full refund.

• Please be wise to protect yourself and purchase a reliable pH indicator (pH testing drops or digital pH meter) and a TDS meter to test the TDS (Total Dissolved Solids) level of the water. Immediately after you purchase the alkaline water pitcher, test your tap water and alkaline water for pH value and TDS value, and compare the results. If the tap water is alkalized, as the manufacturer claims, you should be able to measure the pH level much higher than 7, and if the pitcher is properly adding minerals to filtered water, the TDS value should go up and should be more than 100 ppm or 200 ppm. If the pitcher passes these two tests, then, only then, you start using the pitcher and start drinking alkaline water delivered by the pitcher. If the pitcher fails the test, then you please do not use it and you better return it and get your money back.

• Also please request the water analysis report from the manufacturer to make sure that the filtered and alkalized water has no harmful contaminants in it. If the manufacturer is good, they should be able to provide water analysis report to consumers.

• When using a pitcher for the first time, please get you final product (filtered alkaline water) tested by a certified laboratory in your area, and make sure that the water you drink is one hundred percent free of contaminants. From the water analysis report, you should be able to make sure that there are no contaminants identified in the water sample. If there are contaminants identified, that means that pitcher has a bad filter, and you should not use such a faulty pitcher.

# METHOD 7: PURCHASE AN ALKALINE WATER IONIZER

## HISTORY OF WATER IONIZERS [43, 44]

A water ionizer (also known as alkaline water ionizer) is a home appliance designed to produce alkaline ionized water from tap water by using the principle of electrolysis/electrodialysis. Minerals of tap water become ionized when they either gain or lose electrons during ionization. All water found in nature (natural water) has minerals in it, and is ionized to some extent. In 1880s, a British scientist Michael Faraday discovered the law of electrolysis. The Russians scientists then used Faraday's discovery to invent the first electrolysis machines in the early 1900s.

Japanese scientists further investigated Russian electrolysis technology, and found that electricity could be used to restructure water molecules, thereby recreating what happens in nature when water runs over rocks. That is to say production of alkaline water (pH >7) with a low ORP (oxidation reduction potential). The ionizer machines originally became popular in Japan and other far eastern countries before they became available in the U.S. and Europe.

The Japanese scientists found jaw-dropping links between ionized water and resistance to human diseases. Proponents claimed that consumption of the alkaline ionized water with minerals results in a variety of health benefits including muscle development, increased mental alertness, cancer, heart disease, diabetes and others. However critics speak out loudly that such claims violate basic principles of chemistry and human physiology, and that they are not backed by any proven scientific or medical evidence to believe in any health benefits of alkaline ionized water.

The secret, the Japanese scientists discovery, has been called micro-clustering. They demonstrated that the ionized water actually has smaller molecule clusters than the normal water that comes out of your tap. When you pour a glass of water from the tap or water cooler, the water molecules are clustered together in big groups – usually 10-13 molecules per drop. But in micro-clustered ionized alkaline water, the clusters are made up of only 5 or 6 molecules, allowing the body's cell to absorb them much quicker, and at the same time resulting in nutrients and minerals being absorbed by the body and utilized much faster, making you more concentrated and alert. This breakthrough discovery from Japanese scientists is believed to be the secret behind the incredibly potent hydrating power of alkaline ionized water – and the life-changing health benefits it unlocks. [44]

Water ionizers first appeared in Japanese hospitals and were approved for home use in the 1950s. More than 30 million people have used a water ionizer since then, and they can be found in one out of every five Japanese homes today. Many consumers nowadays in western countries are turning to alkalizer water and/or alkaline ionized water, as they search for ways to be more health conscious. With all the dangers lurking in tap water and bottled water, the massive benefits of ionized water are just a few clicks away if you intend to own a water ionizer and drink alkaline ionized water. Enjoy water as nature intended it.

Demineralized water or deionized water on the other hand is made by ion exchange process, and has no minerals in it. Distilled water and reverse osmosis water (R O water) are also made by removing all minerals. Water with no minerals in it is not natural water, as all water in nature has at least some minerals in it all, and ionized to some extent.

**IMPORTANT NOTE:** You cannot ionize deionized water (distilled water or reverse RO water) without remineralizing it. The water should have minerals in it.

# BASIC PRINCIPLE BEHIND WATER IONIZATION [34]

Please refer to the Faraday's law of electrolysis. The anode is the positively charged electrode, and attracts electrons or anions. On the other hand, the cathode is the negatively charged electrode and attracts cations or positive charge. Please be noted that the electric charge can flow either from positive to negative or from negative to positive! Because of this, the anode could be positively charged or negatively charged, depending on the situation. The same is true for the cathode. [35]

At the anode you have oxidation reaction which produces electrons with negative charge. At the cathode, on the other hand, you have the reduction reaction which consumes electrons. [36]

To ionize means to gain or lose an electron. Direct current (I) flows from anode (positive pole) to cathode (negative pole). It is also correct to say that direct current flows from cathode (negative pole) to anode (positive pole). Whereas electron current (e-) flows in the opposite direction.

**At the Cathode (Negatively Charged Electrode):**
(-) pole gains or receives the electrons          $2 H_2O + 2e^- = H_2 + 2 OH^-$
**At the Anode (Positively Charged Electrode):**
(+) pole loses or gives away the electrons          $H_2O = 2e^- + \frac{1}{2} O_2 + 2H^+$
          $2 H_2O - 4e^- = 4H+ + O_2$

**Net Reactions**          $H^+ + OH^- = H2O$
          $2 H_2O = 2 H_2 + O_2$

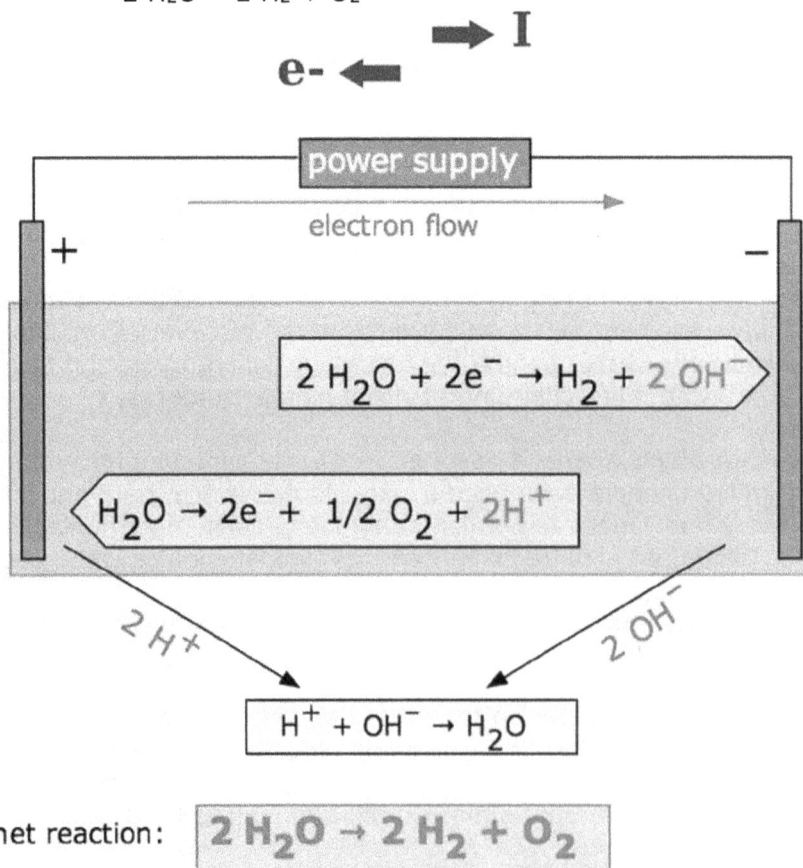

Figure 18.19 Basic principle behind ionization of water.

# HOW DO WATER IONIZERS WORK? [37, 38, 39, 40, 41]

## INTRODUCTION

Home water ionizers use electromagnetic energy to separate the positively charged minerals from the negatively charged bicarbonate components, and produce ionized alkaline water from filtered tap water. Water ionizers are built with charged plates or electrodes. As shown in the diagram, a cathode (negatively charged electrode) and an anode (positively charged electrode) are embedded side by side in an ionization chamber of filtered tap water. These electrodes act like magnets to attract ions that have the opposite charge. Electric current is applied. Positive ions (mineral ions) are attracted to the negative electrode, and negative ions (bicarbonate ions) are attracted to positive electrode. When this occurs, the ions pass through a membrane called "Bipolar Exchange Membrane". This membrane allows only ions (not molecules) of opposite charge to pass through it, but stops other particles, essentially filtering out contaminants. So selecting the appropriate membrane is an important part of this water-ionizer design. Salts and minerals are easily dissolved in water and become ions, and are separated into mineral ions (positively charged) and bicarbonate ions (negatively charged). Water ionizers separate alkaline mineral water from water with bicarbonate ions. Water ionizers also replace the bicarbonate ions with hydroxyl ions ($OH^-$), and produce mineral hydrates. These mineral hydrates raise the water pH, making it alkaline water with healthy properties. The water that contains bicarbonates becomes acidic. Which means that this kind of ion separation process by electrodialysis makes both alkaline water and acidic water at the same time, and are collected into two different reservoirs. The alkaline water is used for drinking and cooking, and acidic water is either discarded or used as a waste byproduct to feed the plants, or as a cleaning agent.

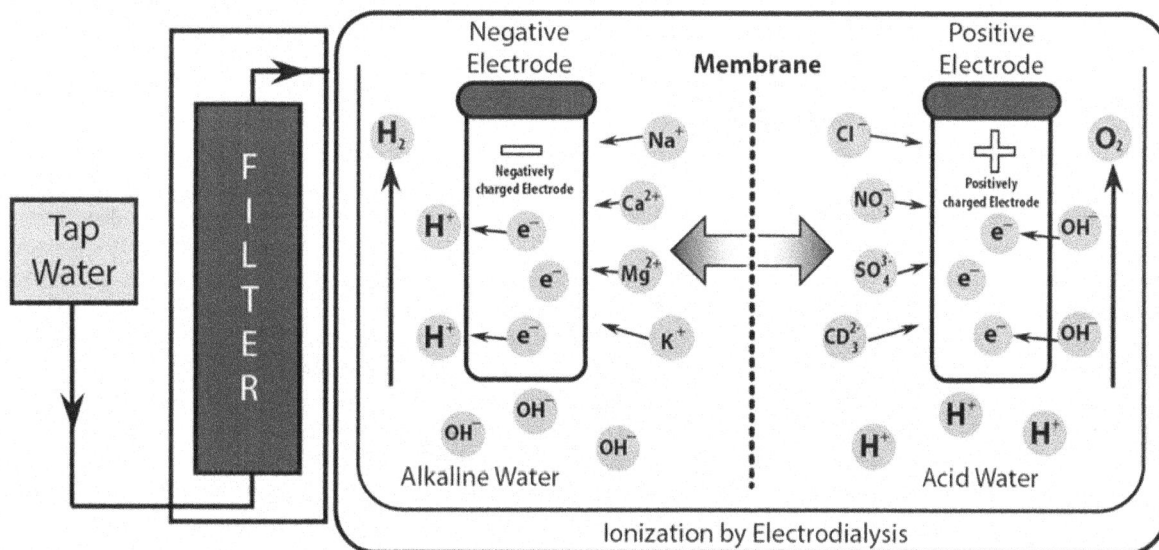

Figure 18.20 Production of ionized alkaline water using ionizers.

## WHAT CHEMICALS ARE ADDED TO TAP WATER IN THE MUNICIPALITY? [41, 42, 43, 44]

Tap water is supplied to your home by the city's local municipality water treatment plants. In those water treatment plants, after passing through several types of filters, they add very many chemicals to treat the unclean or raw water in an attempt to kill and/or destroy toxins, bacteria, unseen viruses, living organisms and microorganisms. The treated water is then distributed to the city's homes. Before it reaches your home, water travels through complex piping systems.

The following is a list of a few chemicals, added to water in the treatment plants:

**Algaecides:** copper sulphate $CuSo_4$, iron salts $FeCl_2$ / $FeBr_2$, rosin amine salts and benzalkonium chloride $C27H42NO2.Cl$.

**Antifoaming Agents:** oils combined with small amounts of silica.

**Coagulants:** aluminum sulphate, aluminum hydroxide, aluminum chloride.

**Corrosion Inhibitors:** compounds of arsenic and antimony, ions such as calcium, zinc or magnesium, may be precipitated as oxides to form a protective layer on the metal pipes.

**Disinfectants:** chlorine, chlorine dioxide, ozone, hydrogen peroxide, uv radiation.

**pH Conditioners:** hydrogen chloride is used to lower pH; lime or calcium hydroxide $Ca(OH)_2$, soda ash or sodium carbonate $Na_2CO_3$, baking soda or sodium bicarbonate $NaHCO_3$ and sodium hydroxide $NaOH$ are used to raise pH.

**Scale Inhibitors:** Some examples of scale formation are calcium carbonate $CaCO_3$, calcium sulphate $CaSo_4$, and calcium silicate $CaSio_3$. Examples of scale inhibitors are phosphate esters, phosphoric acid $H_3PO_4$ and solutions of low molecular weight polyacrylic acid $(C_3H_4O_2)_n$.

In addition they add a variety of other chemicals, not listed here, to treat the water. By the time it travels to your kitchen tap faucet, the water, even though looks clean, crystal clear, transparent, and drinkable, contains many dissolved metals, minerals, chlorides, bicarbonates, nitrates, sulphates and others. All the minerals such as $Fe^{++}$, $Ca^{++}$, $Mg^{++}$, $K^+$, $Na^+$, others are positively charged ions (cations). And all the chlorides, bicarbonates, nitrates, sulphates $Cl^-$, $HCO_3^-$, $NO_3^-$, $SO_4^{--}$, others are negatively charged ions (anions). The tap water is basically a solution of minerals, trace minerals, bicarbonates, chlorides, nitrates, sulphates, other ions and contaminants. If you get your tap water analysed by a certified laboratory, you will see all these components, other minerals, other chemicals and several contaminants such as lead, arsenic, chlorine, fluoride, and other toxins, if present, in the water analysis report.

## IONIZATION OF ELECTRODIALYSIS

As shown in the diagram (see the previous page), the ionization chamber is divided into two compartments by a membrane, and embedded with positively charged electrode (cathode) and negatively charge electrode (anode). When the electric current is applied to the electrodes, the positively charged ions $Fe^{++}$, $Ca^{++}$, $Mg^{++}$, $K^+$, $Na^+$, and others are attracted to negatively charged electrode, pass through the membrane, and the water pH of the left-side compartment increases and becomes alkaline; And negatively charged ions $Cl^-$, $HCO_3^-$, $NO_3^-$, $SO_4^{--}$, and others are attracted to positively charged electrode, pass through the membrane, and the water pH of the right-side compartment decreases, and becomes acidic. The alkaline water in the left compartment contains mostly calcium and magnesium ions. These minerals after they are separated from the bicarbonates, nitrates and sulphates undergo a separate reaction called hydrolysis. They combine with water molecules and pull hydroxyl ions from water molecules. That is the process that forms the mineral hydrates such as calcium hydroxide and magnesium hydroxide - that improves alkalinity. The alkaline water from the left-side compartment is streamed out, stored in a reservoir, and used for drinking and cooking. The acidic water from the right-side compartment is streamed out and either discarded or used for plants or as a cleaning agent. When the ions pass through the membrane, the contaminants are absorbed by the membrane and the water is further purified. The final product "**ionized alkaline water**" is believed to have many health benefits.

| CATIONS (Positively Charged Ions)<br>ALKALINE WATER | ANIONS (Negatively Charged Ions)<br>ACIDIC WATER |
|---|---|
| $Fe^{++}$, $Ca^{++}$, $Mg^{++}$, $K^+$, $Na^+$, others. | $Cl^-$, $HCO_3^-$, $NO_3^-$, $SO_4^{--}$, others |

# OXIDATION REDUCTION POTENTIAL (ORP) [45, 46, 47, 48, 49, 50]

We do not see with our naked eyes, but in the world that surrounds us, there is always a continuous exchange of electrons that takes place between substances in the air, in the Earth, in water, and also in our bodies. This phenomenon is known as ion exchange. In an effort to reach a state of stability, substances that are lacking electrons are desperately seeking out electrons wherever they can, and these substances are referred to as oxidizing agents. On the contrary, substances which have a surplus of electrons are capable of donating their extra electrons, and these substances are referred to as reducing agents, or antioxidizing agents.

The hydrate minerals in alkaline water, as discussed above, are part of the reason why it's good for your health. The alkaline water made by a water ionizer has antioxidant potential. The antioxidant potential of alkaline water, the ability to act as an antioxidant, is measured in millivolts (mV). Scientists call this as the Oxidation Reduction Potential (ORP). Oxidation-reduction potential (ORP) is a measurement that indicates the degree to which a substance is capable of oxidizing or reducing another substance. ORP is measured in millivolts (mV) using an ORP meter.

A positive ORP reading indicates that a substance is an oxidizing agent. The higher the reading, the more oxidizing it is. As such, a substance with an ORP reading of +400 mV is 4 times more oxidizing than a substance with an ORP reading of +100 mV.

A negative ORP reading indicates that a substance is a reducing agent. The lower the reading, the more anti-oxidizing it is. As such, a substance with an ORP reading of -400 mV is 4 times more antioxidizing than a substance with an ORP reading of -100 mV.

Most types of water, including tap water and bottled water, are oxidizing agents as their ORP value is positive. Whereas alkaline ionized water is an antioxidizing agent, and it has a negative ORP value, and it is able to donate extra electrons to neutralize the harmful effects of free radicals on the body. That is why ionized water has health benefits. For example,

**a. Tap water in the USA has positive ORP value between +200 mV and +600 mV.**
**b. The ionized alkaline water has negative ORP value of − 250 mV or lower.**

By having negative ORP value, ionized water produces the "antioxidant" effect in the water through the creation of $OH^-$ ions or the negative hydroxyl ions. As discussed earlier, the minerals in ionized water combine with water molecules and pull hydroxyl ions from water molecules, forming mineral hydrates such as calcium hydroxide and magnesium hydroxide, thereby developing antioxidant properties.

Negative ORP (-ORP) is highly reactive, and dynamic, and does not "stay" in solution for more than a few days before returning to a neutral, or positive state. This is why ionized water is best consumed immediately after it's produced. Ionized water will 'go flat' and loose its antioxidant qualities within a day or few days. If you consume this water immediately after it's produced by the water ionizer machine, you enjoy all benefits of a solution that is substantially high in oxidation reduction potential (free radical neutralizing).

To fully benefit from the ionized alkaline water, and to receive the most therapeutic benefits of your ionized water from any water ionizer device you are planning to own at home, or when you research and purchase a water ionizer, you should verify and choose the machine that fits the following technical criteria.

## WHAT TO DO BEFORE YOU PURCHASE A WATER IONIZER?
(i) Make sure the pH of ionized alkaline water is adjustable between 7.5 and 9.5.
(ii) Make sure it has an abundance of hydrate minerals (TDS is between 200 - 500 ppm).
(iii) Make sure the machine is capable to maintain the negative oxidation reduction potential (ORP) significantly greater than -400 mV (tap water has positive ORP).
(iv) Make sure the final product (ionized alkaline water) has no contaminants. Get the water analysis report from the manufacturer, or get your ionized alkaline water analyzed by a certified laboratory.
(v) Drink ionized alkaline water only when it is fresh, and just came out of the machine or at most within a few hours time. Do not store the ionized alkaline water at home for more than a few hours (or the negative ORP would be neutralized).

## HOW TO PURCHASE AN ORP METER
If you are planning to purchase and own a water ionizer, you should also purchase an ORP meter. There are many ORP meters available on Amazon.com, Amazon.ca, Amazon.co.uk, and also on other marketplaces of Amazon. An example of ORC meter is shown below:

Pinpoint ORP Meter KIT Lab Grade Portable Bench Meter Kit for Alkaline/Hydrogen-Rich/Ionized/Kangen Water, ASIN: B07B35D6HH, Available on Amazon.com.
Click Here to Visit.

https://www.amazon.com/Pinpoint-Portable-Alkaline-Hydrogen-Rich-Ionized/dp/B07B35D6HH/ref=sr_1_3?ie=UTF8&qid=1536000350&sr=8-3&keywords=ORP+meter

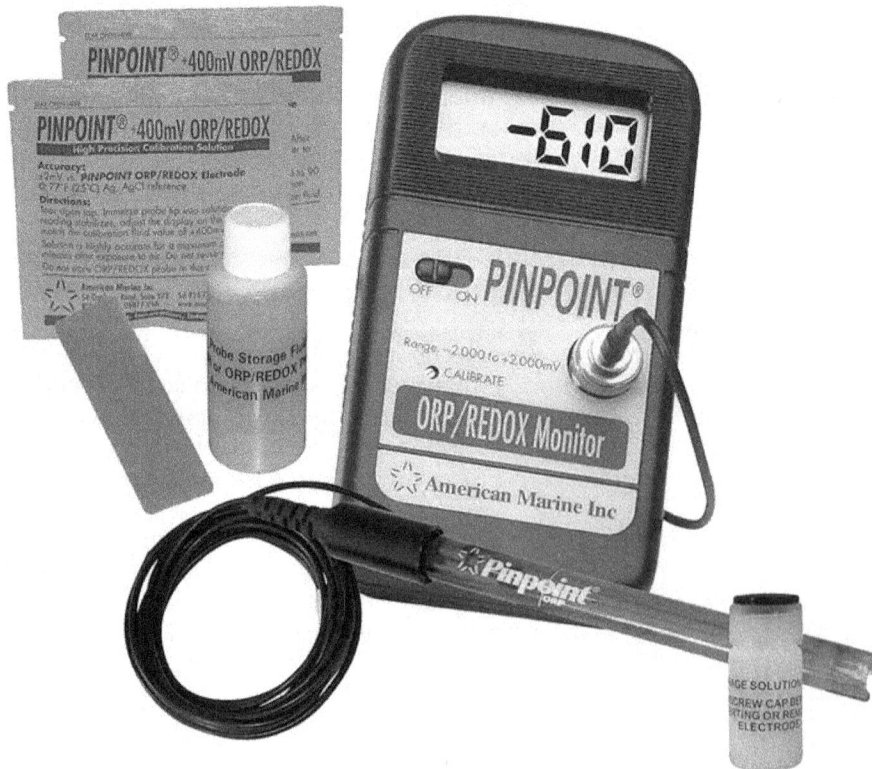

Figure 18.21 ORP meter to monitor oxidation reduction potential.
(Courtesy of American Marine Inc.)

# ELECTROLYZED REDUCED WATER (ERW) [51, 52]

The Japanese scientists discovered that the molecules in tap water (with positive ORP value) are clustered together in big groups – usually 10-13 molecules per drop. But in micro-clustered ionized alkaline water, the clusters are made up of only 5 or 6 molecules groups, allowing the body's cell to absorb them much quicker, and at the same time resulting in nutrients and minerals being absorbed by the body and utilized much faster, which is the major advantage of drinking ionized alkaline water. The ionized alkaline water is therefore called **Electrolyzed Reduced Water (ERW)** because the water of final product from ionization by electrodialysis is transformed into restructured molecules.[34]

This restructure of water molecules creates an abundance of active hydrogen ions (negatively charged) that will seek out, bond with, and neutralize harmful Reactive Oxygen Species (ROS), which are positively charged molecules, more commonly known as "**Free Radicals**". Free radicals are an unstable byproduct of the oxidation process and can be found in tap water and all kinds of bottled water. Free radicals are very unstable and react quickly with other compounds, trying to capture the needed electron to gain stability. These molecules regain balance by stealing electrons from other molecules, resulting in a chain reaction of more unstable free radicals. Once the process begins, it cascades and finally results in the disruption of a living cell. If antioxidants are unavailable, or if the free-radical production becomes excessive, damage can occur. According to the National Cancer Institute, Bethesda, MD, USA, free radicals can be hazardous to the body and damage all major components of cells, including DNA, RNA, proteins, cell membranes, and contributing to the physiology of aging. The damage to cells caused by free radicals, especially the damage to DNA, may play a role in the development of cancer and other health conditions.

Alkaline water acts as an antioxidant, scavenging for and neutralizing harmful free radicals. Because ionized alkaline water has the ability to give up electrons, it can effectively neutralize and block free-radical damage to the body. Ionized alkaline water seeks out free radicals and converts them into oxygen, which your body can use for energy production and tissue oxygenation. Drinking alkaline ionized water regularly may prevent or lower the risk for developing cancerous cells.

## WATER IONIZERS YOU CAN BUY AND OWN

If you are planning to purchase and own a water ionizer, you should first research on Amazon.com, Amazon.ca, Amazon.co.uk, also on other marketplaces of Amazon, and also on Alibaba.com. Read reviews and select the one that best suits your needs. A few water ionizers are shown below:

### 1. Tyent 11-Plate Water Ionizer

Tyent 11-Plate Water Ionizer, Turbo, Lifetime Warranty, Countertop Water Ionizer, Ultra PUREST Filtration, wi.mmp.11-Stainless/Black, Authentic Tyent Brand with Antioxidant Boost™ , ASIN: B00TEFFJP8, Available on Amazon.com, Click Here to Visit.

Alkaline Water Ionizers from Tyent provide pH levels from 2pH to 12pH with TURBO and 1-Touch Technology. 11 Huge Platinum Plates offer DOCTOR RECOMMENDED Antioxidant and -ORP levels. Thin, Sleek Design with Genuine Stainless Steel, UL Listed, FDA approved plastics. Ultra Purest Filtration with 0.01 Micron and Antibacterial Technology (ABT) 75-Day Trial and Lifetime Warranty from Authorized Dealers (longest in the industry).

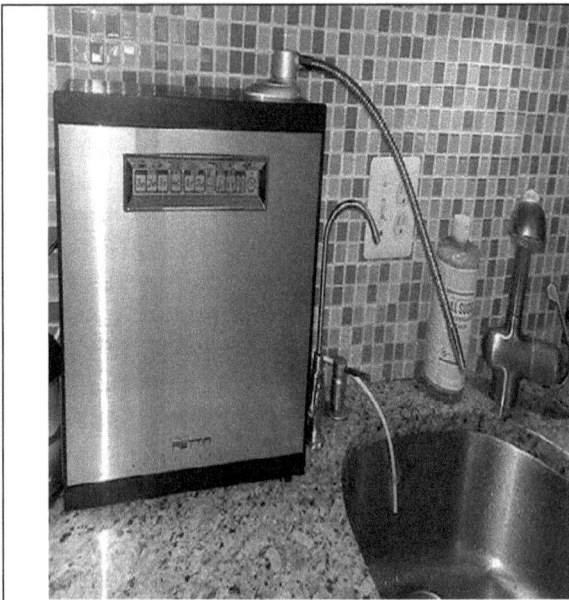

| | |
|---|---|
| Figure 18.22  Tyent 11-Plate Water Ionizer (Courtesy of Tyent 11-Plate Water Ionizer). | Figure 18.23 IntelGadgets Water Ionizer (Courtesy of IntelGadgets). |

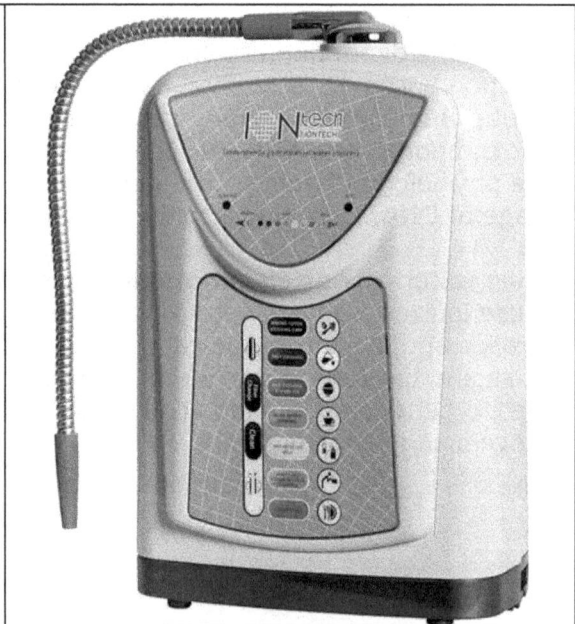

### 2. IntelGadgets NEW Alkaline Water Ionizer Machine

NEW Alkaline Water Ionizer Machine with Filter IONtech IT-580 by IntelGadgets. Powerful, Affordable, FREE Filter by IntelGadgets, ASIN: B00ED2VRAS, Available on Amazon.com. Click Here to Visit.

pH Value Range: 4.5-11 (Max); ORP Value: -850mv (Max) Platinum-titanium electrolysis plates made in Japan Ceramic ion membrane manufactured by Yuasa Japan; Temperature-resistant and non-toxic. Automatic 10-second electrolysis chamber cleansing after each Alkaline water use. 7 selectable levels of water pH values Soft Button Control Panel Built In Activated Carbon Fiber Filter manufactured in USA.

## 3. IntelGadgets Advanced Alkaline Water Ionizer Machine

IntelGadgets IONtech IT-757 Advanced Alkaline Water Ionizer Machine 7 pH Water Levels, Platinum Titanium Electrolysis Plates by IntelGadgets, ASIN: B00E8UC94I, Available on Amazon.com. Click Here to Visit.

pH Value Range 4.5-11 ORP Value -850mv max Platinum-titanium electrolysis plates made in Japan. Ceramic ion membrane manufactured by Yuasa, Japan Temperature-resistant and non-toxic. Automatic 10 second electrolysis chamber cleansing after each Alkaline water use Adjustable filter life settings for various water qualities 7 levels of water pH 7 color LCD display with Soft Button Control Panel; Activated carbon fiber manufactured in USA.

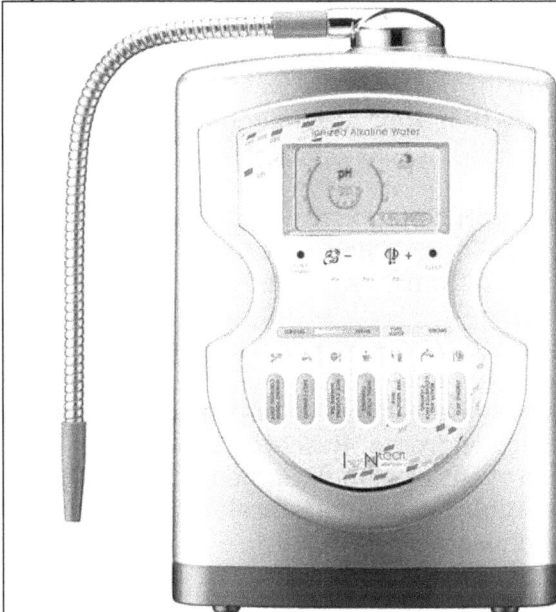

Figure 18.24  IntelGadgets Water Ionizer (Courtesy of IntelGadgets).

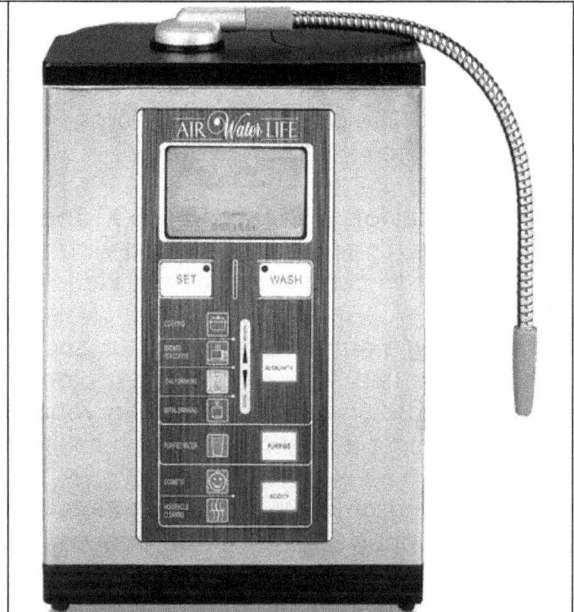

Figure 18.25 Air Water Life Aqua Ionizer (Courtesy of Air Water Life).

## 4. Air Water Life Aqua Ionizer Deluxe 9.0

Air Water Life Aqua Ionizer Deluxe 9.0 | Best Home Alkaline Water Filtration System | Produces pH 3.0-11.5 Alkaline Water | Up to -860mV ORP | 4000 Liters Per Filter | 7 Water Settings by Air Water Life, ASIN: B012E4MURK, Available on Amazon.com. Click Here to Visit.

HAPPY, HEALTHY & HYDRATED: Alkaline water may help detoxify the body, increase energy & hydration. MORE THAN DRINKING WATER: 7 water settings allow you to adjust the alkalinity & add antioxidants. FILTRATION AT ITS FINEST: Advanced filtration technology purifies & ionizes over 4000 liters. ENVIRONMENTALLY FRIENDLY: Ionizer reduces waste from plastic water bottles & is ETL & RoHS certified. 110 VOLTS ONLY - CUSTOMERS SAY: I never realized WATER could taste this good! | Water just became the new soda!

# Benefits of Alkaline Ionized Water, Posted By Life Ionizers [53]
## The Alkaline Ionized Water Manufacturer "Life Ionizers" Posted the following:

**1. Superior Hydration:** Alkaline water has been shown to increase the level of a powerful antioxidant called Superoxide Dismutase (SOD). The function of antioxidant SOD in your liver is to enhance the livers blood cleansing function.

**Oxygen Saturation:** Lactic acid waste in the muscles reduces oxygen uptake. Alkaline water has been shown to counter lactic acid in the muscles which improves the muscles' ability to use oxygen.

**Cleanse Colon:** Ensuring proper hydration keep the colon lubricated. When you are dehydrated, your brain has priority over the rest of your body for the water in your bloodstream. The colon is the first organ in your body that your brain deprives of water, so it dries out when you're dehydrated.

**2. Detoxification & Cleansing in Kidneys:** Alkaline pH bicarbonate ions supplied by alkaline water combine in the blood with acidic toxins. The resulting combined molecule is large enough to get trapped by the kidneys and flushed from your system.

**3. Balancing Your Body's pH:** Your body is not all one pH, some parts are naturally acidic, others naturally alkaline. Your blood maintains a narrow range of 7.35 - 7.45 pH. Maintaining the proper pH balance in your kidneys has been shown to be a preventive measure against a medical condition called metabolic syndrome. Research shows that raising the pH level of your urine by just 1 pH can prevent or eliminate the symptoms of metabolic syndrome. Obesity, High Blood Pressure, High Blood Cholesterol, High Blood Sugar and Kidney Stones can be treated with alkaline water.

**4. Weight Loss and Detoxification:** Fatty acids are poisonous to your body, so it stores the acids it can't get rid of in a protective buffer of fat. Alkaline water can help neutralize these acids and flush them from the body

**Hydration:** Better hydration improves athletic endurance, and helps the body maintain its temperature during workouts.

**pH Balance:** Research published by Harvard University Medical shows that maintaining the body's pH balance with alkaline water reduces your chance of suffering from the symptoms of metabolic syndrome - one of which is weight gain.

**5. Anti-aging:** Aging in the body is a complex process controlled by many factors, one of which is oxidation caused by free radicals. Oxidation occurs when free radicals - also known as oxidants - attack the molecules that make up healthy tissues in the body by stripping them of electrons. Antioxidant alkaline water works to prevent free radicals from attacking your tissues by providing an abundance of excess electrons in the body. These excess electrons neutralize the free radicals that cause cellular and DNA damage that leads to premature aging.

**6. Heart Health & Blood Pressure:** Alkaline ionized water has been shown to reduce blood pressure and lower cholesterol levels in people with mineral deficiencies; a health problem that public health officials estimate is widespread.  One study on alkaline water's ability to reduce blood pressure showed that alkaline water supplied beneficial levels of calcium and magnesium even for people with health problems that impair their ability to absorb those minerals.

**7. Liver Health:** Alkaline water has been shown to reduce oxidative stress in the body that affects the liver. A recent study showed an average 43% reduction in T-BARS (Thiobarbituric Acid Reactive Substances) chemicals in the body that cause liver damage.

Alkaline water has also been shown to increase levels of a critical antioxidant that protect the liver. Superoxide Dismutase (SOD) breaks down bad cholesterol and hydrogen peroxide in the liver. Higher levels of SOD in the liver help it cleanse blood more efficiently.

**8. Bone Health:** Research shows a clear link between alkaline water and bone health. When your body's pH balance becomes acidic, your body will adjust it by taking calcium from your bones. Several studies have shown that drinking alkaline water can significantly reduce the amount of calcium lost due to body acidity, and reduces bone loss. Alkaline water also supplies useful amounts of calcium to your body. Research shows that calcium is easier to absorb from water than it is from food based sources.

**9. Digestive Health:** Alkaline water has an antacid effect which can lead to fewer upset stomachs, and improve overall digestive health. Measurement of stomach pH levels after drinking alkaline water showed that stomach pH increased by .5 to 1 pH. The beneficial antacid effect lasted for a half hour after the water was drunk.

**Digestive Health Tip:** For better digestive health, drink a glass of alkaline water first thing when you get up, and a half hour before meals. That helps get things moving in your intestines, and gently stimulates digestive juices.

**10. Sports Performance:** When exercising, you are consuming more oxygen and metabolizing energy through muscle work. This process creates free radicals, lactic acid and a mild metabolic acidosis. Drinking alkaline, ionized, mineral hydrate water can help ameliorate all three of these byproducts of exercise.

# LISTEN TO WHAT CRITICS SAY ABOUT ALKALINE IONIZED WATER
[54, 55, 56, 57, 58]

The following statements were found in Modern Ghana News: [54]

◉ There is no documented peer-reviewed evidence which has been internationally accepted and endorsed by the World Health Organization (WHO) and/or any accredited Medical Community Association, indicating that drinking water of more alkaline nature impact good health better than regular drinking water, The FDA says.

◉ **Alkaline Ionized Water:** In water ionizers (also in Kangen water machines), they produce artificial alkaline water, splitting the water molecule by applying electricity. Both hydrogen ions and hydroxyl ions travel through a membrane and accumulate on the opposite sides in the process of ionization. The concentration of hydroxyl ions (OH-) travelled to the anode (positive electrode) is responsible to raise the pH of the final product even though no minerals are added to the tap water. Alkaline minerals in the water end up as hydroxides (attached to the OH- ion). These compounds are not recognized by the body. If a person's kidneys are functioning well, they will be excreted in urine. If not, they may end up as arterial plaque or as mineral deposits in joints and other tissues. There are other problems with alkaline ionized water. Nature creates coherent liquid crystalline water using movement and weak electromagnetic fields. Those who sell ionizers believe that the strong electric current used during ionization produces coherent liquid crystalline water. It does not. Although electric current causes water molecules to align in the direction of the electric current, the overall degree of structure in the water is reduced. Water that has been treated in this manner is no longer capable of carrying the finely-tuned signals and other vibratory information that water is intended to carry within the human body. This kind of alkaline ionized water is detrimental to human health.[55, 56]

◉ Alkaline Ionized water is aggressive and imbalanced. In addition, alkaline ionized water has an increased concentration of deuterium, making it heavy water. [55, 56]

◉ Some people experience an initial "high" when they start drinking alkaline water. This can easily be attributed to detoxification, and the fact that they are likely just becoming better hydrated. Detoxification is about the only benefit of alkaline water, and this benefit is limited to very SHORT TERM USE (no more than a week or two). An additional concern is that many individuals have stomach dysfunctions like GERD or ulcers that are largely related to having too little stomach acid. Long-term use of alkaline or ionized water can interfere with your body's natural digestive process by reducing the acid needed to properly break down and absorb food. This could then lead to an upset of your body's good bacteria, which can then open the door to parasitic infection, ulcers and malabsorption. [57]

◉ Alkaline ionizers do not create substantial alkalinity of water. Alkaline ionizers are highly dependent upon the source water. There has to be enough alkaline minerals in the source water supply (e.g., tap water) to create alkalinity of water. Alkaline ionizers do not contribute to acid-alkaline balance in your body (or alkalizing your blood stream). There have to be enough acid-neutralizing minerals to create alkalinity in your body. Alkaline ionizers do not have good filtration. Your drinking water may still contain contaminants that are unsafe to drink. Alkaline ionizers are unnecessarily expensive. Why spend thousands on an inadequate water filter when you can have more success with pure, clean water and a little bit of baking soda? [58]

# METHOD 8: PURCHASE A KANGEN WATER MACHINE KANGEN WATER

## HISTORY OF KANGEN WATER [60, 61, 22]

The word Kangen in Japanese means "return to the origin". During the 1950's Japan was struck by severe acid rains that came from China. Determined to bring healthy pure water to their people, scientists began working on a solution. They searched, far and wide, from Himilayans and throughout India for a natural healing source. Miraculously, they found healing waters that were alkaline and hexagonal. In 1800's, a British scientist Michael Faraday discovered the theory of electrolysis of water. Russians then used Faraday's discovery to invent the first electrolysis machines in the 1940's. Later on, Japanese scientists, armed with the secrets they learned in their travel, returned to Japan and constructed the first commercial water ionizer.

Kangen water is a water that is alkaline, electrolyzed, hexagonal and antioxidant. This means that it contains the same or better healing properties as the natural healing water sources we often heard, and still hear about around the world. This water is unique in the world and is a registered trademark by Enagic – a company based out of Osaka, Japan.

In 1966, the ministry of rehabilitation and health of Japan confirmed that alkaline water was beneficial for one's health and medical use. Since then over one-hundred Japanese hospitals have administered and used this water to their patients. Later they spread out the news.

In 1998, Dr. Shirahata of Kyushu University had discovered the connection between electrolyzed water and Holy water, often called Miracle Water. Holy water is known for its tremendous healing power and has shown that it works against just about any diseases.

In 2001, **Mr. Hironari Oshiro** (the founder of Enagic) emerged with a company in Japan by the name of Toyo Aitex. Up until 2001, Toyo Aitex company was the company producing this amazing medical water in hospitals all over Japan. They even gained a reputation as the best water ionizer company out of 30 other Japanese water ionizer companies. Mr. Oshiro then became the president of the Enagic company and the company was born.

A group of more than 600 Japanese physicians, who are members of the Geriatric Disease Prevention Association, began researching the uses of ionized water in patient treatment. On July 1, 2002 this highly esteemed association presented Enagic with an award of recognition for the quality, safety and efficacy of the LeveLuk series of water ionizers in the role of lifestyle disease prevention. This is the only water ionizing company to receive such an award.

In 2003, Enagic entered the American market through the city of Los Angeles. The first conference was held in Japanese with English translators and all the documents were in Japanese.

Today, over 4,000 Enagic water systems (Kangen Water™) are being sold per month in the USA, and the numbers have been steadily climbing. Known for the Gold Standard, Enagic are certified by ISO 9001 and ISO 14001. They also hold various environmental awards along with medical certificates from Japan.

Enagic introduced Kangen Water™ and the company's "Philosophy of True Health" to the US in 2003 and the response has been remarkable. Physicians and laymen alike have been amazed at the effects Kangen Water™ has been showing on the health of human body.

# KANGEN WATER MACHINES

## What Is Kangen Water™?

The website of Enagic Corporation claims the following information:

For over four decades, Japan-based Enagic International has been the leading manufacturer of alkaline ionizers (Kangen water machines) and water filtration machines in the world. Our passion is to transform the tap water in your home into pure healthy electrolyzed-reduced and hydrogen-rich drinking water. The Enagic Corporation direct sales system empowers hard-working and passionate independent distributors around the world. They fall in love with our products, and they spread the word about the positive changes Kangen Water® has brought into their lives and finances. Since 1974, Enagic has been a pioneer and innovator in alkaline water ionization technologies. By integrating scientific research with superior Japanese craftsmanship Enagic's Kangen Water® enhances and restores your body's most vital life, and is used for various purposes, including drinking, cooking, beauty, and cleaning around the world. [63]

Dr. Hiromi Shinya, a leading endocrinologist, clinical professor of surgery, head of the endoscopic center at Beth Israel Medical Center, Vice-chairman of the Japanese Medical Association in the United States says: Kangen Water® is alkaline rich water (ph 8-9.5), and is considered the very best drinking water because of its incomparable powers of hydration, detoxification, and anti-oxidation. [64]

Kangen Water™ cannot be purchased in bottles from supermarkets. Instead, you need to purchase the Kangen Water machine, and produce your own Kangen water by plugging it to your kitchen sink faucet. Kangen Water™ cannot be bottled and stored for a long time on the shelf or in your fridge, because it will lose its antioxidant value (It has hydrogen in it and hydrogen will slowly dissipate into the atmosphere within 72 hours)!

In Japanese language Kangen is pronounced as "kun-gen", and in Japan Kangen literally means "return to original". Kangen alkaline water has been used in Japan for more than 40 years and has been shown to help restore the body to its healthy and disease-free original condition. Kangen water is alkaline, ionized, antioxidant, electron rich, restructured, micro-clustered, active-hydrogen saturated, oxidation-reduced water. When tested for ORP (oxidizing reduction potential) using an ORP meter, it shows a NEGATIVE reading. The Kangen water pH reading can be adjusted between 8.5 and 9.5, making it alkaline, which is the opposite of acidic. [65]

Kangen Water®, aka electrolyzed reduced water (ERW) or hydrogen-rich water, is antioxidant-rich, healthy water that revitalizes cells and a healthy alternative to regular tap water or bottled water. Kangen Water™ process begins as tap water. The Enagic® machine's carbon filter, embedded in the machine, filters out chlorine and other impurities from the tap water, produces hydrogen and oxygen with a process known as electrolysis, and then separates the hydrogen and oxygen into two different streams. This process adds an electron to the hydrogen, creating a new molecule called diatomic molecular hydrogen gas. When this is added to the alkaline water stream, it produces antioxidant-rich Kangen Water™, which is your healthy drinking water. Oxidant, by definition, is an oxidizing agent, while antioxidant is any substance that acts to slow or prevent the oxidation of another chemical. In the human body, oxidative damage plays a huge role in many of our modern day diseases such as cancer, heart disease, and diabetes. Antioxidants, on the other hand, act to tame the free radicals, which are highly reactive chemicals in the body, that have potential to harm cells and cause disease. [66]

# HOW DOES A KANGEN WATER MACHINE WORK? [65, 66, 67, 68, 69, 70, 71]

**BASIC PRINCIPLE:** The principle based on which the Kanger water is made is that of electrolysis process. You simply connect the Kanger water machine to your kitchen sink faucet, you turn on the power switch, allow the tap water to flow by opening the kitchen sink faucet, and then the magic begins. The regular tap water is initially purified by the internal carbon filter and then ionized via electrolysis process.

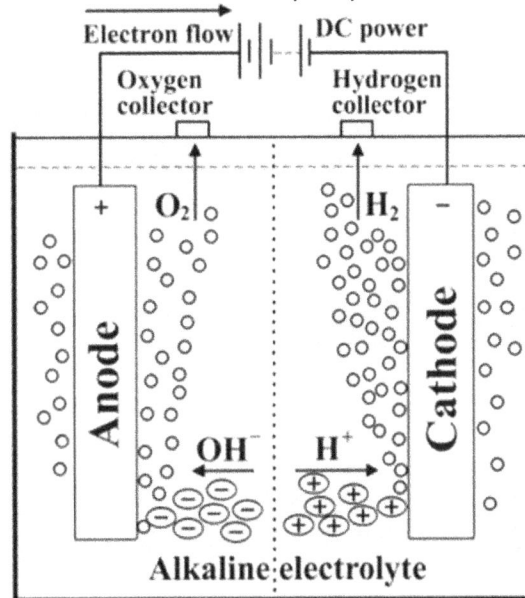

Figure 18.26 Electrolysis of tap water to produce Kangen water.

The electrolysis tank is divided into two compartments by means of a specially designed membrane. Creating an electric potential through water causes positive ions, including the inherent hydrogen ions $H^+$ or $H3O^+$, travel through the membrane towards the cathode (negative electrode). And hydroxide ions ($OH^-$) being negative travel through the membrane in the opposite direction towards the anode (positive electrode). Oxygen can have either a positive or negative charge. Oxygen is two electrons shy of having a full outer electron shell, so in chemical reactions it tends to pick up electrons and become negative. With a sufficient potential difference, this causes electrolysis with hydrogen gas being produced at the cathode and oxygen gas being produced at the anode. The electrolysis of water usually involves dilute or moderately concentrated salt solutions in order to reduce the power loss driving the current through the solution, but the salts and minerals of tap water allow the electrolysis to take place without any addition of salts and minerals. [67]

In the process of ionization, water dissociates into $H^+$ ions and $OH^-$ ions. The $H^+$ ions are attracted to the negative electrode (the cathode) and are converted (or reduced) to hydrogen atoms (H). That is to say $H^+ + e- => H$. Hydrogen atom has a highly unstable configuration, and therefore immediately reacts with another hydrogen atom to produce molecular hydrogen gas ($H_2$) and infuses into the alkaline water being generated. That is why Kangen water is hydrogen-rich water. [68, 69]

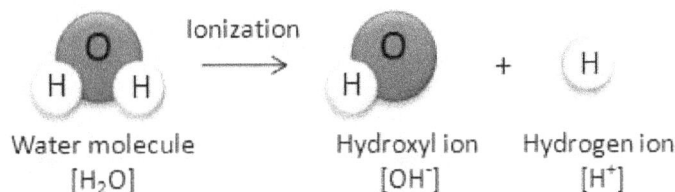

Figure 18.27 Electrolysis of tap water to produce Kangen water.

Both hydrogen ions and hydroxyl ions travel through a membrane and accumulate on the opposite sides. The concentration of hydroxyl ions (OH-) travelled to the anode (positive electrode) is responsible to raise the pH of the final product (Kangen water) even though no minerals are added to the tap water. Hydroxyl ions (OH ions) present in Kangen water are free radical scavengers. That is why Kangen water is called hydrolyzed water as the pH is raised without adding any chemicals or minerals to the tap water. [70]

Antioxidants are important to your body because they neutralize free radicals and stop the harmful damage to your body caused by these renegade cells. Free radicals can be triggered by environmental factors such as sun exposure, pollution, heavy drinking, cigarette smoke, unhealthy eating habits, etc. Free radicals are highly reactive and leave a path of damaged cells and even more free radicals in your body. The damaged cells further create many health problems, including premature skin aging, cancer, diabetes, heart disease and others. You need antioxidants to fight free radical damage. This can be accomplished by drinking Kangen water. [71]

**Electrolyzed Reduced Water (ERW):** Kangen water is produced through a special electrolysis process that changes the pH of the water to alkaline range. Most other water electrolysis equipment will not create active hydrogen in their water and, therefore, the other ionizers merely produce ionized alkaline water that is not true Kangen water. Kangen water is also known to have small clusters of 5 to 6 water molecules, as a result of the special electrolysis process, making it a super hydrating water. You can taste the difference in your first glass. Tap water is typically has 12 to 15 molecules per cluster. That is over double the size of Kangen water. Small clusters also mean that your body can readily absorb the minerals in this water into your cells in mere seconds. That is why Kangen water is called "Electrolyzed Reduced Water (ERW)". [71]

The electrical charge of Kangen machine re-arranges healthy minerals that are naturally included in your tap water as shown in the diagram below. As a result, Kangen water contains essential minerals, such as calcium, magnesium, and potassium, in an ionic form, that can be assimilated immediately into your body. Therefore some people believe that drinking Kangen water is a lot healthier than store-bought mineral water. [71]

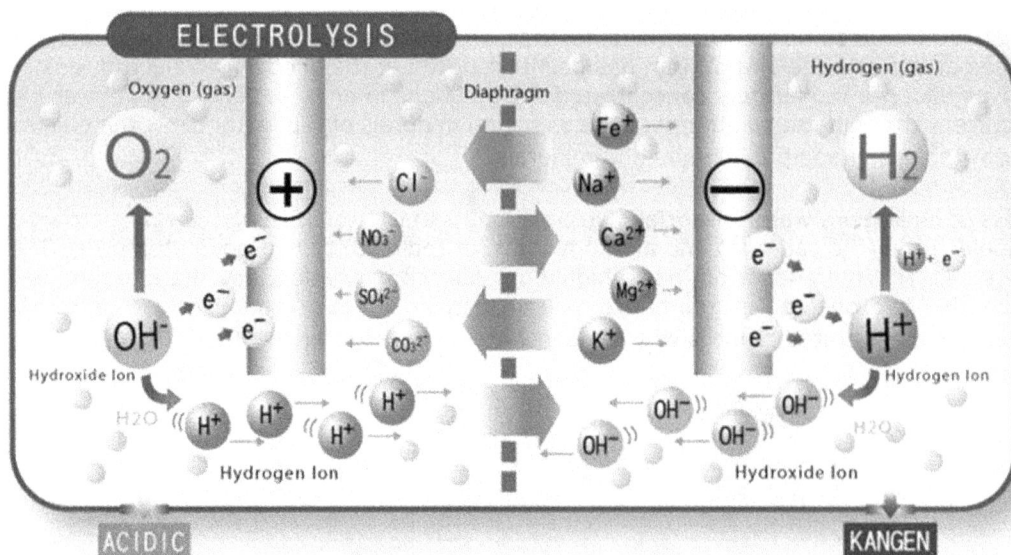

Figure 18.28  Electrolysis of tap water to produce Kangen water.

**Oxidation Reduction Potential (ORP)** of Kangen water is a measurement of voltage. It can be measured by using ORP meter. When the measured value of ORP in water is in negative millivolts, that means the water is electron-rich, healthy and life enhancing. When measured with a positive millivolt it is life depleting. The reading of mV indicates the millivolts (mV) of hydrogen electrons present in the water available to bond with the free radicals and flush them out. Tap water has an ORP of positive value, where as Kangen water has negative ORP. Kangen water machines can produce incredibly functional high pH waters with an ORP below -550 mV for alkaline water, and with an ORP of above +1000 mV for acidic water. [65]

## A REAL KANGEN WATER MACHINE EXPLAINED [65, 72]

The ionizing unit, about 12" high, 11" wide and 7" deep, is a countertop electrical appliance connected to your kitchen water supply to perform electrolysis on tap water before you drink it or use it in the kitchen for cooking or cleaning. The Kangen water contains a lot of hydroxide ions (OH-) and positive ions (such as calcium ions) produced by electrolysis, and it also contains hydrogen. This depends on the choice of resulting water and original water.

A special attachment redirects tap water out of the Kitchen sink faucet through a plastic hose into the unit. Inside the unit, the water is first filtered through activated charcoal. Next, the filtered water passes into an electrolysis chamber, powerful and compact in design, is equipped with 7 platinum-coated electrode plates in which electrolysis takes place.

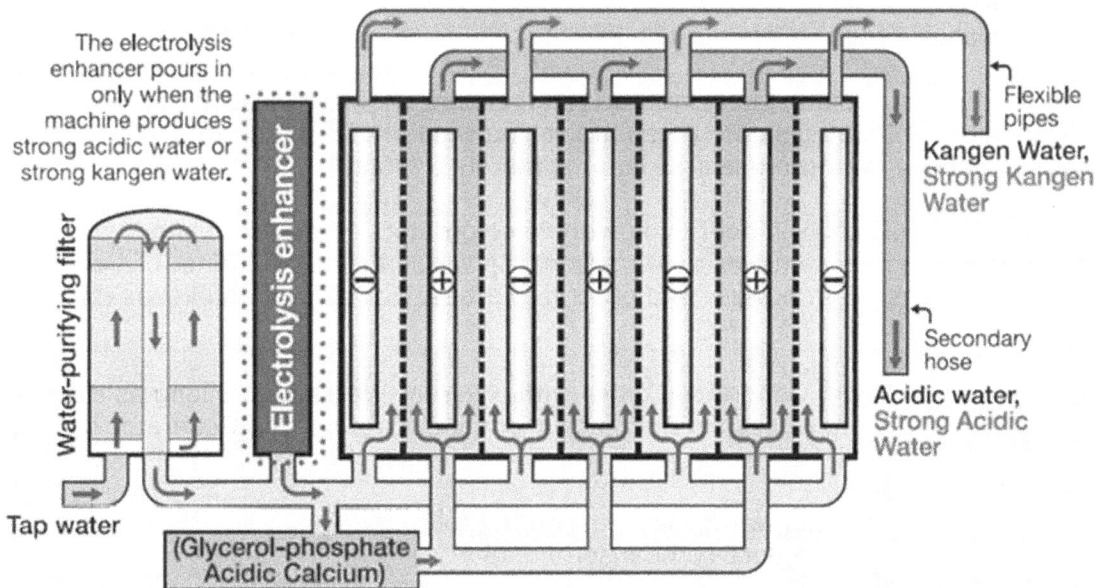

Courtesy of Enagic Corp.
Figure 18.29  Kangen water machine equipped with 7 electrodes.

Cations (positively charged ions) gather at the negative electrodes to create cathodic water or reduced water. Anions (negatively charged ions) gather at the positive electrode to make anodic water (oxidized water). Through electrolysis, reduced water not only gains an excess amount of electrons (e-), but the cluster of $H_2O$ seem to be reduced in size from about 10 to 13 molecules per cluster to 6 molecules per cluster.

This design is made possible by loading an electrolytic cell with seven electrode plates that use electrodes made of platinum plated titanium. The Kangen water side supplies water with a lot of hydroxide ions (OH-) and positive ions (such as calcium ions) produced by electrolysis, and it also contains hydrogen. Therefore Kangen water is also called hydrogen-rich water. The alkaline water stream and acidic water stream are separated by two different outlets.

Electrolysis Enhancer Tank: The unit is equipped with electrolysis enhancer tank. Strong acidic water and strong alkaline water (Kangen water) are produced steadily and continuously. The built-in tank for the electrolysis enhancer fluid makes it easy to supply ample strong acid and strong Kangen water and allows you to produce both kinds of water steadily and continuously. The addition of electrolysis enhancing fluid (440ml) will create 30 liters of strong acidic water in 20 minutes. (Enhancing fluid is available for purchase.)

The unit is designed with a large-sized Liquid Crystal Display (LCD) and the voice prompted guide. It is easy to use with one-touch control panel of "ON" and "OFF" power switch and also it is easy to control to select your desired water type. You can get any desired pH alkaline water for drinking. The LCD Panel with the voice prompts will inform you of the 5 types of water being produced:

a. Kangen Drinking Water (pH 8.5 / pH 9.0 / pH 9.5)
b. Acidic Water (below pH 7)
c. Strong Acidic Water (pH 2.5)
d. Clean Water (pH 7)
e. Strong Alkaline Kangen Water (pH11.5)

You can use your water-cleaning filter until the total amount of waters that the filter has treated reaches around 3,000 gallons. If you are taking the Kangen Water around 16 gallons of water per day, you can use it for approximately 6 months.

The LCD Panel of the machine will notify you with voice prompts and alarm when it is time to change the filter.The filter removes matters from tap water such as chlorine (bleaching), fluoride, effluvium, rusts, lead, powder and other impurities. However, it still keeps the minerals of tap water.

This Ionzed Electrolysis Water Generator Comes with a 5-Year Warranty. As long as the Enagic Kangen Water System is cleaned periodically and consistently, the Generator can last for 15-20 years.

You can find a variety of Kangen water machines on the following link:
https://www.enagic.com/?c=product-comparison

# TYPES OF KANGEN WATER

Kanger water machines produce 5 different types of water as shown in the following table. The type of Kangen water is recognized by its pH value.

Table 18.6  Kangen water machine produces 5 types of Kagen water. [63, 64]

| Type of Kangen Water | pH Range | Application |
|---|---|---|
| 1. Strong Alkaline Water | 11.0 | Should not be used for drinking. Strong cleaning agent for the removal of pesticides and other toxins in raw foods before cooking. Also used for dishwashing, kitchen cleaning, stain removal, etc. |
| 2. Kangen Alkaline Water | 8.5 to 9.5 | Perfect for drinking and cooking with many health benefits (mostly anti-aging and antioxidant). Also used for coffee, tea & all other drinks. This water also gives life and freshness to plants, stimulates germination and improves seedling development. |
| 3. Clean Water | 7.0 | Clean, neutral, delicious & pure drinking water for babies and bady foods. Adults can drink it when taking medications. Free of chlorine, rust and cloudiness. |
| 4. Beauty Water | 4.0 to 7.0 | Not for drinking. This slightly acidic water is recognized for its astringent effects. It's terrific to use for gentle cleaning, beauty care, face wash, hair care, pet care, polishing, and preserving frozen food. |
| 5. Strong Acidic Water | 2.7 | Strong acidic water, and should never be used for drinking. It has disinfecting, sterilising and sanitising properties. It sanitizes kitchen utensils, countertops, and other parts to prevent cross-contamination. Also used for cleaning, disinfecting, hygiene, and commercial operation (beauty salons, hair salons, restaurants, agricultural colleges, daycare centers, pet shops, and nursing homes). |

## Kangen Water pH Cannot Be Measured With pH Strips: [70, 73]

⦿ The mineral salts in tap water consist of alkaline minerals, mostly calcium and magnesium, and bicarbonate. pH test strips can measure the pH of tap water because tap water gets its pH from both the alkaline minerals in it, plus the bicarbonates.

⦿ In Kanger water, particles called hydroxyl ions also raise water pH. Those hydroxyl ions are responsible for some of the most important health benefits of alkaline water. So in order to measure pH of Kangen water, you should use Enagic pH testing drops or a reliable digital pH meter.

# BENEFITS OF KANGEN WATER™

## Benefits of Kangen Water, Posted by Nuoc Kangen ™ [62]
- Abnormal gastrointestinal fermentation
- Rapid Reduction in Blood Sugar Levels in Diabetes Patients
- Rapid Healing of Stomach and Duodenal Ulcers
- Rapid Improvement in High and Low Blood Pressure Levels
- Improvements in Asthma, Skin Rashes, and Dermatitis
- Rapid Improvement in Nasal Allergies
- Improvements in Chronic diarrhea
- Indigestion, Excess Gastric Acid
- Improved Kidney Function and more health benefits

**Please Note:** It should be noted that Kangen Water™ doesn't directly "cure" whatever illness you may have, but instead it safely gets rid of the root of the all evils, the free radicals. When you alkalize your body and rid it of acid wastes, the body returns to homeostasis and can then take care of itself. [62]

## Benefits of Kangen Water Posted By A Water Pollution Filters Company [65]
- Aggressively flush all toxins from your body. Disarms free radicals!
- Restore alkalinity in your body with settings of pH 8.5, pH9, or pH 9.5!
- Reduces the high levels of toxins we take in daily is crucial for optimal health and well being. VOC's, organic, and inorganic material alike are rendered harmless as the Kangen water machine is equipped with the carbon pre-filter and subsequent electrolysis process!
- Better Hydration! Drinking micro-clustered water helps keep the body properly hydrated and assist with colon function better than plain tap, filtered, bottled, distilled, RO, or ozonated waters.
- Increase stable (dissolved!) oxygen in your body. Needed by every cell in your body for respiration and nutrient breakdown. Enhances delivery of nutrients! For taking supplements. Alkaline water has outstanding dissolving, extracting and anti-oxidizing properties that will enhance the effectiveness of any supplements you may be taking.
- Cooking with Kangen alkaline water improves the nutritional value and the taste of food and drinks such as tea and coffee. It makes acidic foods and drinks more alkaline. Kangen also has stronger heat conduction than regular water, effectively cutting as much as 30% from cooking times. There are an estimated 30,000 restaurants and eateries in Japan already using Kangen alkaline water to prepare their food, and the quality and cleanliness of Japanese food is world-renowned.
- Use mild acid 5.5 pH water as a skin toner to give your skin a healthy, radiant shine.
- After consuming alcohol. Dilute the acidity of the alcohol and prevent hangovers. Use alkaline water ice cubes with your drinks and ingest a sufficient quantity of alkaline water before bed to prevent a hangover.
- For drinking during meals. When eating acidic foods such as meat, egg yolks, white bread, etc, drinking Kangen water will help balance the pH. For brewing tea and coffee. Alkaline water prevents tannin in the tea and allows the tea to infuse fully, creating a rich color and taste. In coffee, Kangen brings out the aroma, color and natural flavor, while reducing acidity taste. Only half the amount of coffee beans are required to create the same full taste.
- For cut flowers and plants. Plants experience great results when watered with ionized water. The life of cut flowers can be lengthened and health restored to sick plants.
- For pets: Unpleasant odors from both their bodies and waste will be eliminated. They will also experience the same great health benefits as humans.
- For artists and painters, Kangen alkaline water is exceptional when mixing paints. Colors are more vibrant and a smoother texture is created.

⏺ Use the the acidic water setting to create a 100% safe and natural anti-bacterial cleaner. Kills 99.9% of bacteria on contact. Can also be sprayed directly onto the skin and into the throat to prevent a cold. Also ideal as a 100% safe alternative for bathrooms, baby areas and toys.

⏺ As an all-purpose cleaner. Use the the strong alkaline water setting to create a natural, chemical free cleaner for glass, tiles, bench tops, etc.

⏺ The single overall greatest benefit is improved intestinal and colon health. A large portion of the free radicals in your body are created by a toxic colon. Free radicals also account for 70% of chronic diseases, such as cancer and diabetes. Every day you remain dehydrated and every day you don't take action against the free radicals and acid build-up throughout your bowels and body, you are basically encouraging disease in your body.

## National Institute of Health (NIH) Reported The Following: [66]

A scientific study conducted by the National Institute of Health (NIH) revealed that the consumption of hydrogen rich water (similar to Kangen water) for 8 weeks resulted in a 39% increase ($p<0.05$) in antioxidant enzyme superoxide dismutase (SOD) and a 43% decrease ($p< 0.05$) in thiobarbituric acid reactive substances (TBARS) in urine. Further, subjects demonstrated an 8% increase in high density lipoprotein (HDL) cholesterol and a 13% decrease in total cholesterol/HDL cholesterol from baseline to 4 weeks. What does this mean? According to this study, those who drank hydrogen-rich water showed a substantial increase in their antioxidant enzymes and a massive decrease in acid in the urine. Further, participants showed a significant increase in HDL (the good cholesterol) and a significant decrease in LDL cholesterol (the bad cholesterol). Kangen Water® aka Electrolyzed Reduced Water or hydrogen water has been used in hospitals in Japan for decades.

## Benefits of Kangen Water, Posted by OM Kanger Water Center: [71]

⏺ Drinking plenty of alkaline-micro clustered water helps to keep the our bodies hydrated. This means that the water molecules are smaller than other types of drinking water. Our bodies can easily and quickly absorb those smaller molecules of water keeping us well-hydrated. Drinking enough alkaline water also helps to detoxify our bodies by improving digestion and elimination.

⏺ Alkaline water has a higher pH level than plain tap water.  This helps neutralize acid in your bloodstream, boosts your metabolism and helps your body absorb nutrients more effectively.  It can prevent disease and slow the aging process.

⏺ Kangen Water® lubricates joints and muscles to help prevent injuries. This can benefit those who are susceptible to sprains or may suffer from arthritis.  Dehydration can cause organs, such as the heart, to have to work harder and leave you feeling exhausted.  Drinking Kangen Water® eliminates harmful substances and leaves you feeling more energetic.

## Benefits of Kangen Water, Posted by Eagic Corp [74]

**Kangen Alkaline Water:** Hydration and drinkability, micro Clustering, free radical scavenging, encouraging longevity, detoxification.

**Kangen Acidic Water :** Toxic-free cleaning, personal hygiene, environmentally green.

# KANGEN WATER AND KANGEN-WATER MACHINES HAVE BEEN CRITICISED!
## DISADVANTAGES OF KANGEN WATER
### LIFE IONIZERS, A COMPETITOR IN THE FIELD, POSTED THE FOLLOWING STATEMENTS: [75]

**Too Expensive:** Kangen water is the most expensive alkaline water available on the market. At a pH of 10, Kangen water simply doesn't have enough acid-fighting alkalinity to tackle the toughest health problems, and athletes looking to improve their performance would also be better served with a more powerful machine.

**Weak Filtration:** The Kangen machine has only a single filter, and it's inadequate for dealing with many of the toxins found it tap water. The filter in the Kangen machine doesn't reduce levels of heavy metals or salt. This means that if a heavy metal like lead is found in your water (lead contamination in the US is widespread) then that lead will be in your Kangen water.

**Underpowered:** One of the main selling points Enagic representatives use to promote the Kangen machine is that it has large plates. The problem is that the machine doesn't have enough power for those large plates. The lack of power is why the Kangen machine struggles to reach over a pH of 10, and why some people have to add calcium glycerophosphate (a drug compound) as an enhancer to their Kangen machine to get acceptable pH levels.

**Multi-Level Marketing (MLM):** One of the questions you hear all the time about the Kangen machine is: "Why is it so expensive?" The reason the Kangen machine is very expensive is that it's sold through multi-level marketing (MLM). This kind of marketing makes things more expensive than they should be because a whole lot of people in the pyramid get paid commissions anytime a product is sold through MLM. The consumer's money goes to very many pockets, not just the manufacturer of Kangen machine.

### Alkaline Water Has Been Criticized By Healthline [28]
• Alkaline water is somewhat controversial. Many health professionals argue against its use by saying that there isn't enough research to support the many health claims made by users and sellers. According to the Mayo Clinic, there is no scientific evidence that fully verifies the claims made by supporters of alkaline water.
• Drinking alkaline water may produce negative side effects by lowering of natural stomach acidity. Acidity in the stomach is of upmost importance to human body as it helps kill bacteria and expel other undesirable pathogens from entering your bloodstream.
• An overall excess of alkalinity in the body may cause gastrointestinal issues and skin irritations. Too much alkalinity may also agitate the body's normal pH, leading to metabolic alkalosis, a condition that may produce the following symptoms:
- Nausea & vomiting
- hand tremors
- muscle twitching
- tingling in the extremities or face
- confusion
- a decrease in free calcium in the body

• There is no documented peer-reviewed evidence which has been internationally accepted and endorsed by the World Health Organization (WHO) and/or any accredited Medical Community Association, indicating that drinking water of more alkaline nature impact good health better than regular drinking water, The FDA says. [54]

# METHOD 9: PURCHASE A HYDROGEN WATER GENERATOR
# HYDROGEN WATER | H2 WATER

## About Hydrogen Water [85, 86, 87]

● Hydrogen water, hydrogen-rich water, water enriched with hydrogen gas, or hydrogen-infused water are synonyms of H2 water, which is the  drinking water saturated with molecular hydrogen ($H_2$). Hydrogen water is filled with antioxidants, and possesses anti-inflammatory and anti-allergic properties. Hydrogen water stimulates the metabolism and hydrates the organs which lead to great health benefits for humans as well as animals. It is a natural remedy  for health, youth and beauty. It is perfect for every person of any age category, including babies, pregnant women, and athletes.

● H2 water contains a high concentration of molecular hydrogen (H2). H2 water contributes to the proper functioning and rejuvenation of the cells in the body. It helps dissolve and flush out acid solid waste and toxins that accumulate in the body.

● H2 has four main properties and abilities: anti-oxidative, anti-inflammatory, anti-apoptotic and cell-repairing. Anti-apoptotic means ability to prevent cell damage. Apoptosis is a form of programmed cell death that occurs in multicellular organisms. Biochemical events lead to characteristic cell changes (morphology) and death.

● H2 selectively neutralizes harmful free radicals in the body converting them into water. Oxidative stress occurs when an oxygen molecule splits into single atoms with unpaired electrons, which are called free radicals. Free radicals are the natural byproducts of chemical processes, such as metabolism. Free radicals are some kind of  waste products from various chemical reactions in the cells that when built up, harm the cells of the body. Free radicals are unstable molecules or atoms that lack one or more electrons. They have increased activity and are very actively trying to make up for the loss, taking away the missing electron from nearby molecules. Once an electron is taken from the molecule, it is converted into free radicals. This triggers a chain reaction and the oxidation process. This leads to damage in the proteins, cell membrane and DNA. As a result, diseases may emerge.

● The strongest oxidant is hydroxyl-radical (OH), which is a byproduct of the metabolism involving oxygen. It can oxidize protein and lipid molecules, especially by actively attacking membrane lipids that contain unsaturated double bonds. This process leads to the formation of lipid hydroperoxides and a change in the properties of cell membranes. The hydroxyl radical causes a break in the bonds in the DNA molecule, which can cause deep damage to the genetic apparatus of cells.

● In 1950, scientist Danham Harman published the theory of free radicals. In this theory, he explained that the deterioration of human health and its aging is due to the accumulation of toxins – damage in cells, caused by free radicals over time.

● As a result of the aggressive action of free radicals, cell walls are damaged, as well as their important internal structures that lose their function, which disrupts the process of nutrition, elimination of toxins and the production of the skin's primary protein, collagen, responsible for skin elasticity. Thus, our body quickly wears out and grows old. The muscles begin to lose elasticity which then causes wrinkles, pigmentation and flabbiness of the skin to appear. In other words, the body goes through an aging process. In the process of cells being damaged by free radicals, oxidative stress occurs, which can cause a number of diseases, including atherosclerosis, Parkinson's disease, Alzheimer's disease, stroke, diabetes, autoimmune diseases, arthritis, various forms of cancer, and many others.

● The remarkable feature of Molecular Hydrogen is that it can selectively eliminate only toxic free radicals such as hydroxyl and lipid radicals. This selective neutralization allows the body to balance the number of free radicals and boost its protection functions.

● Molecular hydrogen is absorbed into the intestine within one minute and spreads through the whole body within ten minutes. It eliminates free radicals and prevents cellular damage. There is no toxicity in molecular hydrogen (H2) because the byproduct of the free-radical neutralizing reaction is water. Each molecule of H2 will neutralize itself to hydroxyl radicals which are the two molecules of H2O that hydrate your cells. The water then will be flushed out through urine and sweat, eliminating any unnecessary toxins. Hence, the effects of consuming Molecular Hydrogen are not only safe but are also very positive and effective in helping the body function at an optimal level.

● Hydrogen is 100% safe and has no negative side effects. H2 can be effectively consumed through drinking, inhalation or the other ways.

● According to 500 scientific studies since 2007, it has been revealed that molecular hydrogen has great therapeutic potential to treat and heal more than 150 diseases. As it enters our body, it instantly starts to repairing and recover the tissues and organs at a cellular level.

● Hydrogen water carefully cares for the skin and increases the synthesis of collagen which contributes to the deceleration of the aging process, hence allows you to enjoy your youth and beauty for longer than you imagine.

● Hydrogen water generators/machines produce hydrogen rich water – water that contains molecular hydrogen. These particular generators work from electrolysis that breaks the molecular of H2O (water) into H2 (Molecular Hydrogen) and O (Oxygen) and release large quantities of H2 into the water.

● PEM (Proton Exchange Membrane) type of hydrogen water generators are well known for producing safe hydrogen water for drinking. PEM separates hydrogen from oxygen and discharges oxygen from the water. When oxygen is discharged by-products such as oxygen and chlorine can not be formed in the water.

● **Latest Wellness Trend:** Hydrogen water is the latest wellness trend to hit the US, UK and Asian markets. After vitamin-fortified water, health and fitness gurus are now switching to hydrogen-enriched water with much-touted benefits such as reducing inflammation, wrinkles, and bone loss, and some people believe that the hydrogen water also helps metabolise fat and glucose faster than the regular water. These benefits can be achieved by chugging just about 500 ml (two glasses) of hydrogen-enriched water a day, much less than the recommended 8 to 10 glasses a day of regular water as some studies suggested. However much research is needed to confirm these wellness benefits. [87b]

## Alkaline Warer Vs Hydrogen Water [88]
● **Alkaline Water:** Improves hydration, increases performance and lowers fatigue, rich in minerals and improves gut health, disinfects the body and fights chemical byproducts, reduces risk of diabetes, improves athletic performance, and protects the body from harmful effects.

● **Hydrogen Water:** Fights free radicals by being antioxidant rich, may or may not contain minerals, reduces blood pressure, promotes healthy blood circulation, detoxes the body, protects from sunlight, promotes good health and healthy cell structure throughout the body, boosts energy and boosts collagen production (collagen is well-recognized for the elasticity it provides to skin).

# HOW DOES A HYDROGEN WATER GENERATOR WORK?

## BASIC PRINCIPLE BEHIND: PEM Technology [89, 90, 91, 92]

Proton Exchange Membrane (PEM) Diagram is the heart of a hydrogen infusion machine (HIM) electrolytic cell is the proton exchange membrane (PEM) with solid polymer electrolyte (SPE), a very different type of membrane from that used in a standard alkaline ionizer. The electrolysis process in the production of H2 gas in water is described below:

1. Water at the anode provides source of H+ ions.
2. PEM (membrane) permits migration of H+ ions from anode to cathode.
3. At cathode, H$^+$ ions combine with electrons from the power supply (reduction reaction) to form H atoms which pair-up (two hydrogen atoms become one hydrogen molecule) to form H$_2$ gas.

$$\text{Anode Reaction:} \quad 2H_2O \rightarrow O_2 + 4H + + 4e-$$
$$\text{Cathode Reaction:} \quad 4H + + 4e- \rightarrow 2H_2$$

4. Oxygen is two electrons shy of having a full outer electron shell, so in chemical reactions it tends to pick up electrons and become negative. With a sufficient potential difference, this causes electrolysis with hydrogen gas being produced at the cathode and oxygen gas being produced at the anode (through oxidation of hydroxide). Oxygen gas must be vented out. Alternatively, chlorine gas may be produced instead of oxygen, depending on source water chloride levels.
5. PEM contains an electrolyte (SPE, solid polymer electrolyte, an electrical conductor), and therefore electrolysis is not dependent on source water minerals.
6. Lower electrical resistance between anode & cathode results in less voltage drop and more efficient electrolytic production of H$_2$.
7. Because pH of the drinking water is not raised, this design does not encourage the precipitation of calcium which greatly reduces the degree of lime-scale buildup within the system.

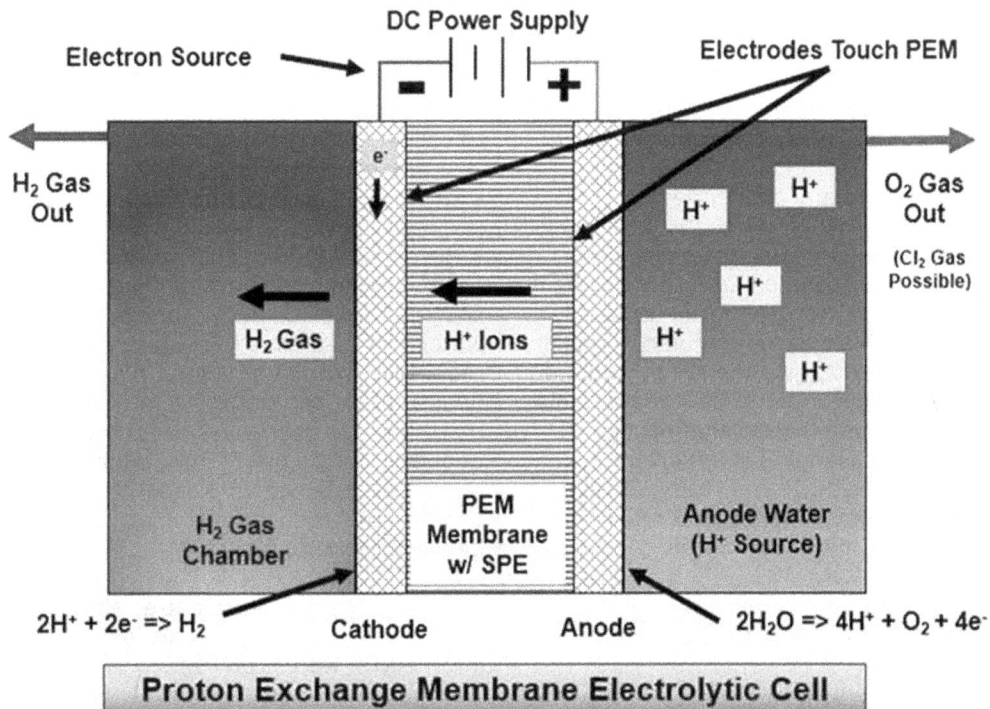

Figure 18.30  Basic principle behind hydrogen water generator.

# WATER IONIZERS VERSUS HYDROGEN WATER GENERATORS
[93, 94, 95, 96]

The major differences between water ionizers and hydrogen water machines are described below:

Table 18.7  Water ionizers versus hydrogen water machines.

| WATER IONIZERS | HYDROGEN WATER MACHINES |
|---|---|
| ◉ Water ionizers use the same process called electrolysis or electrodialysis to generate their healthy drinkable water. | ◉ Hydrogen machines use the same process called electrolysis or electrodialysis to generate their healthy drinkable water. |
| ◉ The machines run water over electrically charged platinum-coated titanium plates separated by a membrane to produce drinkable water. The machines use bidirectional ion-permeable membrane. | ◉ The machines run water over electrically charged platinum-coated titanium plates separated by a membrane to produce drinkable water. The machines use unidirectional proton exchange membrane. |
| ◉ Water ionizers purify the water by means of a filter embedded within the machine, and raise the pH of water to an alkaline level, and enrich the water with antioxidant potential. Enagic's Kangen water machines make alkaline hydrogen-rich water. | ◉ A hydrogen machines do not filter or purify the water, and  may or may not make water alkaline, but instead generate a small amount of molecular hydrogen and infuse with purified water, and enrich the hydrogen water with antioxidant potential. |
| ◉ Advocates of both machines claim similar health benefits. However, alkaline water has superior antioxidant radical scavenging activity, and it can neutralize acidity. | ◉ Advocates of both machines claim similar health benefits. Hydrogen water (also known as hydrogenated water) doesn't neutralize acidity. |
| ◉ Water ionizers produces the antioxidant hydroxyl ion and  small amount of antioxidant molecular hydrogen! | ◉ Hydrogen machines don't generate any antioxidant hydroxyl ions. They pump antioxidant molecular hydrogen into the water. |
| ◉ Water ionizers have two outlets, one for alkaline water and the other for acidic water. And they have many settings to choose from. pH can be adjusted to any desired level. | ◉ Hydrogen water generators do not have many settings to choose from, just one outlet to collect hydrogen-enriched water. Just one pH level that is close to 7 (though some brands do produce alkaline water). |
| ◉ ROS (Reactive Oxygen Species) molecules attack and oxidize tissues and DNA, destroying cells. Scavenging is a process that neutralizes ROS, taking away those harmful molecules ability to oxidize and destroy tissue and DNA. Oxidation caused by ROS is considered to be a major factor in premature aging and the development of diseases. So ROS scavenging is important for maintaining good health. In the study, alkaline water showed four times higher ROS scavenging activity compared to hydrogen water. | ◉ Research suggests that while inhalation and saline injection of hydrogen gas are better sources of molecular hydrogen, drinking it in water is the safest and easiest way to consume molecular hydrogen. It improves your heart health, brain health, and it may be an effective treatment for psoriasis and arthritis. It is also beneficial for recovery from injuries, and many other health benefits.  Research showed that pre-exercise reduced blood lactate levels and improved muscle function. |
| ◉ Molecular hydrogen antioxidant is consumed through highly alkaline water that is produced from a water ionizer. | ◉ Some people do a lot better after getting their molecular hydrogen antioxidants pumped into neutral water (pH=7). |

# HYDROGEN WATER GENERATORS YOU CAN BUY AND OWN

If you are planning to purchase and own a hydrogen water generator, you should first research on Amazon.com, Amazon.ca, Amazon.co.uk, also on other marketplaces of Amazon, and also on Alibaba.com. Read reviews and select the one that best suits your needs. A few hydrogen water generators are shown below:

**1. The Ultrastream Water Filter and Alkalizer:** UltraStream is the world's most advanced natural water filter. It purifies, alkalizes, ionizes and infuses your home water with beneficial molecular hydrogen. https://alkaway.com/the-ultrastream/   Click Here to Visit

**About the Product:** Removes heavy metals, toxins, bacteria, chlorine, chloramines and fluoride plus hundreds more toxins in our water. Tested for the life of the filter. Advanced alkalizing, adds essential calcium, magnesium, and trace minerals to ultra purified water for perfect pH balance. Continues to outperform electric ionizers costing thousands with more molecular hydrogen. The is the best hydrogen-enriching water generator. Over 700 scientific studies validate health benefits from infused hydrogen!

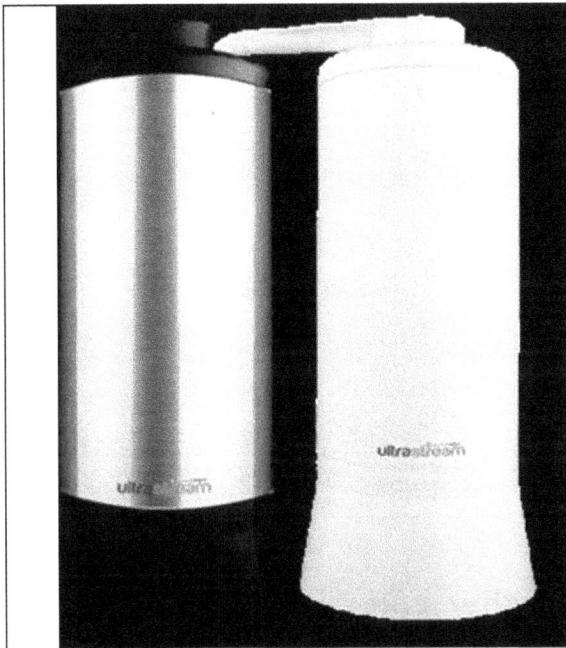

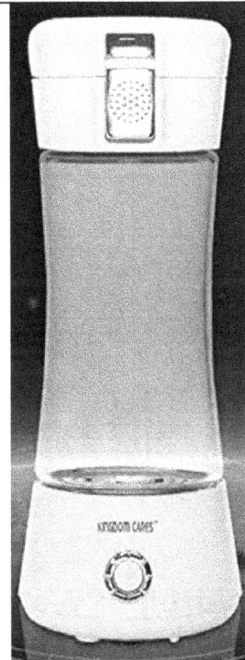

| Figure 18.31 Ultrastream hydrogen water maker. Courtesy of Alkaway | Figure 18.32 Kingdombeauty hydrogen water maker. Courtesy of Kingdom |

**2. KINGDOMBEAUTY Portable Hydrogen Water Bottle Cup:** Recharge Hydrogen Rich Water Ionizer Maker Generator With Large Capacity Battery Colorful Light by Kingdom, ASIN: B06WWHS41G, Available on Amazon.com, Price; $87.99   Click Here to Visit

**About the Product:** High end hydrogen water ionizer: It comes with world class extreme filtration, remove impurities, reduces the water molecular size which allows it to be more easily absorb by your body and also contains minerals. A few minutes can produce a cup of hydrogen rich water which can be directly drunk. Portable hydrogen rich water ionizer provides more healthy water for you. This Hydrogen Rich Water Bottle is made of food-grade PC material, high quality and safe to use.

### 3. Davidlee Hydrogen-Rich Generator Water Bottle: PEM Technology Ionizer
High Concentration Discharge Ozone and chlorine by DavidLee, ASIN: B07CWP7MVM, Available on Amazon.com, Price: $159.          Click Here to Visit

**About the Product:** Suits for most types of drinking water (distilled water, RO purified water, mineral water, tap water). Distinguishing from other machines in the market which cannot process with distilled water or purified water. Ultra-high purity hydrogen-rich water - Electrolysis 1 time can produce hydrogen water contains hydrogen ion upto 1400ppb. Equipped with high-quality ion-exchange membrane, which can remove impurities, absorb the residual chlorine ozone, discharge water contains ozone, hydrogen peroxide, chlorine from the bottom.

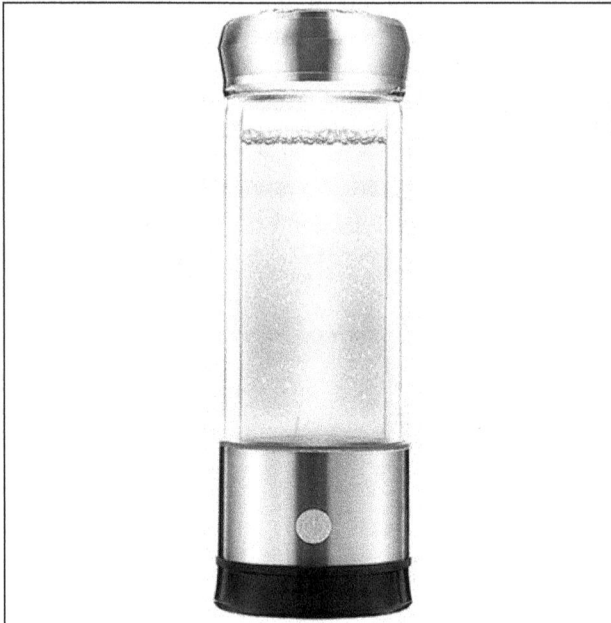

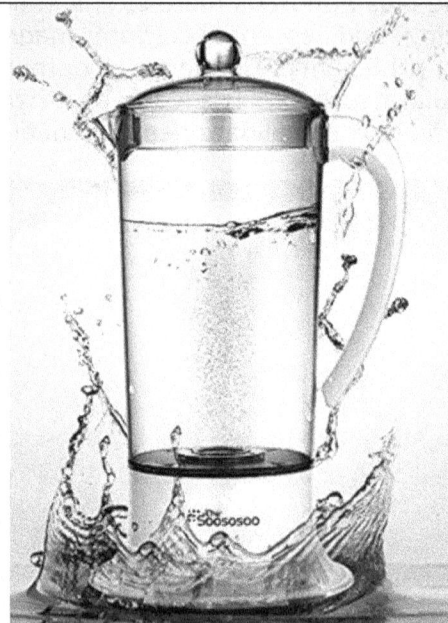

| Figure 18.33 Davidlee hydrogen water maker. Courtesy of Davidlee | Figure 18.34 Hyzen hydrogen water maker. Courtesy of Hyzen |

### 4. Hyzen Hydrogen Water Generator Pitcher 1.2L: Hydrogen water can
offer many health benefits. Fast hydrogen generation means hydrogen-enriched water whenever you need it. Highly dissolved hydrogen to ensure you're actually reaping the benefits of hydrogen water. Easy to use and easy to clean, recommended deep cleaning only twice a month. Proven quality by the high demand in Asia. Made in Korea. ASIN: B071R86FRY, Available on Amazon.com. Price: $259.99. Click Here to Visit

## 5. New 2018 Lourdes Hydrofix Hydrogen Water & Inhalation Machine:

The most advanced technology from Japan with separate chamber electrolysis system. Pure (99.999%) molecular H2 Water 1.2 ppm - 1.537 ppm. 10-min mode for 500 ml, 30-min mode for 1.5L, longest lasting H2 Water on the market! H2 Gas Inhalation 26ml -120ml/min = 780 L/206 Gal of 1.0ppm H2 Water in 30-min!! ASIN: B07C838CBS, Available on Amazon.com, Price: $2000. Click Here to Visit

Also available on https://holyhydrogen.com/

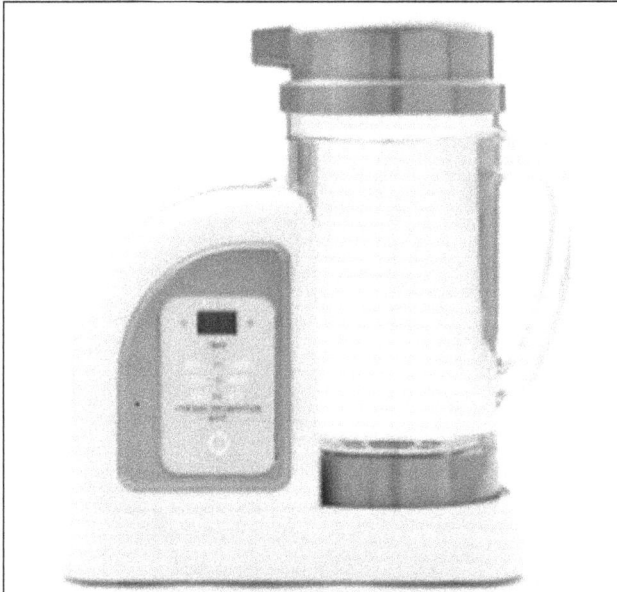

| Figure 18.35 Lourdes hydrogen water machine. Courtesy of Lourdes | Figure 18.36 Hydrogen water testing drops. Courtesy of Miz Company |

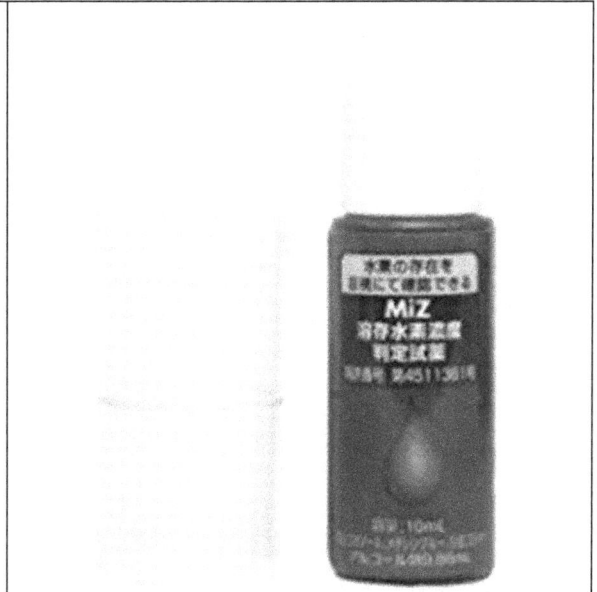

**Hydrogen Water Testing Drops:** H2 Blue Drops Reagent or H2 Blue Test Reagent or Miz Blue Drops or Dissolved Hydrogen Level Testing Reagent or H2 Blue Test Kit or Hydrogen Water Tester Better Than Trustlex H2 Meter ENH-1000, ASIN: B07F66ZH5Z, Available on Amazon.com. Price: $39. Click Here to Visit.

## How To Test Hydrogen Water For The Presence of Hydrogen Gas?

To make sure that the dissolved hydrogen is still present in the hydrogen water you drink, you need to test the water by means of "Miz testing drops" every now and then. The package comes with a small measuring flask (bottle), 6 mL in volume. Fill up this flask precisely to the 6 mL mark with hydrogen water, and start adding Miz drops one by one until the water is fully saturated and turns blue in color. Always count the number of Miz drops being added. One drop dissolves in 0.1 ppm concentration of H2 in the water. If you added 15 drops, the H2 concentration in hydrogen water would be 1.5 ppm. Just follow the instructions on the Miz drops bottle you purchased. You can also purchase more expensive and more accurate "hydrogen meter" to monitor hydrogen concentration in drinking water.

**PLEASE NOTE:** You can drink hydrogen water with as much hydrogen as you want. There is no upper limit. You don't overdose hydrogen.

# METHOD 10: PURCHASE AN RO ALKALINE WATER SYSTEM [REVERSE OSMOSIS REMINERALIZATION SYSTEM]

It is known that purified water produced by reverse osmosis has been criticized because it is demineralized water, meaning that there are no minerals or trace minerals present in the drinking water. But this drawback has been corrected, and some companies such as KENT came up with a new technology to produce "Alkaline RO Water" by the purification and remineralization of tap water at the touch of a button. There are many machines, but a few are described below:

**1. Reverse Osmosis Water System by Max Water Limited, 8-Stage Alkaline Water Producer, Adds Minerals to RO  Purified Water,** Price: $325 CAD. https://www.maxwaterflow.com/maxwater8stagereverseosmosissystem101080?gclid=EAIaI QobChMIvfG9quDH3QIVg8JkCh3jiQY6EAQYAiABEgIdJfD_BwE

**8-Stage Reverse Osmosis System with 3-in-1 pH+ Filter:** Our 8-stage under-sink reverse osmosis system gives you pure, fresh tasting water. Like all of our RO systems this one removes silt, dirt and chlorine and also filters out 95% of impurities including lead and mercury, but our 3-in-1 Alkaline/Far Infrared/Remineralization Filter also changes the pH of the water to be more alkaline and adds back in essential minerals like magnesium and calcium. The Far Infrared media in our 3-in-1 filter also has anti-bacterial/biotic properties to further purify the water.

**Features:** Our Alkaline/Far Infrared/Remineralization filter optimizes the pure water from our reverse osmosis process to make it the best possible water for drinking. Our filters do many tasks:
- Changes the pH to be slightly alkaline, which has several health benefits.
- Adds several minerals including calcium and magnesium, which promote healthy bones and teeth.
- Activates the water creating smaller water clusters. These smaller clusters are easier for your body absorb and providing better hydration for your skin.
- Generates powerful antioxidants, which can remove free radicals, considered to the source of many diseases and premature aging.

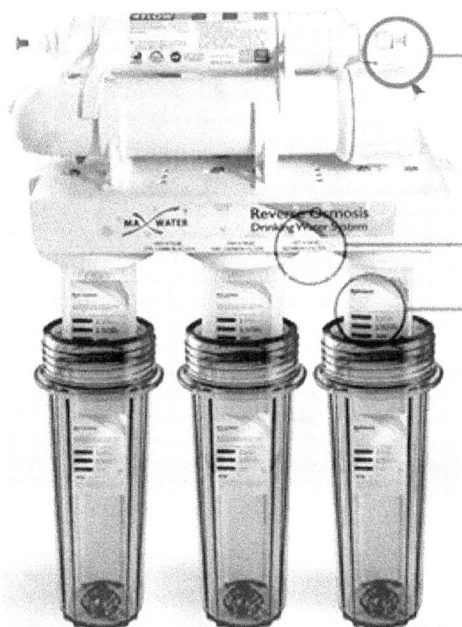

Courtesy of Max Warer Limited.
Figure 18.37 Reverse Osmosis Water System by Max Water Limited.

## 2. KENT QNET SMART ALKALINE-MINERAL RO WATER PURIFIER by KENT (India):

http://products.qnetindia.in/Productdetail.aspx?prodcode=8800003292&lang=en&planid=8
https://www.kent.co.in/water-purifiers/ro/

**KENT and QNET India** have collaborated to bring to the fore an exclusive solution for water purification — the brand new KENT-QNET SMART Alkaline-Mineral RO Water Purifier. This water purifier ensures the right pH levels in your water, and removes dissolved impurities like arsenic, rust, bacteria and viruses, providing you with pure water for a healthy lifestyle.

**RO TECHNOLOGY:** At the heart of the KENT-QNET SMART Alkaline-Mineral RO Water Purifier is a Reverse Osmosis membrane which has capillaries as small as 0.0001 microns, which helps reduce dissolved impurities (salts and heavy metals,) and converts hard water to sweet and pure drinking water.

**What Makes The KENT-QNET SMART Alkaline-Mineral RO Water Purifier Unique?**
A first of its kind in any RO water purifier system in India, the KENT-QNET SMART Alkaline Mineral RO Water Purifier has Alkaline 8+ pH water, which has powerful antioxidant properties, and promotes better hydration, improves bowel conditions, improves energy and metabolism, and increases blood oxygen levels.

**Key Features:** Unique Reverse Osmosis + Ultrafiltration + Ultraviolet + Alkaline with Total Dissolved Solids (TDS) Controlled water purification system. Patented mineral retention technology. Pure and healthy alkaline water that maintains pH levels of 8+. Tamperproof RO membrane. Interactive Touch Screen Display with Real Time monitoring of purity, performance, and service history. Fully automatic operation. 9-liters storage tank with water level indicator. Comes with one-year onsite warranty.

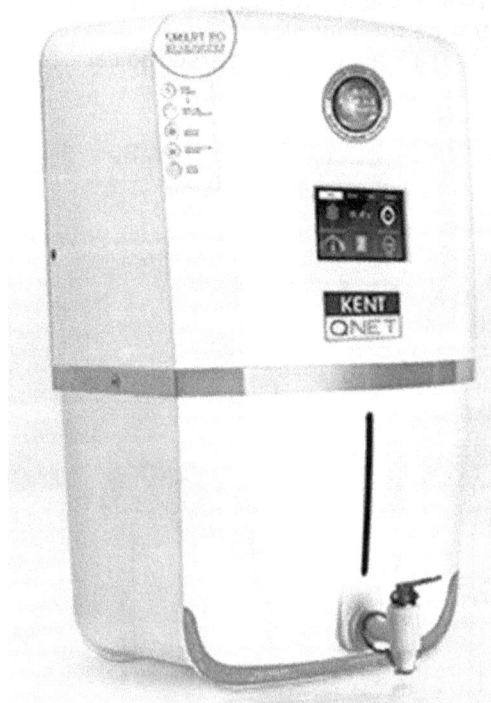

Courtesy of Kent-Qnet
Figure 18.38 Reverse Osmosis Water System by Max Water Limited.

# RANODOMIZED RESEARCH STUDIES ON ALKALINE WATER
## [SCIENTIFIC RESEARCH STUDIES]

### National Institute of Health (NIH) Reported The Following: [66]

A scientific study conducted by the National Institute of Health (NIH) revealed that the consumption of hydrogen rich water (similar to Kangen water) for 8 weeks resulted in a 39% increase (p<0.05) in antioxidant enzyme superoxide dismutase (SOD) and a 43% decrease (p< 0.05) in thiobarbituric acid reactive substances (TBARS) in urine. Further, subjects demonstrated an 8% increase in high density lipoprotein (HDL) cholesterol and a 13% decrease in total cholesterol/HDL cholesterol from baseline to 4 weeks. What does this mean? According to this study, those who drank hydrogen-rich water showed a substantial increase in their antioxidant enzymes and a massive decrease in acid in the urine. Further, participants showed a significant increase in HDL (the good cholesterol) and a significant decrease in LDL cholesterol (the bad cholesterol). Kangen Water® aka Electrolyzed Reduced Water or hydrogen water has been used in hospitals in Japan for decades.

In recent years, alkaline water has become popular among business and health enthusiasts and professional athletes. They have been researching to find out the health effects of alkaline water on body's hydration, especially for those athletes who need to hydrate their bodies during their athletic performances. These people claim that some NBA stars "LeBron James and Carmelo Anthony" have been drinking electrolysed alkaline water often to maintain proper hydration in order to perform well.

We all know that water is essential for survival. It explains how dehydration can affect the physical health and body function. The problem is that it's easy for the body to become dehydrated when working out, performing strenuous physical activity on a daily basis. Every time the athletes perform, the body loses water through sweating. Losing even 2% of body mass from sweating can impair the physiological performance. It can also reduce aerobic function. Over time, dehydration can lead to lowered metabolic function and reduced neurological function. It may also increase the risk of heat strain. Dehydration can also cause cardiac drift. This occurs when the heart rate rises while the amount of blood pumped out of the heart decreases due to dehydration. So the health enthusiasts have been looking for a solution to this problem.

### RANDOMIZED RESEARCH STUDY-I [101a, 101b]

The most compelling evidence comes from a 2016 study, which led to a scientific journal publication. The research included 100 athletic participants, who performed a mild exercise routine. They reported that the exercise led to a 2% loss in body mass through perspiration or sweating.

After the exercise, 50 participants (half of them) were asked to hydrate their bodies with alkaline water at a pH between 8 and 9 (electrolysed high pH water), which was remineralized with essential minerals such as calcium, magnesium, potassium and sodium. All these minerals play an important role in the hydration. Potassium and sodium, in particular, are critical for balancing the hydration levels. The other 50 participants received regular water (purified water without minerals). The researchers then measured the thickness of the blood or so called blood viscosity. They learned from the blood test results that those who drank alkaline water had a lower blood viscosity than those who had regular water. The blood viscosity dropped by 6.3% with the group who drank alkaline water with minerals. The blood viscosity dropped by only 3.36% with the other group who drank regular purified water without minerals.

The researchers interpreted that the blood viscosity (thickness of the blood) is a measure of hydration. The lower the thickness of the blood, the higher the hydration level would be. They concluded that the hydration level can be improved by consuming alkaline water with minerals in it. However it was unclear whether the electrolysed alkaline water at high pH or the presence of minerals in that alkaline water was responsible for the drop in blood viscosity. This research somehow demonstrated that the alkaline water's superior hydrating effects, and published a paper in the Journal of the International Society of Sports Nutrition.

## RANDOMIZED RESEARCH STUDY-II [102a, 102b]
Another research study conducted in February 2017 reported that favorable changes in the rehydration status among athletes who drank remineralized alkaline water after high intensity exercise. These results suggested that electrolyzed alkaline water (similar to ionized alkaline water or Kangen water) may be better for rehydrating after exercise. However, the study consisted of fewer than 40 participants, and was not confirmed by conducting more studies on athletic performance. This paper was published in the Biology of Sport.

## RANDOMIZED RESEARCH STUDY -III [103]
Abstract: Another study suggested that drinking alkaline water may have benefits for people who have high blood pressure, diabetes, and high cholesterol. See details in the reference.

## RANDOMIZED RESEARCH STUDY-IV [104]
Several scientific papers were referenced in this article posted by Bawell Water Ionizers. The article confirms that scientific proof exists that alkaline ionized water benefits human health. See details in the reference.

- Many diseases such as obesity & inflammatory bowel disease could be caused by an imbalance in the human microbiome. Articles published on Electrolyzed Reduced Water's ability to act as an antioxidant protecting against oxidative damage to DNA, RNA, and protein.

- Drinking alkaline ionized water significantly reduced the blood glucose concentration and improved glucose tolerance in both type 1 and type 2 diabetes cases. Medical scientist have even advocated its use as an anti-diabetic agent after discovering that "Electrolyzed Reduced Water (ERW) with Reactive Oxygen Species (ROS) scavenging ability reduced the blood glucose concentration, increased blood insulin level, improved glucose tolerance and preserved beta-cell mass in db/db mice.

- Electrolyzed Reduced Water (ERW) protects pancreatic beta-cells from alloxan-induced cell damage by preventing alloxan-derived ROS generation. Reduced water may be useful in preventing alloxan-induced type 1-diabetes mellitus.

## RANDOMIZED RESEARCH STUDY -V [105]
Abstract: In 2012, a research study found that drinking alkaline water with a pH of 8.8 may help deactivate pepsin, which is the main enzyme that causes acid reflux. See details in the reference.

Similar scientific research studies can be found in the articles described in the references 106 through 113.

# HOW TO ACCOMPLISH ACID-ALKALINE BALANCE?

ACID-ALKALINE BALANCE WRITTEN BY ALKALIFE AND POSTED BY NATIONAL NUTRITION [121]
Over acidity has been linked to cancer, indigestion, osteoporosis, tooth decay, headaches, fatigue, candida, & others. The function of human body is optimized when the body's tissues and fluids are at a pH between 6.3 and 6.8 (optimal range). Acidosis occurs when the body is overly acidic (pH below 6.3). Alkalosis occurs when the body is overly alkaline (when the blood pH rises greater than 6.8, and switches to beyond 8, 9 or 10).

A problem with the pH of the body is not a disease in itself. Rather, it is always a sign that there is dysfunction in a part or several parts of the body. Different parts of the human body have different optimal ranges of pH. Acidosis can result from asthma, bronchitis, diabetes, stomach ulcers, some cancers, liver, kidney, or adrenal dysfunction. Stress, anger, poor diet, aspirin, alcohol and coffee can also contribute to acidosis.

Alkalosis can result from diarrhea, vomiting, poor diet, high cholesterol or osteoarthritis. Alkalinizing drugs for treatment of stomach ulcers can also contribute to alkalosis. In the general population everyday imbalances in pH are usually due to improper diet and stress.

The symptoms of acidosis are variable depending on the cause of the imbalance. They can include everything from insomnia, migraines and difficulty swallowing to strong smelling or burning breath, stool and perspiration. The symptoms of alkalosis usually begin with an excitation of the nervous system. This can lead to hyperventilation and seizures. Other symptoms of alkalosis are variable and can include sore muscles and joints, bone spurs, high blood pressure, allergies, indigestion, menstrual problems or prostatitis.

Treating the root cause is the best way to deal with pH imbalance. Conventional treatment is only used when the imbalance is severe enough to be life threatening. By maintaining a healthy, internal environment, you can prevent future illness. This works by maximizing your body's potential for regulation of natural processes that aid in good health, especially if osteoporosis is of concern to you. The air we breathe in is a vital part of maintaining acid/base balance. Proper breathing from the diaphragm, yoga and other activities that promote proper breathing are important. Since the food that we eat directly contributes to our body pH, well-balanced diet at optimal pH is extremely essential.

Naturopathic doctors and some health care professionals normally give patients a list of foods that are both acidic and alkaline, and recommend eating mainly foods of alkaline nature. Some people prefer to test their urine or saliva pH using litmus paper or pH strips throughout the day. They then choose their diet accordingly. High amounts of raw foods, chewing properly and eating small meals have been shown to help the body maintain its healthy pH balance.

**Here are some examples of acid forming foods:** alcohol, meat, fish, dairy products (unfermented), coffee, tea, soft drinks, any food with added sugar, breads, noodles and other flour products, vinegar, most legumes, most nuts and seeds, dried fruits, most pharmaceutical drugs.

**Here are some examples of alkaline forming foods:** most fresh vegetables and fresh fruits (including citrus fruits, citrus is acidic but it neutralizes the body and urine), soy products, honey, molasses, maple syrup, horseradish, almonds, brazil nuts, millet, lima beans, fermented dairy products like yogurt.

## Blood pH Fluctuates Due to Acidosis and Alkalosis [122]

No matter what kind of water he/she drinks, the human body has an amazing ability to maintain normal blood pH between 7.35 to 7.45 if he/she is healthy. This means that blood is naturally slightly alkaline or basic. The stomach pH is always acidic ranging between 1.5 to 3.5. A low pH in the stomach is essential for digesting food and destroying any bacteria, viruses and germs that get into the stomach while eating.

**But the following health conditions could cause blood pH go out of normal range "7.35 to 7.45" to some people:** asthma, diabetes, heart disease, kidney disease, lung disease, gout, infection, shock, hemorrhage (bleeding), drug overdose, poisoning, and other diseases or conditions. Acidosis develops when the blood pH goes below 7.35, and alkalosis develops when the blood pH goes above 7.45.

**Lungs and kidneys** are two main organs in your body that are responsible to regulate the blood pH. Lungs help remove the waste gas "carbon dioxide", and kidneys help remove acid waste by pumping it through the urine. Both acidosis and alkalosis can be controlled and cured by adjusting the eating and water-drinking habits.

## Acid-Alkaline Balance Can Be Accomplished By Doing The Following: [Written by Dr. RK]

๏ Eat well-balanced meals every day, with appropriate proportions of protein, fat & carbohydrate. Make sure there is some protein in every meal you consume.

๏ Eat one lemon a day including pulp, and learn how to neutralize your urine pH. Eat whole foods only with fresh organic vegetables, legumes, dark-leafy greens, nuts & seeds, and fruits. Please do not consume processed foods, refined foods and deep-fried foods. Always eat oven-baked skinless chicken, turkey or fish with a variety of vegetables, and limit eating out in restaurants.

๏ Don't drink too much coffee. Limit your coffee drinking to 1 or 2 cups before noon.

๏ Limit or quit intake of pop, diet pop and soda. Limit or quit alcohol intake and smoking.

๏ Quit intake of regular vinegar, and consume the "organic apple cider vinegar with mother, unfiltered and unpasteurized" a few times a day instead.

๏ Exercise every day (either walking outdoors, or in a mall, or working out in a gym).

๏ Practice deep breathing and/or meditation every day, and go to swimming and sauna.

๏ Take high quality multivitamins and minerals on a regular basis, and make sure that your mineral levels are normal and kidneys are functioning properly by taking routine blood tests.

๏ Please always drink purified water (RO water, distilled water, or zero water). Please do not drink tap water, well water or bottled water of any kind without knowing how pure it is. Drinking purified water is always far better than drinking any water that is not purified.

๏ Remineralize the purified water up to a TDS level of 200 ppm by adding a pinch of Himalyan pink salt or Celtic sea salt to purified water. Learn how to monitor TDS level with a TDS meter.

๏ Or, remineralize and slightly alkalize the purified water by adding a few ConcenTrace mineral drops to a cup of purified water. Learn how to monitor the drinking water pH. Get your drinking water tested by a certified laboratory once or twice a year, and make sure that those drops did not release any contaminants into your drinking water.

๏ Drink alkaline water periodically in limited and prescribed amounts only. Please do not drink alkaline water at a high pH throughout the day. Please get your blood pH tested routinely if you are drinking or planning to drink alkaline water at a high pH frequently.

๏ Purified water that is either neutralized or slightly alkalized, and remineralized up to a TDS level of 200 ppm is the healthy drinking water. Learn how to make that kind of water at home, and always drink only that king of water at least 8 cups a day. This book teaches how to make and drink that kind of water at home (Refer to Chapter 14, Chapter 17, Chapter 18 & Chapter 19).

## ALKALINE WATER BASICS
## Understanding the Water pH, Alkalinity, Alkaline & Buffers

### The pH of Water: [123]

The pH of water or any other solution is a measure of the acid–base equilibrium on a scale between 0 and 14. The water pH is a measure of how acidic or basic (or alkaline) the water is. In most natural waters, the pH is controlled by the presence of carbon dioxide, bicarbonate and carbonate. When an acid such as carbonic acid or hydrochloric acid is added to water, pH decreases. And when a base such as sodium hydroxide, sodium bicarbonate or calcium carbonate is added to water, the pH increases. When carbon dioxide dissolves in water, carbonic acid is formed by a chemical reaction [ $CO_2 + H_2O = H_2CO_3$ ], and the presence of this acid causes the water pH go down. On the other hand, when sodium bicarbonate dissolves in water, sodium hydroxide is formed by a chemical reaction [ $NaHCO_3 + H_2O = NaOH + CO_2$], and the presence of the strong base sodium hydroxide causes the water pH to go up.

**Scientific Definition of pH:** The pH of a solution is expressed as the negative logarithm of the hydrogen ion activity. In dilute solutions, the hydrogen ion activity is approximately equal to the hydrogen ion concentration. Therefore the pH is defined as:
pH = -log [$H^+$]

a. For example, some acidic water has a pH of 2. What is the hydrogen ion concentration [$H^+$]?
pH = - log [$H^+$]
2.0 = -log [$H^+$]
Therefore [$H^+$] = $10^{-2.0}$ = 1/100 = 0.01 mol/L

b. For example, some acidic water has a pH of 4. What is the hydrogen ion concentration [$H^+$]?
pH = - log [$H^+$]
4.0 = -log [$H^+$]
Therefore [$H^+$] = $10^{-4.0}$ = 1/10000 = 0.0001 mol/L

From these 2 examples, one can understand that as the hydrogen ion concentration increases, the water pH goes down, and as the hydrogen ion concentration decreases, the water pH goes up. The US Environmental Protection Agency (EPA) warns that the drinking water must have a pH value of 6.5-8.5 to fall within EPA standards. However, the pure water should have a pH of 7.

### The Alkalinity of Water: [124, 125, 126]

The alkalinity is a measure of the buffering capacity of water, or its ability to resist dramatic or sudden changes in pH. Buffers can react with both strong acids and strong bases to minimize and stabilize the large changes in pH. Therefore buffering agents are the pH stabilizers. In general alkaline water (with pH above 7) would neutralize the acids or acid waste in the stomach, but is not always the case with artificial alkaline water.

For example the overly cooked meat before consumption is very alkaline (pH is over 7), but after consuming cooked meat contributes to acidity in the tissues of the body. That is why, people are told that eating meat products could make your body too acidic. On the other hand, an acidic citrus fruit such as lemon contributes to neutralizing the body after it is consumed and digested. That is why it is recommended to drink lemon water, which neutralizes acids, and assists the body to drain the acid waste through urine.

## Adding Minerals to Water Does Not Neutralize Acids

In the same manner, the addition of alkaline minerals to water (such as calcium, magnesium, sodium, potassium, etc.) raises the pH and makes the water more alkaline, but this kind of alkaline water does not contribute to the neutralization of acids. Alkaline water made by adding minerals improves the TDS (Total Dissolved Solids) level as well as pH in drinking water, but some scientists say that it does not contribute to the neutralization of acids.

## IMPORTANCE OF BUFFERS IN THE ALKALINE WATER

Only Buffers Can Neutralize Acids. Neutralization of acids needs the presence of buffers. For example, if you add a weak acid to a glass of alkaline water at pH=8 that has no buffering capacity, the pH will immediately drop significantly. On the other hand if you add the same amount of the same acid to a glass of buffered water at pH=8, the pH will barely change. That is to say that the buffer or buffering agent neutralizes the acid, resists a dramatic change in pH, leaving the solution's pH unchanged. Buffers contribute to alkalinity which is defined as the ability to neutralize acids. Alkalinity is different from the term **"alkaline"** which simply refers to a pH over 7. In the drinking water and also in the human body, buffers are predominantly bicarbonates. These buffers neutralize acids by scavenging hydrogen ions ($H^+$). Alkalinity should therefore be the ability to neutralize acids.

Alkalinity is often measured in $CaCO_3$ equivalents (ppm or mg/L CaCO3). Alkalinity values of 20-200 ppm are common in freshwater ecosystems. Alkalinity levels below 10 ppm indicate poorly buffered streams, which are the least capable of resisting changes in the water pH, and in assisting the neutralization of acids. [104]

**IMPORTANT NOTE:** If the water you drink is alkaline because of the presence of bicarbonates, it's alkaline pH represents alkalinity which is the ability to neutralize acids. Even if this kind of water is only slightly alkaline, because of its buffering capacity it will neutralize the acids, and assists the body in the removal of acidic waste through urine. On the other hand, if the water you drink is alkaline without bicarbonates, it has little alkalinity or buffering capacity and so it does not contribute to resisting the pH and to neutralize acids. Some scientists say that drinking this kind of alkaline water could be detrimental to the human body.

## Alkaline Ionized Water & Kangen Water Are Criticised Based On the Aforementioned Discussion:
Alkaline ionized water or Kangen water is produced by electrolysis in an ionization machine by splitting the water molecule into hydrogen ions ($H^+$) and hydroxyl ions ($OH^-$). Alkaline minerals in the water end up as hydroxides (attached to the $OH^-$ ions). Some scientists argue that these compounds are not recognized by the body and if a person's kidneys are functioning well, these compounds will be excreted through the urine. If they are not excreted through the urine, then they may end up as arterial plaque or as mineral deposits in joints and other tissues. [124]

The aforementioned discussion highlights the fact that when a person drinks alkaline water, the presence of buffering agents such as bicarbonates in it is of utmost important in order to neutralize acids and to get rid of acid waste through the urine.

# RECOMMENDATIONS ON ALKALINE WATER (by Dr. RK)

## ACIDITY IN THE STOMACH IS VERY IMPORTANT! [127]
◦ The stomach of a human body has a naturally low pH level that varies from 1 to 2 immediately after a large meal consumption, as the stomach secretes hydrochloric acid and releases enzymes in order to aid digestion. However the buffers present in the same stomach quickly raise the pH of the stomach to 3 or 4, or somewhere in between. After that, the stomach pH naturally raises further to a resting level 4 or 5 until we eat next time.

◦ That beneficial acidity at a very low pH level of 1 or 2 in the stomach not only helps with the food digestion, but also kills bacteria, viruses and germs instantly while we consume meals.

## HUMAN BODY HAS AN AMAZING ABILITY TO MAINTAIN STEADY BLOOD pH
◦ No matter what kind of water you drink, the human body has an amazing ability to maintain a steady pH in the blood between 7.35 and 7.45, which is perfectly normal.

## ACIDIC WATER IS HARMFUL TO YOUR HEALTH [128, 129]
◦ Acidic water while traveling through pipes make them corrode and cause them leach heavy metal contaminants such as lead, iron, copper, zinc, manganese and others into the water. These contaminants, more particularly the lead, cause illness and poisoning. Acidic water could be fatal or debilitating for children. Vomiting, diarrhea, kidney disease, liver disease, stomach cramps, and nausea are among the leading health issues caused by the consumption of acidic water. Acidic water can also have a rather metallic and unsavory taste when drinking.

◦ Brushing your teeth every morning with acidic water could encourage bacteria growth in most instances, cause cavities, and ultimately corrode and damage your teeth. Acidic water can have negative side effects on your hair and will make it become more brittle over time. Since acidic water is more likely to be contaminated with heavy metal pollutants, and these are going to get into your bathtub and shower water, resulting in negative side effects. You may notice rashes developing on your skin if you bath in acidic water that was filled with the contaminants and pollutants.

## DRINKING PURIFIED WATER THAT IS EITHER NEUTRALIZED (pH=7) OR SLIGHTLY ALKALIZED (pH=7 to 7.25) IS GOOD FOR YOU!
◦ Even the purified water such as distilled water and RO water in almost all instances exists in acidic state. When you purchase purified water in supermarkets, and measure pH, you will be surprised to learn that the the pH could be between 6 and 6.5 (never more than 6.5), which is seriously acidic. You need to take action, and should not drink it as purchased, but should try to neutralize it or slightly alkalize it before drinking.

◦ Even though the human body has an amazing ability to maintain steady pH between 7.35 and 7.45, when you drink water that is acidic, you body has to work harder to neutralize it. If you drink purified water that already neutralized, then you would be doing a favor to your body.

## DRINKING HIGHLY ALKALIZED WATER EVERY DAY IS NOT RECOMMENDED!
◦ There is no credible evidence thus far that drinking highly alkalized water (at a pH of 8, 9 or 10) every day has any reported health benefits. Many people have been drinking this kind of alkaline water daily, and nobody knows what could happen to their health in a long run. It would be scaring to drink that kind of alkaline water at that kind of high pH level. Those people who drink that kind of alkaline water at high pH don't realize the fact that "the normal blood pH should be between 7.35 and 7.45".

If a person constantly drinks alkaline water at a pH 8, 9 or 10 every day,
(i) What will happen to the acidity in the stomach that is desperately needed? and
(ii) What will happen to that normal blood pH (7.35 to 7.45) that is essential?
Think about it seriously before drinking alkaline water frequently at high pH.

If you have already been drinking or planning to drink alkaline water at high pH every day for therapeutic purposes or for athletic performance enhancement, you should get your blood pH tested routinely and make sure it is always normal.

## DRINKING ALKALINE WATER PERIODICALLY IS GOOD FOR YOU
Considering the randomized research studies and the scientific journal publications, if you are an athlete, you can drink alkaline water when you work out or perform high-intensity exercise a few times a week or periodically. But it would be inappropriate to consume all 8 cups of alkaline water per day, every day because there is no credible evidence that suggests that alkaline water is not harmful to your health in a long run. Alkaline water does have some therapeutic benefits and athletic performance benefits, but you should not overconsume alkaline water that is at a high pH.

## ACID-ALKALINE BALANCE IS IMPORTANT! [130]
● People consume beverages of acidic and/or alkaline nature all the time. According to the Merck Manual (which is the world's most widely used medical reference guide), the human body naturally buffers to balance the pH. For example if you consume something acidic, your blood would produce more bicarbonate and less carbon dioxide to neutralize the acidity. Likewise, if you consume something alkaline, your blood would produce more carbon dioxide and less bicarbonate to balance out the pH.

● However, this natural process of human body's acid-alkaline balance could be interrupted if you consume too much alkaline water at a high pH continuously every day.

## BEWARE OF ALKALOSIS
● Drinking alkaline water continuously makes it difficult for your body to maintain the stomach pH in the very low acidic range. Very low stomach pH level is essential for the food digestion, and to kill bacteria, viruses and germs that may be present in the stomach through food consumption.

● The human body has an amazing ability to maintain a steady blood pH between 7.35 and 7.45, no matter what kind of water you drink. There are no long-term research studies that suggest that drinking of alkaline water at a high pH is not harmful to health. However, if you drink too much alkaline water at high pH of 9, 10 or more every day for a long time, it becomes very difficult for the body to maintain blood pH between 7.35 and 7.45, and eventually you could develop alkalosis (a condition developed due to the presence of excess base), and this condition could affect the proper functioning of lungs, kidneys & liver. You should maintain a healthy acid-base balance for your body by not consuming too much alkaline water, but by consuming the right quantity of alkaline water periodically. That right quantity of alkaline water has to determined by trial and error until you feel healthy with alkaline water in a long run (not just consuming it for a week or month time). Please get your blood pH tested routinely if you are planning to drink highly alkaline water every day.

# REFERENCES

## ALKALINE WATER
1. Acids, Bases and Metals, Chemical Material Behavior, Bitesize of BBC, UK.
http://www.bbc.co.uk/bitesize/ks3/science/chemical_material_behaviour/acids_bases_metals/revision/4/

2. Hydrion Ph paper (93) with Dispenser and Color Chart - Full range Insta Chek ph- 0-13, ASIN Number B005FYGXUC, Available on Amazon.com.

3. HM Digital PH-80 pH HydroTester, 0-14 pH Range, 1 pH Resolution, 2% Readout Accuracy , ASIN Number B0096N8OWI, Available on Amazon.com.

4. Drinking Water Regulations and Contaminants, Posted by United Stares Environmental Protection Agency (EPA).
https://www.epa.gov/dwregdev/drinking-water-regulations-and-contaminants

https://www.watersystemscouncil.org/download/wellcare_information_sheets/potential_groundwater_contaminant_information_sheets/9709284pH_Update_September_2007.pdf

4b. pH in Drinking Water by World Health Organization, Geneva, Switzerland, 1996.
http://www.who.int/water_sanitation_health/dwq/chemicals/ph.pdf

5. pH and Alkalinity by Nova Scotia Environment of Canada.
http://www.evowater.ca/uploads/ph_alkalinity_well_water.pdf

6. What should be the pH value of drinking water? by Star Health Desk, Posted on September 06, 2015.
https://www.thedailystar.net/health/what-should-be-the-ph-value-drinking-water-138382

7. What pH Should My Drinking Water Be? by Healthline.
https://www.healthline.com/health/ph-of-drinking-water#takeaway

8. pH Values of Water Completely Explained by APEC Water Systems.
https://www.freedrinkingwater.com/water-education/quality-water-ph.htm
https://www.freedrinkingwater.com/water-education/quality-water-ph-page2.htm

9. How to Increase the Alkalinity of Your Water? by E.C. LaMeaux.
https://www.gaiam.com/blogs/discover/how-to-increase-the-alkalinity-of-your-water

10. How to Drink Water With High pH by Ireland Wolfe, Posted on Oct. 03, 2017.
https://www.livestrong.com/article/487702-how-to-drink-water-with-high-ph/

11. Amazing Alkaline Lemons by Chronicle Flask, Posted on August 28, 2013.
https://chronicleflask.com/2013/08/28/amazing-alkaline-lemons/

12. Journal Publication (Influence of Lemon Juice on Urine pH)
In vitro and in vivo study of effect of lemon juice on urinary lithogenesis, Authors: Oussama A1, Touhami M, Mbarki M., Arch Esp Urol. 2005 Dec;58(10):1087-92.
https://www.ncbi.nlm.nih.gov/pubmed/16482864

## URINE pH (Normal Range)

13. Urine pH by RnCeus Interactive™, LLC.
https://www.rnceus.com/ua/uaph.html

14. 4 Steps to Achieve Proper pH Balance by Dr. Axe.
https://draxe.com/ph-balance/

15. How to balance your pH and find out if you're too acidic by Natasha Turner, ND, Published on Sep 13, 2014 Updated on Jun 27, 2017.
https://www.chatelaine.com/health/diet/tired-overweight-you-might-be-too-acidic/

16. What Are the Factors That Influence Urine pH? by SHARON PERKINS, Posted on Aug 14, 2017.
https://www.livestrong.com/article/526347-what-are-the-factors-that-influence-urine-ph/

## BENEFITS OF LEMON

17. YouTube Video Title: How to Prepare Alkaline Water at Home, Home Yog, Publishied on March 14, 2017.          https://www.youtube.com/watch?v=J1F72B0-eqI

18. YouTube Video Title: pH 7 to 14: Nobel Prize Winner Says "Alkaline Water Kills Cancer" - Here's How You Can Prepare It!, AJA Ancestral Healing, Published on Oct 2, 2017.
https://www.youtube.com/watch?v=0gyN_bov-OE

19. 6 Evidence-Based Health Benefits of Lemons by Healthline.
https://www.healthline.com/nutrition/6-lemon-health-benefits#section2

20. What Are the Health Benefits of Citrus Pulp? by Jonathan Thompson, Posted Oct. 03, 2017.
https://www.livestrong.com/article/429208-what-are-the-health-benefits-of-citrus-pulp/

21 Things That Happen to Your Body When You Eat Lemons by Christina Stiehl, Posted on February 23, 2017.
https://www.eatthis.com/benefits-of-lemon/

22. What Is the Benefit of Eating Whole, Fresh Lemons?, Written by Sara Ipatenco; Posted on December 11, 2017.
https://healthyeating.sfgate.com/benefit-eating-whole-fresh-lemons-4390.html

23. 10 Benefits of Drinking Warm Lemon Water in the Morning by La Jolla Mom, Posted on January 11, 2011.
https://lajollamom.com/drink-warm-lemon-water-in-the-morning/

24. What is the pH level of Baking Soda? by Samuel Markings, Posted on April 26, 2018.
https://sciencing.com/ph-level-baking-soda-5266423.html

25. Sodium bicarbonate Side Effects by Drugs.Com, Medically Reviewed on June 7, 2018.
https://www.drugs.com/sfx/sodium-bicarbonate-side-effects.html

26. How Baking Soda Can Improve Athletic Performance by Darla Leal, Reviewed by a board-certified physician, Posted on November 11, 2017.
https://www.verywellfit.com/how-baking-soda-can-improve-athletic-performance-4057192

27. Alkaline Drops, Alkaline Water Machine Reviews, by Jessica Roberts.
http://alkalinewatermachinereviews.com/alkazone-alkaline-booster-drops-reviewed/

28. Alkalife pH Booster Drops.
http://www.alkalife.com/
https://alkalifestore.myshopify.com/

29. Alkazone pH Booster Drops.
https://alkazone.com/alkaline-drops/

30. Alkavision Plasma pH Drops.
https://alkavision.com/
https://alkavision.com/plasma-ph-drops/

31. Piping Rock Booster pH Drops, Piping Rock Health Products, LLC.
https://ca.pipingrock.com/alkaline/alkaline-booster-ph-protector-drops-2-fl-oz-59-ml-dropper-bottle-40646

32. Alkaline Water Drops With Natural Antioxidant 2oz (from HeatthyWiser), ASIN: B01M337KL3, Available on Amazon.com.
https://www.amazon.com/Alkaline-Antioxidant-Purifier-Filtration-Supports/dp/B01M337KL3/ref=sr_1_5_a_it?ie=UTF8&qid=1535506650&sr=8-5&keywords=ph+booster+drops

## ALKALINE WATER PITCHERS
33. Water Ionizers, from Free Wikipedia.
https://en.wikipedia.org/wiki/Water_ionizer

## WATER IONIZERS (ALAKALINE IONIZED WATER)
34. How It Works: The History of Water Ionizers and How Ionized Water is Made by Chanson Alkaline Water.
https://chansonalkalinewater.com/how-it-works-the-history-of-water-ionizers-and-how-ionized-water-is-made/

35. How to Define Anode and Cathode? by Anne Marie Helmenstine, Ph.D., Posted on September 21, 2017.
https://www.thoughtco.com/how-to-define-anode-and-cathode-606452

36. Positive or Negative Anode/Cathode in Electrolytic/Galvanic Cell by Chemistry Stackexchange.
https://chemistry.stackexchange.com/questions/16785/positive-or-negative-anode-cathode-in-electrolytic-galvanic-cell

37. What is Ionized Water? by Life Ionizers.
http://www.lifeionizers.com/water-facts/ionized-water.html

38. Alkaline Water Science | Hydroxyl Ions by Leo McDevitt, Life Ionizers, Posted On March 1, 2013.
http://www.lifeionizers.com/blog/alkaline-water-hydroxyl-ions/

39. How Ionizers Work! by Life Ionizers.
http://www.lifeionizer.com.au/water-facts/ionizer-how.html

40. How Does A Water Ionizer Work? by Water Ionizer Expert, Posted on Sept 03, 2015.
https://www.waterionizerexpert.com/blogs/news/43703681-how-does-a-water-ionizer-work

**WHAT CHEMICALS ARE ADDED?**
41. Water Treatment Chemicals by Lenntech.
https://www.lenntech.com/products/chemicals/water-treatment-chemicals.htm#Boiler%20water%20chemicals

42. Stages in typical municipal water treatment by Filtronics, Posted on September 25, 2013 .
http://www.filtronics.com/blog/tertiary-treatment/stages-in-typical-municipal-water-treatment/

43. 8 Chemicals from Water Treatment and Distribution by World Health Organization (WHO).
http://www.who.int/water_sanitation_health/dwq/cmp130704chap8.pdf

44. YouTube Title: Water Ionizer Fundamentals of Water Ionizer by Alkalinewaterchannel, Malaysia, Published on Dec 10, 2012.
https://www.youtube.com/watch?v=W4eDhm-U93w

**OXIDATION REDUCTION POTENTIAL**
45. Understanding pH and Oxidation Reduction Potential (ORP) by Aqua Health Products.
http://www.aquahealthproducts.com/understanding-ph-and-orp

46. Question 24, What is ORP?, Ionlife Water Ionizer FAQs.
https://ionizers.org/faq.php

47. What is +ORP and −ORP? by Air Water Life Water Ionizers.
https://airwaterlife.com/what-is-alkaline-water/

48. pH and Oxidation Reduction Potential (ORP) by Aqualife.
https://www.aqualife.ca/en/ph-orp/

49. Alkaline Water and Oxidation Reduction Potential (ORP) by Alkaway.
https://www.alkaway.com.au/learning-centre/alkaline-water/alkaline-water-and-oxidation-reduction-potential-orp/

50. What Is Alkaline Water?, Alkaline Water & Ionized Alkaline Water – What's The Difference? by Air Water Life.
https://airwaterlife.com/what-is-alkaline-water/

**ELECTROLYZED REDUCED WATER (ERW)**
51. Scientific Proof of alkaline Ionized Water Benefits by Bawell Water Ionizers.
http://www.bawellwaterionizers.com/benefits.html

52. Ionized Water by Nashville's First Alkaline Ionized Water Store.
http://nashvillealkalinewaterstore.com/alkaline-ionized-water/ionized-water-orp/

**BENEFITS OF ALKALINE IONIZED WATER**
53. YouTube Title: Alkaline Water Benefits - 10 Benefits of Alkaline Water in just 3 Minutes by Life Ionizers, Published on Apr 17, 2014.
https://www.youtube.com/watch?v=XucJa5RpmQE
http://www.lifeionizers.com/        http://www.lifeionizer.ca/

## LISTEN TO WHAT CRITICS SAY ABOUT ALKALINE IONIZED WATER

54. Alkalinity Water and FDA: Is it All Hype? by Raphael Nyarkotey Obu, Posted on April 26, 2018.
https://www.modernghana.com/news/849886/alkalinity-water-and-fda-is-it-all-hype.html
https://www.modernghana.com/news/847621/a-quick-response-to-the-fda-alkalinity-water-statement.html

55. Alkaline Water Why Not? by Dancing With Water, The New Science of Water, Updated October 1, 2019.
http://www.dancingwithwater.com/articles/alkaline-water-not/

56. Microfiltered Seawater by Rene Quinton, Website of Dancing With Water.
http://www.dancingwithwater.com/microfiltered-seawater/

57. Different Types of Water by Heartland Springs.
http://www.heartlandsprings.com/different-waters/

58. Scientists say don't be duped by alkaline water by Mark Timmons, Posted on on August 30, 2017.
https://www.uswatersystems.com/blog/2017/08/scientists-say-dont-be-duped-by-alkaline-water/

There is no Reference # 59.

## KANGEN WATER

60. The History of Kangen Water, The History of Kangen Water by KangenWaterHQ, Kangen Water Distributor, December 21, 2014.
http://kangenwaterhq.com/history-of-kangen-water/

61. The History of Kangen Water.
http://www.nettxus.com/healthsolutions/id70.html

62. The History of Kangen Water by Nuoc Kangen, Kangen Water Distributor.
https://kangenshui.wordpress.com/water/

63. The website of Enagic Corp.
https://www.enagic.com/

64. Doctors, Scientists and Nutritionists on Kangen Water.
https://www.overvoedingengezondheid.nl/wp-content/uploads/2015/10/Doctors_Scientists_and_Nutritionists_on_Kangen_water-2.pdf

65. Kangen Healing Water, Frequently Asked Questions by Water Pollution Filters Company.
http://waterpollutionfilters.com/kangen-water-FAQs.htm

66. Hydrogen-Rich Kangen Water, People everywhere are discovering the life-changing power of Kangen Water® by Roger & Sabine Gaudette, Kanger Water distributors in BC, Canada.
https://www.worldofhydration.com/?_vsrefdom=p.2833&gclid=EAIaIQobChMIg4CPurav3QI VkWF-Ch0jMw_BEAAYBCAAEgJbLvD_BwE

67. Electrolysis of Water, Water Structure and Science by Martin Chaplin, BSc, PhD, CChem FRSC.
http://www1.lsbu.ac.uk/water/electrolysis.html

226

68. Electrolysis by Molecular Hydrogen Institute.
http://www.molecularhydrogeninstitute.com/electrolysis

69. How An Ionizer Works by Aqua Health Products, 2018.
http://www.aquahealthproducts.com/how-ionizer-works

70. YouTube Title: Dr Michael explains the difference between AlkaLINE and alkaLYZED water by Abigail Donaldson, Published on Aug 22, 2013.
https://www.youtube.com/watch?v=t-mUB2yiPzQ

71. Kanger Water Explained at OM Kangen Wellness Center.
http://omkangenwellnesscenter.com/water/

72. Healthy Ionized Alkaline Kangen Water by Healthy Living Water.
https://healthylivingwater.wordpress.com/2013/08/22/how-to-obtain-healthy-living-water/

73. pH test strips: Why you can't test alkaline water with them by Leo McDevitt, Posted On January 11, 2018.
http://www.lifeionizers.com/blog/ph-test-strips-why-you-cant-test-alkaline-water-with-them/

74. Benefits of Kangen Water, Posted by Eangic Corp.
http://www.enagic-asia.com/en/water_benefit.php

75. Kangen Water Pros & Cons: Will it really change your life? By Leo McDevitt Posted On February 28th, 2017.
http://www.lifeionizers.com/blog/kangen-water-pros-and-cons/

There are no references between 76 and 84.

**HYDROGEN WATER**
85. H2 Miracle Water.
https://h2miraclewater.com/

86. Free Radicals and Antioxidants, Posted by H2 Miracle Water.
https://h2miraclewater.com/free-radicals/

87. Frequently Asked Questions (FAQ) About Hydrogen Water, Posted by H2 Miracle Water.
https://h2miraclewater.com/hydrogen-water/

87b. Why hydrogen water is the new health fad by Megha Sharma, Posted on May 21, 2017.
https://timesofindia.indiatimes.com/life-style/health-fitness/health-news/why-hydrogen-water-is-the-new-health-fad/articleshow/58772035.cms

88. The Ultimate Guide to Alkaline Water Vs Hydrogen Water, Westcom Solutions, Posted on Oct 13, 2017.
https://www.westcomsolutions.com/ultimate-guide-alkaline-water-vs-hydrogen-water/

89. What is PEM Technology? by AlkaVoda, Posted on October 2, 2017.
http://www.alkavoda.com/news/PEM-technology.html

90. The Best Water For Your Health by HYBON.
http://www.gz-hibon.com/Products/Show_60.html

91. Hydrogen Rich Water Bottle With PEM-SPE Technology by HHO Gas Technology.
http://hhogastechnology.weebly.com/store/p20/____HYDROGEN_RICH_WATER_BOTTLE_W
ITH_PEM_-_SPE_TECHNOLOGY.html

92. Hydrogen Water, SPE/PEM Electrolysis by H2 For Life.
https://19l.ro/hydrogen/2017/10/23/spepem-electrolysis/

93. Alkaline Water vs. Hydrogen Water: Which is best? By Leo McDevitt, Life Ionizers,
Posted on May 26th, 2017.
http://www.lifeionizers.com/blog/alkaline-water-vs-hydrogen-water-which-is-best/

94. Alkaline Water vs Hydrogen Water by Leo McDevitt, Life Ionizers, Posted On January
20th, 2016.
http://www.lifeionizers.com/blog/alkaline-water-vs-hydrogen-water/

95. Difference Between Hydrogen Water Machines and Water Ionizers by Alkaline Water Plus.
https://www.alkalinewaterplus.com/our-products/hydrogen-water-machines/

96. What Is the pH of the Stomach? A Breakdown of the Acidity Inside the Stomach by
Anne Marie Helmenstine, Ph.D., Updated on July 03, 2019.
https://www.thoughtco.com/ph-of-the-stomach-608195

There are no references between 97 and 100.

## RANDOMIZED RESEARCH STUDIES (SCIENTIFIC PAPERS)

101a. Why Alkaline Water Is Better For Hydration by The Tyent Team, Posted on January 24, 2019.
https://www.tyentusa.com/blog/hydration-alkaline-water/

101b. Journal Publication: Effect of electrolyzed high-pH alkaline water on blood viscosity in
healthy adults, Authors: Joseph Weidman, Ralph E. HolsworthJr., Bradley Brossman, Daniel
J. Cho, John St.Cyr and Gregory Fridman, Journal of the International Society of Sports
Nutrition 201613:45.
https://jissn.biomedcentral.com/articles/10.1186/s12970-016-0153-8

102a. Health Effects of pH on Drinking Water by Ariana DiValentino, Reviewed by Claudia
Thompson, Updated on August 15, 2019.
https://www.livestrong.com/article/214475-health-effects-of-ph-on-drinking-water/

102b. Journal Publication: The effect of mineral-based alkaline water on hydration status
and the metabolic response to short-term anaerobic exercise, Jakub Chycki,1 Tomasz
Zając,2 Adam Maszczyk,corresponding author and Anna Kurylas, Biology of Sport, Published
online on Feb 19, 2017.
https://www.ncbi.nlm.nih.gov/pmc/articles/PMC5676322/

103. Preliminary observation on changes of blood pressure, blood sugar and blood lipids
after using alkaline ionized drinking water, Authors: WANG Yu-lian, First Hospital of Shanghai
Textile, Shanghai 200060, Published in Shanghai Journal of Preventive Medicine, China.
http://en.cnki.com.cn/Article_en/CJFDTOTAL-SHYI200112005.htm

228

104. Scientific Proof of Alkaline Ionized Water Benefits by Balwell Water Ionizers.
http://www.bawellwaterionizers.com/benefits.html

105. Potential benefits of pH 8.8 alkaline drinking water as an adjunct in the treatment of reflux disease, Published in US National Library of Medicine, National Institutes of Health Authores: Koufman JA1, Johnston N.
https://www.ncbi.nlm.nih.gov/pubmed/22844861

106. Selective stimulation of the growth of anaerobic microflora in the human intestinal tract by electrolyzed reducing water. Author: Vorobjeva NV1., Med Hypotheses. 2005;64(3):543-6.
https://www.ncbi.nlm.nih.gov/pubmed/15617863

107. Humans Have Ten Times More Bacteria Than Human Cells: How Do Microbial Communities Affect Human Health?, American Society for Microbiology, June 5, 2008.
https://www.sciencedaily.com/releases/2008/06/080603085914.htm

108. Electrolyzed-reduced water protects against oxidative damage to DNA, RNA, and protein, Authors: Lee MY1, Kim YK, Ryoo KK, Lee YB, Park EJ., Appl Biochem Biotechnol. 2006 Nov;135(2):133-44.
https://www.ncbi.nlm.nih.gov/pubmed/17159237?ordinalpos=13&itool=EntrezSystem2.PEn trez.Pubmed.Pubmed_ResultsPanel.Pubmed_DefaultReportPanel.Pubmed_RVDocSum

109. Enhanced induction of mitochondrial damage and apoptosis in human leukemia HL-60 cells due to electrolyzed-reduced water and glutathione, Authors: Tsai CF1, Hsu YW, Chen WK, Ho YC, Lu FJ., Biosci Biotechnol Biochem. 2009 Feb;73(2):280-7. Epub 2009 Feb 7.
https://www.ncbi.nlm.nih.gov/pubmed/19202298

110. Inhibitory effect of electrolyzed reduced water on tumor angiogenesis, Authors: Ye J1, Li Y, Hamasaki T, Nakamichi N, Komatsu T, Kashiwagi T, Teruya K, Nishikawa R, Kawahara T, Osada K, Toh K, Abe M, Tian H, Kabayama S, Otsubo K, Morisawa S, Katakura Y, Shirahata S., Biol Pharm Bull. 2008 Jan;31(1):19-26.
https://www.ncbi.nlm.nih.gov/pubmed/18175936

111. Anti-diabetic effects of electrolyzed reduced water in streptozotocin-induced and genetic diabetic mice, Authors: Kim MJ1, Kim HK., Life Sci. 2006 Nov 10;79(24):2288-92. Epub Aug 2, 2006.
https://www.ncbi.nlm.nih.gov/pubmed/16945392?ordinalpos=7&itool=EntrezSystem2.PEntr ez.Pubmed.Pubmed_ResultsPanel.Pubmed_DefaultReportPanel.Pubmed_RVDocSum

112. Preservative effect of electrolyzed reduced water on pancreatic beta-cell mass in diabetic db/db mice, Authors: Kim MJ1, Jung KH, Uhm YK, Leem KH, Kim HK., Biol Pharm Bull. 2007 Feb;30(2):234-6.
https://www.ncbi.nlm.nih.gov/pubmed/17268057

113. Protective mechanism of reduced water against alloxan-induced pancreatic beta-cell damage: Scavenging effect against reactive oxygen species, Authors: Li Y1, Nishimura T, Teruya K, Maki T, Komatsu T, Hamasaki T, Kashiwagi T, Kabayama S, Shim SY, Katakura Y, Osada K, Kawahara T, Otsubo K, Morisawa S, Ishii Y, Gadek Z, Shirahata S., Cytotechnology, 2002 Nov;40(1-3):139-49. doi: 10.1023/A:1023936421448.
https://www.ncbi.nlm.nih.gov/pubmed/19003114

There are no references from 114 to 120.

## ACID-ALKALINE BALANCE
121. Acid Alkali Balance, Alkalife pH Booster Drops, Written by Alkalife, Posted by National Nutrition.Ca.
https://www.nationalnutrition.ca/Detail.aspx?ID=6777

122. What's a Normal Blood pH and What Makes It Change? by Healthline.
https://www.healthline.com/health/ph-of-blood#takeaway

## Understanding the Water pH, Alkalinity, Alkaline & Buffers
123. pH in Drinking Water by World Health Organization, Geneva, Switzerland, 1996.
http://www.who.int/water_sanitation_health/dwq/chemicals/ph.pdf

124. Alkaline Water Why Not? by Dancing With Water, The New Science of Water, Updated October 1, 2019.
http://www.dancingwithwater.com/articles/alkaline-water-not/

125. Microfiltered Seawater by Rene Quinton, Website of Dancing With Water.
http://www.dancingwithwater.com/microfiltered-seawater/

126. Acid Mine Damage: Alkalinity, Exploring the Environment Water Quality by Wheeling Jesuit University/NASA-supported Classroom of the Future, Posted on Nov 10, 2004.
http://www.cotf.edu/ete/modules/waterq/wqalkalinity.html

## RECOMMENDATIONS ON ALKALINE WATER (by Dr. RK)
127. What Is the pH of the Stomach? A Breakdown of the Acidity Inside the Stomach by Anne Marie Helmenstine, Ph.D., Updated on July 03, 2019.
https://www.thoughtco.com/ph-of-the-stomach-608195

128. 7 Reasons Why Acidic Water Is Bad For You by The Tyent Team, Posted on February 19, 2019.
https://www.tyentusa.com/blog/acidic-water-negative-effects/

129. Acidic Water by All About Water Filters.
http://all-about-water-filters.com/acidic-water-bad-for-you/

130. Can Pure Water Be Acidic And Harmful To Your Health? Is pure water acidic and harmful to your health?, Posted by Water Depot.
https://www.waterdepot.com/faq/reverse-osmosis-questions/74-is-pure-water-acidic-and-harmful-to-your-health

# CHAPTER 19: DRINKING WATER GUIDE IN A NUTSHELL QUICK-REFERENCE AND DO-IT-YOURSELF GUIDELINES

## TABLE OF CONTENTS

# CHAPTER 19: DRINKING WATER GUIDE IN A NUTSHELL QUICK-REFERENCE AND DO-IT-YOURSELF GUIDELINES

## THIS IS YOUR DRINKING WATER GUIDE IN A NUTSHELL!

ALL YOU NEED DO IS JUST FOLLOW THESE SIMPLE INSTRUCTIONS DESCRIBED IN THIS SHORT CHAPTER, AND YOU WILL REWARD YOURSELF FOR DOING A FAVOR TO YOURSELF!

+++++++++++++++++++++++++++++++++++++++++++++++++++++++++++

## PURCHASING EXPENSIVE WATER PURIFICATION SYSTEMS IS UNNECESSARY!

PURCHASING EXPENSIVE WATER PITCHERS, AND INSTALLING COMPLEX WATER PURIFICATION SYSTEMS AT HOME IS UNNECESSARY. MAINTENANCE OF THESE UNITS AT HOME IS FRUSTRATINGLY TEDIOUS, AND THE WATER PURIFICATION SYSTEM AT HOME IS A HASSLE. YOU NEVER KNOW IF THE SYSTEM IS WORKING PERFECTLY OR BROKE DOWN. YOU NEED TO TEST THE DRINKING WATER EVERY DAY IN ORDER TO MAKE SURE THAT IT IS WORKING, WHICH IS A NUISANCE!

⏺ Some people purchase expensive water-filtering pitchers to produce purified water, remineralization pitchers, alkaline water pitchers, water ionizers, Kangen water machines, RO water systems to produce purified water or alkaline water, and use them at home to drink the water for daily use without knowing whether the unit is working perfectly or not. Those people don't even know how to test the final product (purified water), and make sure that the unit they purchased is indeed working, and the water they drink is indeed purified or not, remineralized or not, or alkalized or not. Please do not get into that kind of dilemma. Some people don't bother monitoring and testing the unit, and just drink that water without exercising caution. They don't even notice if they were drinking contaminated tap water.

⏺ Those machines are untrustworthy. Maybe there are some good machines out there, but you never know which one is good and which one is bad, or you never know if the machine you purchased is working perfectly or broke down. If the machine broke down, you would be unknowingly drinking contaminated tap water! You can easily get into that kind of situation if you purchase and use a water purification system at home.

## INSTEAD OF PURCHASING THOSE EXPENSIVE PURIFICATION SYSTEMS, PURCHASE PURIFIED WATER HASSLE-FREE FROM LOCAL VENDORS, OR MAKE YOUR OWN, AND LEARN HOW TO REMINERALIZE IT & ALKALIZE IT. ALL YOU NEED DO IS:

1. Learn how to monitor the TDS level of drinking water (Please refer to Chapter 17).
2. Purchase a digital kitchen scale that can measure weights in 0.01 g (10 mg) increments.
3. Learn how to measure the drinking water pH & urine pH (Please refer to Chapter 18).
4. Learn how to purchase purified water from supermarkets or local vendors, or make your own.
5. Learn how to remineralize the purified water up to a TDS level of 200 ppm (Chapter 17).
6. Learn how to neutralize or slightly alkalize the purified water (Chapter 18).

⏺ **THIS BOOK TEACHES THAT:** Purified water that is either neutralized (pH=7) or slightly alkalized (pH=7 to 7.25), and remineralized up to a TDS (Total Dissolved Solids) level of 200 ppm is the healthy drinking water.

⏺ This chapter is designed to give you guidelines on how to obtain that kind of clean and healthy drinking water at the comfort of your home without purchasing expensive purification systems or machines, or installing sophisticated filters. Please proceed and read further!

**1. LEARN HOW TO MONITOR TDS LEVEL (Chapter 17):** Learn how to monitor TDS (Total Dissolved Solids) level of drinking water or any water by using a TDS meter. You can purchase TDS meter on Amazon.com. Please refer to Chapter 17 for details. Everything is explained there on how to purchase and how to use a TDS meter.

**2. PURCHASE A DIGITAL KITCHEN SCALE**: Purchase digital scale that can measure weights in 0.01 g (10 mg) increments. You can purchase this digital scale on Amazon.com. You should be able to measure weights as small as 10 mg. Please refer to Chapter 17 for details. Everything is explained there on how to purchase it.

**3. LEARN HOW TO MONITOR WATER pH AND URINE pH (Chapter 18):**
Learn how to measure water pH using pH testing drops and/or digital pH meter. You can purchase those pH testing drops in a pet store or aquarium store. Enagic pH testing drops (of Kangen Water Company) work perfectly well, but these drops indicate only whole numbers of pH. If you want to measure the pH with fraction such as 6.5 or 7.5, you better use digital pH meter. And also purchase a pH paper roll to measure the urine pH. Genuine Health pH paper roll is a reliable one. Please read through the beginning part of Chapter 18, where everything is explained on how to purchase pH drops, digital pH meter, pH roll, and how monitor water pH and urine ph.
If you master the above-mentioned three instructions and have a thorough understanding on how to use them, then you can easily become a drinking water expert.

**4. LEARN HOW TO PURCHASE OR MAKE YOUR OWN PURIFIED WATER**
(i) Learn where and how to purchase the RO water at Refill Yourself Stations in the nearby supermarket. **The vendors test this purified water routinely and make sure that the unit is working perfectly. Therefore this RO water is reliable and trustworthy!** Whenever you purchase RO water, test it with TDS meter. The TDS level of RO water should be below 5 ppm (Most of them have TDS level from zero to 2 ppm).
(ii) Learn how to purchase distilled water in BPA-free plastic bottles in a local pharmacy, or from local vendors. When you purchase distilled water, test it with a TDS meter.
The TDS level of distilled water is precisely zero.
(iii) After purchasing purified water (RO water, distilled water, or zero water), boil it using a large electric kettle or on the stove. After boiling, store the boiled water in a large stainless steel container or stockpot until it cools down to room temperature, and then transfer the boiled water to BPA-free plastic bottles, and refrigerate it before drinking. Boiling kills pathogens (all kinds of bacteria, viruses, fungi, parasites), microorganisms and E. coli and so you can drink that purified water worry-free and hassle-free. Always close the purified water bottle tightly with a cap.
(iv) OR, MAKE YOUR OWN DISTILLED WATER: Purchase a "Countertop Water Distiller" that distills 1 gallon of tap water in 5.5 hours. This topic is explained in detail in Chapter 13 of the original book "Drinking Water Guide".

**5. LEARN HOW TO REMINERALIZE THE PURIFIED WATER**
Purchase Himalayan pink salt, Celtic sea salt or ConcenTrace drops in any health food store.
- Himalayan pink salt contains 88 trace minerals in it. (See Chapter 17).
- Celtic sea salt contains over 70 trace minerals. (See Chapter 17).
- ConenTrace mineral drops contains 73 trace minerals in it. (See Chapter 17).

Please read Chapter 17 thoroughly, and learn how to remineralize the purified water (or RO water, distilled water, or zero water) up to a TDS level of 200 ppm. You can remineralize a batch of purified water (2 liters or 8 cups) sufficient for a day. There are many easy-to-understand experiments conducted in Chapter 17. Please read it thoroughly. You will enjoy Chapter 17.

## **6.** LEARN HOW TO NEUTRALIZE OR SLIGHTLY ALKALIZE THE PURIFIED WATER
## PLEASE READ THE BEGINNING SECTION OF CHAPTER 18

⊛ Pure water has a pH of 7 and is considered "neutral" because it has neither acidic nor basic qualities. But the purified water (RO water, distilled water, or zero water), because of its high purity, quickly reacts with the carbon dioxide if exposed to the atmospheric air, and forms carbonic acid [ $CO_2 + H_2O = H_2CO_3$ ], thereby lowering the pH level to below 7 (it may drop to a pH of 6 or even below 6).

⊛ When you purchase purified water in supermarkets, and measure pH, you will be surprised to learn that the the pH could be between 6 and 6.5 (never more than 6.5), which is seriously acidic. You need to take action, and should not drink it as purchased, but should try to neutralize it or slightly alkalize it before drinking. The following options are being proposed to neutralize or slightly alkalize the purified water.

## OPTION # 1  ADD LEMON JUICE TO PURIFIED WATER OR CONSUME ONE LEMON A DAY, AND THIS HABIT NEUTRALIZES YOUR URINE

Learn how to remineralize the purified water up to a TDS level of 200 ppm as explained earlier.  Always use this remineralized purified water. Please read through the beginning part of Chapter 18 to understand how to neutralize your body by consuming a lemon and by doing urine tests. Even though lemon juice is acidic, it increases pH after consumption as your body reacts with the lemons' anions during the digestive process, and neutralizes your body shifting you from acidic state. Eat one or two lemons, and monitor your urine pH once every hour or every 2 hours. You should use the right pH paper or pH strips to do this. For example, **Genuine Health** pH paper roll works perfectly well, and is designed to monitor urine pH only (not water pH). If your urine pH stays through out the day close to 7, that means your body was in the neutralized state (neither acidic not alkaline), which is a great achievement. If you can do this every day, you don't need to drink any alkaline water.

## OPTION # 2  LEARN HOW TO NEUTRALIZE OR SLIGHTLY ALKALIZE THE PURIFIED WATER BY ADDING THE TRACE AMOUNT OF BAKING SODA

Learn how to remineralize the purified water up to a TDS level of 200 ppm (please refer to Chapter 17). Always use this remineralized purified water. Please read through the beginning part of Chapter 18 to understand how to increase the pH of purified water by adding only a tiny bit of baking soda. In Chapter 18, when Dr. RK conducted experiments, he was able to neutralize 1 liter of purified water by adding only trace amount 0.01 g (10 mg) of baking soda. 10 mg of baking soda is trace amount, and you won't confront any negative side effects of baking soda.

Table 19.1 The pH of purified water (RO water) can be increased by adding baking soda.

| Baking Soda Added To 1 Liter of RO Water | pH of RO Water Measured (pH) |
|---|---|
| 0 g | 6.0 to 6.5 |
| 0.010 g (10 mg) | 7.0 (turned green) |
| 0.020 g (20 mg) | 7.5 (turned pale blue) |
| 0.040 g (40 mg) | 8.0 (turned light blue) |

**How Much Baking Soda?** On the Internet, you can find articles, suggesting that "simply add ½ a teaspoon of baking soda to a gallon of purified water" to alkalize it. ½ Teaspoon = 2.84 g = 2840 mg; 1 Gallon = 3.78 Liters; Per Liter = 2840/3.78 =751 mg/L

That means the articles suggest that add 0.751 g (751 mg) of baking soda per liter of water, which is inappropriately too much! That much baking soda is unnecessary! If you drink that kind of alkaline water by adding that much baking soda, you will face adverse side effects, and in a very short time, you will quit using baking soda.

Dr. RK was able to neutralize 1 liter of purified water by adding only a trace amount of 10 mg of baking soda (see the table shown above).

If this option does not work for you, please choose Option # 3.

**OPTION # 3** LEARN HOW TO NEUTRALIZE OR SLIGHTLY ALKALIZE A CUP OF PURIFIED WATER JUST BY ADDING ONLY 1 OR 2 CONCENTRACE MINERAL DROPS
Please read Chapter 17 thoroughly, and learn how to remineralize the purified water (RO water, distilled water, or zero water) up to a TDS level of 200 ppm, and at the same time alkalize it by simply adding a few ConcenTrace mineral drops. It is very easy to do that. Please read the whole Chapter 17, and you will enjoy it.

---

## IMPORTANT MESSAGE

If genuine distilled water and RO water are not available in the market, this book suggests that a consumer must switch to zero water. Make your own purified water using a ZeroWater pitcher. And learn how to remineralize and slightly alkalize the zero water at home.

Please refer to Chapter 14, and read through the topic:"WHY IS ZERO WATER PREFERABLE, COMPARED TO DISTILLED WATER AND RO WATER?

# ADDITIONAL RECOMMENDATIONS (by Dr. RK)

## 1. WHILE COOKING MEALS

● Of course you should always cook your meals only with purified water. There are some unconfirmed reports in the scientific community such as: Cooking foods in purified water (RO water, distilled water, zero water) pulls the essential minerals (iron, calcium, magnesium, potassium and others ) out of foods and lowers the nutrient value of the cooked foods we consume.

● This claim has been disputed by some other scientists by saying that: This problem can be easily prevented, if needed, by adding a pinch of Himalayan pink salt, Celtic sea salt or a few drops of ConcenTrace minerals to purified water while cooking.

● Therefore to be on the safe side, you should develop a habit of adding a tiny bit of Himalayan pink salt (only a few kernels) to purified water whenever you cook meals with purified water (RO water, distilled water, zero water). Please always cook your meals with purified water. Please do not cook your foods with tap water (you could consume harmful contaminants).

**2**. RO water, distilled water, and zero water are your choices. You can choose either one or the other depending on the circumstances and comfortability. Distilled water is usually more expensive than RO water. You can make your own zero water by purchasing a ZeroWater pitcher.

**3**. It would be a good idea to install a faucet filter and use that filtered water from your kitchen sink for all non-drinking purposes (dish washing, cleaning, etc). Please do not use filtered water from faucet filter for drinking and cooking unless you know that the filtered water is one 100% safe and contaminants-free, and was confirmed by a certified laboratory. Always use purified water (RO water, distilled water, or zero water) for drinking and cooking. Never drink any kind of water that is not purified. Protect your health before it is too late.

4. Stop eating all those greasy foods in restaurants. Eat at home well-balanced meals throughout the day. Make sure that every meal you consume (either small meal or big meal), there is some protein in it. Consume whole foods only, and avoid processed foods and refined foods. Consume well-balanced meals with oven-baked skinless & boneless chicken, turkey or fish, a variety of organic vegetables and dark-leafy greens, legumes, a variety of organic fruits, grains, nuts and seeds so that your body would get sufficient amount of protein, fat and carbs, all kinds of vitamins, minerals and fiber. Consume plenty of organic egg whites to boost your protein consumption (Avoid processed meat products). Did you know egg-white is one 100% protein?

**5. IMPORTANT!** Take high-quality multivitamins and minerals (calcium, magnesium, potassium and others) so that your body would not suffer from any mineral deficiency. Request your doctor to take routine blood tests at least once or twice a year for iron deficiency, minerals deficiency, and make sure that all mineral levels in your blood are within the optimal ranges, or at least normal. And make sure by taking a kidney test that your kidneys are functioning properly.

**6.** Most pH meters, pH drops, pH strips and pH paper being sold in shops don't work properly. You got to be very careful, and purchase a high quality and reliable pH indicator that comes with calibration solutions. Test your pH indicator by comparing the pH of a reliable solution (of known pH), and make sure that the pH indicator works perfectly. You should also make sure that your TDS meter is working perfectly by using calibration solutions every now and then.

# THE PURPOSE OF THIS BOOK "DRINKING WATER GUIDE-II" FULFILLED
## How to Remineralize and Alkalize the Purified Water at Home!

OUR UNIVERSE, OUR STARS, OUR MILKY WAY GALAXY, OUR SOLAR SYSTEM, OUR SUN, OUR PLANET EARTH, OUR MOON & OUR WATER: How Were They Created?
This book has answered that question in a simple layperson's language!

• The purpose of Chapter 1 is to let everybody know where exactly our planet Earth is located in our Universe, and how exactly our planet Earth possessed that much liquid water that we drink to survive today. This objective has been fulfilled through an extensive research, innovative depictions, mindful clarification, and the scientific evidence gathered by astronomers, cosmologists, space scientists and researchers. The Origin of the Earth's Water revealed!
• **In Chapter 14,** this book suggests that if genuine RO water and distilled water are not available in the market, a consumer must switch to zero water. Make your own purified water using a ZeroWater pitcher. And learn how to alkalize and remineralize the zero water at home. Everything is explained clearly in Chapter 14. Just by reading the instructions provided in 2 pages only, you will be able to remineralize and alkalize the purified water (RO water, distilled water, or zero water) like a layperson.
• **In Chapter 17 & Chapter 18**, There are More Than 10 Scientific Experiments Conducted at Home with easy-to-follow instructions on how to correctly and precisely remineralize the purified water (RO water and distilled water) up to a TDS level of 200 ppm by adding precisely measured amount of Himalayan pink salt, Celtic sea salt, or ConcenTrace mineral drops.
• **All You Need Are:** TDS meter, digital kitchen scale, digital pH meter, and measuring spoons.
• Any reasonable person with minimal scientific background would be able to read and understand these experiments, and would be able to remineralize and alkalize the purified water to any desired level comfortably at home.
• **In Chapter 18**, this book teaches how to make your own alkaline water at home by adding precisely measured amount of baking soda or ConcenTrace mineral drops. There are several experiments conducted at home.
• **In Chapter 18**, this book also details how a person can purchase an appropriate machine and produce alkaline water at home. This book explains basic principle behind each process and how each unit functions, and also details how to purchase and use Water Ionizers, Kangen water machines, Hydrogen water machines and RO water machines that produce alkalized and remineralized water at home. When you use a machine, you need to test the final product using a TDS meter & digital pH meter, and make sure the machine is indeed working.
• **Chapter 19** Is Your "Drinking Water Guide In A Nutshell". All you need do is just follow these simple instructions described in a few pages, and you will reward yourself for doing a favor to yourself!

## LIVE LIKE AN ADVANCED HUMAN BEING!
• Please do not drink tap water, well water, or bottled water of any kind directly without knowing how pure it is. Please always drink purified water (reverse osmosis water, or distilled water, or other), and learn how to neutralize it or slightly alkalize it, and remineralize it before drinking.
• Purified water that is either neutralized (pH=7) or slightly alkalized (pH=7 to 7.25), and remineralized up to a TDS (Total Dissolved Solids) level of 200 ppm is the healthy drinking water.

• **REMEMBER:** More than 99% of your amazing body's molecules are water molecules, and 55% to 60% of your body weight is water. You therefore should make sure that the water in your body is clean, healthy and nutritious, and more importantly you should make sure that the water you drink is one hundred percent free of contaminants! This book is designed to help you achieve that goal!

# About the Author

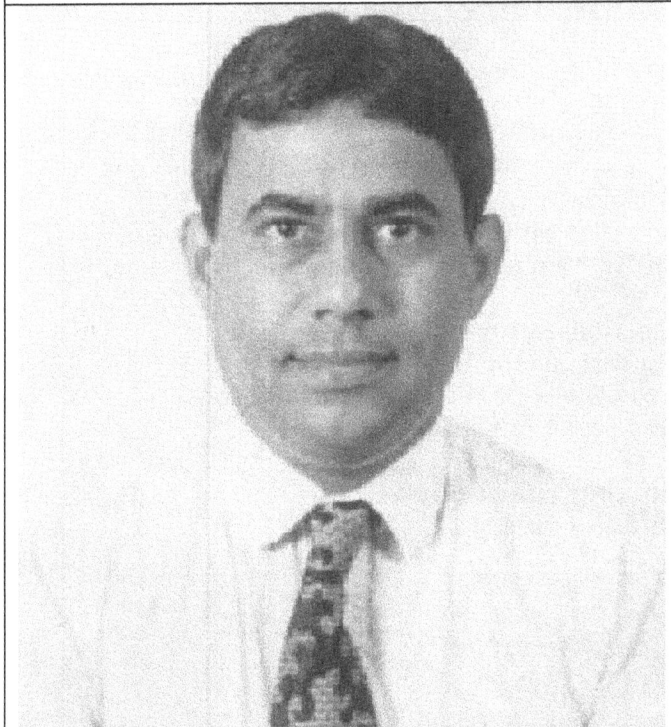

Dr. Rao M Konduru was a Chemical Engineer, and held two Master's degrees and two doctorates and two post-doctoral titles, all in chemical engineering. He published a book in 2003 titled "Permanent Diabetes Control," which earned immense respect and appreciation. Many people said it was a wonderful book. After suffering from a sudden heart attack in 1998, even though his left artery was 75% clogged with severe angina, he said "NO" to bypass surgery. He did what none of us would even think of doing. He simply relied on his natural self-prevention diet and exercise, and with it he reversed his critical diabetic heart disease in a matter of months, and developed a method to accomplish Permanent Diabetes Control. He also came up with a trial-and-error procedure to determine the optimal insulin dose that would tightly control diabetes, and would allow a diabetic person to live like a normal person for the rest of his/her life.

Dr. Rao M Konduru maintained his hemoglobin A1c level under 6.0% consistently. His personal best hemoglobin A1c level of 5.0% was an extraordinary result any diabetic person would hope to accomplish in a lifetime. Perhaps Dr. Rao M Konduru was the only diabetic person lived in this world with "Permanent Diabetes Control".

Once again, health demons such as uncontrollable weight gain, sleep apnea and chronic insomnia came his way. He did not give up, but persisted on discovering new, natural and effortless treatments of his own in reversing these most difficult disorders. His extensive scientific research experience and his powerful knowledge helped him battle and combat these life challenges. He figured out their root causes, and developed natural yet powerful techniques to cure these health disorders himself. After losing 40 pounds of weight and 12 inches around the waist, he successfully reversed his obesity, obstructive sleep apnea and chronic insomnia. He carefully created and published the following excellent guidebooks on Amazon so that others can benefit and be inspired to achieve similar results. His most recent book "Drinking Water Guide" is a 540-page book of wealth of information on drinking water for the rest of us.

1. Permanent Diabetes Control — www.mydiabetescontrol.com
2. The Secret to Controlling Type 2 Diabetes — www.mydiabetescontrol.com
3. Reversing Obesity — www.reversingsleepapnea.com/ebook2.html
4. Reversing Sleep Apnea — www.reversingsleepapnea.com
5. Reversing Insomnia — www.reversinginsomnia.com
6. Reversing Insomnia in 3 Days — www.reversinginsomnia.com
7. Drinking Water Guide — www.drinkingwaterguide.com
8. Drinking Water Guide-II — www.drinkingwaterguide.com
9. The Origin of the Earth's Water — www.drinkingwaterguide.com
10. Autobiography Of Dr. Rao M Konduru — www.mydiabetescontrol.com/Bio/

- Prime Publishing Co.

## PLEASE WRITE A REVIEW ABOUT THIS BOOK

Now that you have read this book, please write a review about this book, and post your review on Amazon.

a. Please log into your Amazon account,
b. Search for this book "Drinking Water Guide-II (Author: Rao Konduru, PhD)", or by using ISBN # 9780973112078, and click on the book cover & scroll down,
c. Click on "Customer Reviews", click on "Write a customer review" button, and "Create Review" box pops up.
d. Kindly write your REVIEW in the Write-Your-Review box, type a Headline, and click on 5 stars overall rating (you can give up to 5 stars).
e. Click on "Submit" button, and your review will be registered on Amazon.
f. Amazon will acknowledge your review with an email confirmation!

**Thanks for posting your review!**
**Your opinion counts!**

YOUR OPINION
**COUNTS!**

## Kindle eBook Is Available on Amazon

You can read this book on your computer, laptop, tablet, e-reader, iPhone, or any Kindle device by purchasing Kindle eBook. It is available on Amazon. Please log into your Amazon account, and search for "Drinking Water Guide-II, Kindle eBook" or by using ASIN # B07ZDHHGFZ.

## THE END OF THE BOOK "DRINKING WATER GUIDE-II"!

## BEST WISHES!

www.ingramcontent.com/pod-product-compliance
Lightning Source LLC
Chambersburg PA
CBHW081147270326
41930CB00014B/3062